Quality in Gastroenterology

Joseph D. Feuerstein • Daniel J. Stein
Editors

Quality in Gastroenterology

A Concise Guide to Establishing High Value Clinical Care

Springer

Editors
Joseph D. Feuerstein
Harvard Medical School
Beth Israel Deaconess Medical Center
Boston, MA, USA

Daniel J. Stein
Harvard Medical School
Brigham and Women's Hospital
Boston, MA, USA

ISBN 978-3-031-58491-6 ISBN 978-3-031-58492-3 (eBook)
https://doi.org/10.1007/978-3-031-58492-3

This Springer imprint is published by the registered company Springer Nature Switzerland AG
The registered company address is: Gewerbestrasse 11, 6330 Cham, Switzerland

Preface

Quality in gastroenterology is an evolving field. Quality metrics serve as a measure by which the quality of care can be assessed and standardized. Quality measures should be focused on patient-important outcomes and ideally should provide high-quality, cost-effective care. In gastroenterology, quality metrics are needed in both clinical care and endoscopy. We are excited that this book *Quality in Gastroenterology: A Concise Guide to Establishing High Value Clinical Care* provides the reader with expert reviews on critical topics pertaining to quality standards in gastroenterology. This book will serve as a primer for providing high-quality cost-effective care in gastroenterology.

The book includes chapters focused on both endoscopic management and clinical patient care in gastroenterology. Each chapter is written by renowned experts focused on how to provide high-quality care in gastroenterology. We believe this book will provide the reader with a thorough review of the latest evidence on quality in gastroenterology.

Boston, MA, USA — Joseph D. Feuerstein
Boston, MA, USA — Daniel J. Stein

Contents

Chapter 1
Quality in Gastroenterology

David I. Fudman, Shaharyar Zuberi, and Joseph D. Feuerstein

Table of Quality Measures/Metrics

Key Points

- Quality in gastroenterology is evolving.
- Gastroenterology societies are working to establish quality standards; however, only a limited set of accepted metrics now exist.
- Quality measures need to be patient-focused and proven to improve patient important outcomes.

D. I. Fudman (✉)
Division of Digestive and Liver Diseases, University of Texas Southwestern Medical Center, Dallas, TX, USA
e-mail: David.Fudman@UTSouthwestern.edu

S. Zuberi
Department of Medicine, Beth Israel Deaconess Medical Center, Boston, MA, USA
e-mail: szuberi@bidmc.harvard.edu

J. D. Feuerstein
Harvard Medical School, Beth Israel Deaconess Medical Center, Boston, MA, USA
e-mail: jfeuerst@bidmc.harvard.edu

J. D. Feuerstein, D. J. Stein (eds.), *Quality in Gastroenterology*,
https://doi.org/10.1007/978-3-031-58492-3_1

Over the past decade, medicine has had an increasing focus on defining quality of care and how to objectively measure the quality of care in clinical practice. Suboptimal quality of healthcare can lead to increased morbidity and mortality. The World Health Organization (WHO) reports that 5.7–8.4 million deaths are attributed to suboptimal quality care every year in low- and middle-income countries [1]. To reduce these harms and financial burden, the quality of health services provided needs to be improved. The WHO identifies three key components that define quality health services: effectiveness at providing evidence-based healthcare, provide healthcare in a safe fashion avoiding harm when caring for patients, and the care must be people centered responding to individual preferences of the patients. To achieve these goals, healthcare must be provided in a timely and equitable fashion, and disparities in care need to be eliminated [1].

One way to establish such systems is to provide objective quality measures or indicators that can be reported [2, 3]. Multiple gastrointestinal societies have published standard quality measures for clinical practice [4–8]. The evidence supporting these recommendations has varied in underlying quality and supporting evidence. Not every measure has a robust evidence basis [9, 10]. As a result, quality measures have not always been shown to improve clinical outcomes of importance to patients. Nonetheless, organizations have still pushed forward with attempts at codifying quality in gastroenterology and standardized what is considered high-quality care [2, 3]. Ideally, to establish an ideal quality measure/indicator, it must be one that improves clinical care, reduces ineffective care, reduces disparities in care, is cost-effective, and provides outcomes that are of importance and of high relevance to patients.

In 2015 the American College of Gastroenterology and the American Society for Gastrointestinal Endoscopy published joint papers on quality in endoscopic procedures [4, 5, 7, 11–13]. These papers have been used to set the standard quality measures and expectations when performing endoscopy. However, there is a paucity of similar publications for other gastrointestinal diseases despite evidence of care gaps for a multitude of conditions under the care of gastroenterologists [14–16]. The Centers for Medicare and Medicaid Services have also attempted to establish quality measures over the last two decades [16]. In 2012 the American Gastroenterological Association established a series of quality measures in inflammatory bowel disease (IBD) referred to as the Bridges to Excellence IBD Care Recognition. These measures were used to comply with the CMS Physician Quality Reporting System (PQRS). However, reporting on these measures was variable, and the measures lacked data to show that they improved patient outcomes [17]. CMS discontinued the PQRS program in 2016 and replaced it with the Merit-Based Incentive Payment System (MIPS) and in 2017 established the quality payment program (more details can be obtained from the CMS website: https://qpp.cms.gov/mips/explore-measures). The number of GI-relevant quality-based MIPS measures is limited due to the strict requirements for establishing quality metrics for CMS. In 2012, the Choosing Wisely campaign was initiated by the American Board of Internal Medicine (ABIM). This campaign focuses on reducing overused and unnecessary medical tests, treatments, and procedures, including avoiding overuse of endoscopic procedures, acid suppressive medications, and CT scans in patients with functional abdominal pain [18–20]. However, while rooted in evidence, a reporting system on adherence to these quality-based recommendations was never established.

Despite this paucity of metrics, the literature is consistent that variation in care practices, including under- and overuse, is a marker of suboptimal care quality and is present across many disease states in gastroenterology [21–23]. In inflammatory bowel disease, for example, there is variation in treatment selection between practice settings and among individual physicians that cannot be explained by patient-level factors, in knowledge regarding recommendations for preventive actions such as vaccinations and venous thromboembolism prophylaxis in hospitalized patients, and there are disparities among racial and socioeconomic groups with regard to care access [24]. Moreover, emergency rooms and CT imaging are overused in IBD, while early effective therapy, inflammatory monitoring, and IBD-specific health maintenance activities remain underutilized [25, 26]. Although societies have updated practice guidelines to provide clear evidence-based recommendations for these clinical situations, real-life clinical practice remains incongruent with present practice guidelines [27–29]. Guidelines are an important aspect in developing quality standards, but they alone are not considered quality metrics [30–32].

Stool-based colon cancer screening tests also carry examples of both overuse and underuse [33]. Fecal occult blood testing is frequently used inappropriately in the hospital for the evaluation of anemia or overt gastrointestinal bleeding despite its high false negative and positive rates in these settings, leading at least some institutions to eliminate the test's availability for inpatients [34, 35]. Even when noninvasive colon cancer testing is used appropriately for colon cancer screening, unfortunately a substantial proportion of positive tests are not followed by colonoscopy evaluation, and it is not uncommon for such evaluation to be excessively delayed when performed [36].

In endoscopy, the most studied area in gastroenterology with regard to quality, variations exist in its diagnostic use. The inappropriate overuse of upper endoscopy has been well described in patients presenting with vague upper abdominal symptoms such as dyspepsia [22, 37]. Many patients are referred for endoscopy prior to any further workup or therapeutic trials, potentially due to the relative safety of the procedure as well as unfamiliarity with guidelines and uncertainty about etiology of symptoms. While most studies have focused on the overutilization of upper endoscopy, underuse in patients with dysphagia or dyspepsia refractory to antisecretory treatment has also been found [38, 39].

Presently, most established quality metrics in gastroenterology focus on endoscopy [4, 11]. A number of quality measures have been established including cecal intubation, withdrawal time, quality of bowel preparation, and others [4]. Most notable among these is the adenoma detection rate, which measures the proportion of screening colonoscopies during which an adenoma is removed [40]. This metric has been associated strongly with the risk of interval colorectal cancer [41]. Although this measure is widely accepted as valid and important, its uptake has been mixed, largely due to the administrative burden of collecting the data required to report it [42]. Additionally, as evidence continues to evolve, the optimal thresholds for adenoma detection have changed [43]. Like many areas in quality, quality metrics are not static and require continued reassessment for relevance and accuracy.

However, measures are more limited outside of the endoscopic arena. There have been efforts to establish condition-specific quality metrics, often published as consensus documents. While gastroenterology societies have taken a lead in trying to establish quality metrics, there still remains a paucity of non-endoscopic quality measures. The gap between the present state of condition-specific metrics and the need for valid measures that can be leveraged to close quality gaps remains broad. This gap reflects multiple factors, including an evidence base that must expand further to support high-quality metrics, concerns regarding metric feasibility (i.e., the administrative burden of reporting the metric), and concerns regarding metric implementation including questions of their impact on a practice's bottom line.

Nonetheless, there is reason to be very optimistic for the future of quality in gastroenterology. The advent of natural language processing as well as machine learning and artificial intelligence approaches will offer ways to measure quality without manual input, thus automating the process of metric reporting. Although this will come with its own challenges, removing the need for personnel hours to implement a metric will allow for a great expansion not only of the breadth of a metric's adoption but also the number of metrics a practice can feasibly measure and report. For example, machine learning platforms can utilize so-called big data within an institution's electronic health record to populate numerators and the denominators for a variety of metrics without a clinician's input. Such approaches are already here: the use of natural language processing to automate adenoma detection rate reporting is now available in commercial platforms and also has been developed internally at academic institutions [44, 45].

However, technology alone will not be a panacea for increasing the quality of care in gastroenterology. The underpinnings of shared knowledge, not just of the literature but of implementation science, and the incentives to put this knowledge into action must form the bedrock of quality improvement. Implementation science, still a relatively new field, has been expanding at an encouraging clip, providing the tools to identify best practices.

Quality in gastroenterology is still in its infancy. Gastroenterology societies are working to establish quality metrics and standards, but further data on patient-focused outcomes on how these measures improve outcomes of importance to patients are needed. Establishing quality standards throughout gastroenterology including both endoscopic and clinical care will ultimately improve patient-centric care.

References

1. National Academies of Sciences, Engineering, and Medicine; Health and Medicine Division; Board on Health Care Services; Board on Global Health; Committee on Improving the Quality of Health Care Globally. Crossing the global quality chasm: improving health care worldwide. National Academies Press (US); 2018.
2. Kane S, Leighton J, Kefalas C, et al. Quality commitment: the newly established American College of Gastroenterology quality council to meet the needs of clinical gastroenterology. ACG. 2013;108:7–9.
3. Brotman M, Allen JI, Bickston SJ, et al. AGA Task Force on Quality in Practice: a national overview and implications for GI practice. Gastroenterology. 2005;129:361–9.
4. Rex DK, Schoenfeld PS, Cohen J, et al. Quality indicators for colonoscopy. ACG. 2015;110:72–90.
5. Rizk MK, Sawhney MS, Cohen J, et al. Quality indicators common to all GI endoscopic procedures. Gastrointest Endosc. 2015;81:3–16.
6. Beg S, Ragunath K, Wyman A, et al. Quality standards in upper gastrointestinal endoscopy: a position statement of the British Society of Gastroenterology (BSG) and Association of Upper Gastrointestinal Surgeons of Great Britain and Ireland (AUGIS). Gut. 2017;66:1886–99.
7. Rex DK, Schoenfeld PS, Cohen J, et al. Quality indicators for colonoscopy. Gastrointest Endosc. 2015;81:31–53.
8. Hung KW, Maratt JK, Cho WK, Shah BJ, Anjou CI, Leiman DA. AGA Institute Quality measure development for the management of gastric intestinal metaplasia with Helicobacter pylori. Gastroenterology. 2022;163:3–7.
9. Weissman S, Aziz M, Baniqued MR, et al. Quality measures in endoscopy: a systematic analysis of the overall scientific level of evidence and conflicts of interest. Endosc Int Open. 2022;10:E776–E86.
10. Weissman S, Goldowsky A, Mehta TI, Sciarra MA, Feuerstein JD. Are quality metrics in inflammatory bowel disease rooted in substantial quality evidence? A systematic review. J Crohn's Colitis. 2021;15:326–34.
11. Park WG, Shaheen NJ, Cohen J, et al. Quality indicators for EGD. Am J Gastroenterol. 2015;110:60–71.
12. Adler DG, Lieb JG II, Cohen J, et al. Quality indicators for ERCP. Gastrointest Endosc. 2015;81:54–66.
13. Wani S, Wallace MB, Cohen J, et al. Quality indicators for EUS. Gastrointest Endosc. 2015;81:67–80.
14. Pinto-Sanchez MI, Silvester JA, Lebwohl B, et al. Society for the study of celiac disease position statement on gaps and opportunities in coeliac disease. Nat Rev Gastroenterol Hepatol. 2021;18:875–84.
15. Egberg MD, Gulati AS, Gellad ZF, Melmed GY, Kappelman MD. Improving quality in the care of patients with inflammatory bowel diseases. Inflamm Bowel Dis. 2018;24:1660–9.
16. Kanwal F, Tapper EB, Ho C, et al. Development of quality measures in cirrhosis by the Practice Metrics Committee of the American Association for the Study of Liver Diseases. Hepatology. 2019;69:1787–97.
17. Feuerstein JD, Castillo NE, Siddique SS, et al. Poor documentation of inflammatory bowel disease quality measures in academic, community, and private practice. Clin Gastroenterol Hepatol. 2016;14:421–8.
18. Born K, Kool T, Levinson W. Reducing overuse in healthcare: advancing choosing wisely. BMJ. 2019;367:6317.
19. Levinson W, Born K, Wolfson D. Choosing wisely campaigns: a work in progress. JAMA. 2018;319:1975–6.
20. https://www.choosingwisely.org/societies/american-gastroenterological-association/. Accessed 3 January 2023.

21. Murphy CC, Sandler RS, Grubber JM, Johnson MR, Fisher DA. Underuse and overuse of colonoscopy for repeat screening and surveillance in the Veterans Health Administration. Clin Gastroenterol Hepatol. 2016;14:436–44.
22. de Jong JJ, Lantinga MA, Drenth JP. Prevention of overuse: a view on upper gastrointestinal endoscopy. World J Gastroenterol. 2019;25:178.
23. Jatoi I, Sah S. Clinical practice guidelines and the overuse of health care services: need for reform. CMAJ. 2019;191:E297–E8.
24. Weizman AV, Nguyen GC. Quality of care delivered to hospitalized inflammatory bowel disease patients. World J Gastroenterol. 2013;19:6360.
25. Gashin L, Villafuerte-Galvez J, Leffler DA, Obuch J, Cheifetz AS. Utility of CT in the emergency department in patients with ulcerative colitis. Inflamm Bowel Dis. 2015;21:793–800.
26. Yarur AJ, Mandalia AB, Dauer RM, et al. Predictive factors for clinically actionable computed tomography findings in inflammatory bowel disease patients seen in the emergency department with acute gastrointestinal symptoms. J Crohn's Colitis. 2014;8:504–12.
27. Dong J, Wang LF, Ardolino E, Feuerstein JD. Real-world compliance with the 2020 US Multi-Society Task Force on Colorectal Cancer polypectomy surveillance guidelines: an observational study. Gastrointest Endosc. 2022;97(2):350–6.
28. Clarke WT, Satyam VR, Fudman DI, et al. Antibiotic prophylaxis and infectious complications in patients on peritoneal dialysis undergoing lower gastrointestinal endoscopy. Gastroenterol Rep. 2020;8:407–9.
29. Hart L, El-Matary W. Poor clinician adherence to inflammatory bowel disease guidelines: how do we remedy the situation? Crohn's Colitis. 2022;5(3):31.
30. Clarke K, Adler N, Agrawal D, et al. Reducing overuse of proton pump inhibitors for stress ulcer prophylaxis and nonvariceal gastrointestinal bleeding in the hospital: a narrative review and implementation guide. J Hosp Med. 2021;16:417–23.
31. Hoffmann F, Glaeske G, Schmiemann G. Underuse of proton-pump inhibitors in older patients newly starting NSAID treatment. Int J Clin Pract. 2015;69:791–5.
32. Dharmarajan TS. The use and misuse of proton pump inhibitors: an opportunity for deprescribing. J Am Med Dir Assoc. 2021;22:15–22.
33. Burke CA, Lieberman D, Feuerstein JD. AGA clinical practice update on approach to the use of noninvasive colorectal cancer screening options: commentary. Gastroenterology. 2022;162:952–6.
34. Bangaru S, Tang D, Agrawal D. Inappropriate use of fecal occult blood testing. JAMA Intern Med. 2018;178:1702–3.
35. Mathews B, Ratcliffe T, Sehgal R, Abraham J, Monash B. Fecal occult blood testing in hospitalized patients with upper gastrointestinal bleeding. J Hosp Med. 2017;12:567–9.
36. Said H, Dong J, Miller S, Systrom H, Feuerstein JD. S296 appropriateness and completion of multitarget stool DNA testing in primary and subspecialty care. ACG. 2022;117:e214–e5.
37. Rubenstein JH, Pohl H, Adams MA, et al. Overuse of repeat upper endoscopy in the veterans health administration: a retrospective analysis. ACG. 2017;112(11):1678–85.
38. Seematter-Bagnoud L, Vader J-P, Wietlisbach V, Froehlich F, Gonvers J-J, Burnand B. Overuse and underuse of diagnostic upper gastrointestinal endoscopy in various clinical settings. Int J Qual Health Care. 1999;11:301–8.
39. Gawron AJ, Cole G, Hu N, Thompson WK, Fang J, Samore M. Regional variability of repeat esophagogastroduodenoscopy use in the national veteran population. Dig Dis Sci. 2017;62:2303–10.
40. Keswani RN, Crockett SD, Calderwood AH. AGA clinical practice update on strategies to improve quality of screening and surveillance colonoscopy: expert review. Gastroenterology. 2021;161:701–11.
41. Corley DA, Jensen CD, Marks AR, et al. Adenoma detection rate and risk of colorectal cancer and death. N Engl J Med. 2014;370:1298–306.
42. Jones B, Scott FI, Espinoza J, et al. Leveraging electronic medical record functionality to capture adenoma detection rate. Sci Rep. 2022;12:1–5.

43. Shaukat A, Holub J, Pike IM, et al. Benchmarking adenoma detection rates for colonoscopy: results from a US-based registry. ACG. 2021;116:1946–9.
44. Tinmouth J, Swain D, Chorneyko K, et al. Validation of a natural language processing algorithm to identify adenomas and measure adenoma detection rates across a health system: a population-level study. Gastrointest Endosc. 2023;97:121–9.
45. Nayor J, Borges LF, Goryachev S, Gainer VS, Saltzman JR. Natural language processing accurately calculates adenoma and sessile serrated polyp detection rates. Dig Dis Sci. 2018;63:1794–800.

Chapter 2
Quality in Colonoscopy

Emery Lin, Ranjan Mascarenhas, and David Lieberman

Table of Quality Measures/Metrics

E. Lin · D. Lieberman (✉)
Division of Gastroenterology, Department of Medicine, Portland Veterans Affairs Hospital, Oregon Health Science University, Portland, OR, USA
e-mail: emery.lin@va.gov; lieberma@ohsu.edu

R. Mascarenhas
Division of Gastroenterology, Department of Medicine, Dell Medical School, The University of Texas at Austin, CTVHCS, Austin OPC, Austin, TX, USA
e-mail: ranjan.mascarenhas@austin.utexas.edu

J. D. Feuerstein, D. J. Stein (eds.), *Quality in Gastroenterology*,
https://doi.org/10.1007/978-3-031-58492-3_2

Key Points

- High-quality colonoscopy improves patient outcomes, whereas poor quality is associated with a higher risk of post-colonoscopy colorectal cancer
- If quality is not measured, it is unknown
- Key elements of high quality colonoscopy include:
  - Pre-procedure metrics including appropriate indication and assessment of co-morbidity
  - High-quality report which includes key intra-procedure quality metrics such as bowel prep quality, exam completeness and polyp descriptors
  - Adenoma detection rate (ADR) determined for each endoscopist
  - Post-procedure recommendations for follow-up, which are consistent with guidelines
  - Ongoing research will determine if technical aids such as artificial intelligence improve colonoscopy quality

Introduction

Colorectal cancer (CRC) is the third most common cancer and second leading cause of cancer death worldwide. In the United States, CRC is the third most common cancer by incidence and third leading cause of cancer death among both men and women [1]. Declining rates of colon cancer in the past two decades have been attributed in part to screening and removal of precancerous polyps via colonoscopy and finding colorectal cancer at an earlier stage, which has a more favorable prognosis. However, although the overall death rate has continued to drop, deaths from CRC among people younger than 55 have increased 1% per year from 2008 to 2017. This has led to a revision of screening guidelines from the United States Preventive Services Task Force and from major gastroenterology societies which now recommend that average-risk individuals begin colon cancer screening at the age of 45 years instead of 50 years [2]. Colonoscopy is presently the gold standard screening modality for CRC and evaluation of lower gastrointestinal symptoms. Therefore, it is important to understand and evaluate indicators of a high-quality colonoscopy which has led to better patient outcomes by minimizing interval CRC, minimizing complications, and increasing patient satisfaction. A 2015 consensus statement released from the American Society for Gastrointestinal Endoscopy (ASGE) and the American College of Gastroenterology identified several indicators of high-quality colonoscopy which were divided by interval into pre-procedure, intra-procedure, and post-procedure (Table 2.1) [3].

Table 2.1 Quality indicators for colonoscopy with measurable performance targets

Quality measure	Performance target
Pre-procedure	>80%
Appropriate indication documented	>98%
Informed consent obtained	≥90%
Appropriate colorectal screening/surveillance interval	≥90%
Appropriate inflammatory bowel disease surveillance interval	
Intra-procedure	>98%
Documentation of bowel preparation quality	>85%
Adequate bowel preparation to perform adequate examination	≥90% all, ≥95% screening
Documentation of cecal intubation	>98%
Documentation of withdrawal time	≥6 min
Average withdrawal time for negative examinations	≥30% males, ≥20%
Adenoma detection rate	females, ≥25% combined
Biopsies for indications of chronic diarrhea	>98%
Tissue sampling for inflammatory bowel disease	>98%
Attempted endoscopic removal of polyps <2 cm before surgical removal	>98%
Post-procedure	<1:500
Monitor complications	<1:1000
(a) Perforation in all examinations	
(b) Perforation in screening examinations	
Managing bleeding	
Recommendations for surveillance interval of repeat colonoscopy, including histology	
Patient satisfaction	

Adapted from the ASGE/ACG Task Force on Quality in Endoscopy, 2015, with permission from the American College of Gastroenterology [3]

Pre-procedure Quality Metrics

Appropriate Indication for Colonoscopy

The first step in a high-quality colonoscopy is ensuring that the patient has been referred for a colonoscopy for a necessary indication. The American Society for Gastrointestinal Endoscopy (ASGE) has published on appropriate indications for colonoscopy, which are detailed in Table 2.2 [3]. Present guidelines recommend that the appropriate indication is documented in at least 80% of procedures. A systemic review of 12 cohort studies comprising 14,160 patients, based on both ASGE and European Panel on the Appropriateness of Gastrointestinal Endoscopy (EPAGE) guidelines, revealed that 26% of colonoscopy indications were categorized as inappropriate, although there was significant heterogeneity among the 12 studies with an inappropriateness rate ranging from 14% to 37% [4]. The use of decision support tools, like the EPAGE online decision tool (www.epage.ch), can help improve on the appropriateness of patient selection.

Colorectal cancer screening and surveillance is one of the most common indications for referral for colonoscopy, but it is also one of the most difficult areas to adhere to guidelines, particularly in this era of open access endoscopy where

Table 2.2 Appropriate indications for colonoscopy

Evaluation of an abnormality on barium enema or other imaging study that is likely to be clinically significant, such as a filling defect or stricture
Evaluation of unexplained GI bleeding
Hematochezia
Melena after an upper GI source has been excluded
Presence of fecal occult blood
Unexplained iron deficiency anemia
Screening and surveillance for colon neoplasia
Screening of asymptomatic, average-risk patients for colon neoplasia
Examination to evaluate the entire colon for synchronous cancer or neoplastic polyps in a patient with treatable cancer or neoplastic polyp
Colonoscopy to remove synchronous neoplastic lesions at or around the time of curative resection of cancer followed by colonoscopy
at 1 year, if examination is normal, and then 3 years, if normal, and then 5 years thereafter to detect metachronous cancer
Surveillance of patients with neoplastic polyps
Surveillance of patients with a significant family history of colorectal neoplasia
For dysplasia and cancer surveillance in select patients with long-standing ulcerative or Crohn's colitis
For evaluation of patients with chronic inflammatory bowel disease of the colon, if more precise diagnosis or determination of the extent
of activity of disease will influence management
Clinically significant diarrhea of unexplained origin
Intraoperative identification of a lesion not apparent at surgery (e.g., polypectomy site, location of a bleeding site)
Treatment of bleeding from such lesions as vascular malformation, ulceration, neoplasia, and polypectomy site
Intraoperative evaluation of anastomotic reconstructions (e.g., evaluation for anastomotic leak and patency, bleeding, pouch formation)
As an adjunct to minimally invasive surgery for the treatment of diseases of the colon and rectum
Management or evaluation of operative adverse events (e.g., dilation of anastomotic strictures)
Foreign body removal
Excision or ablation of lesions
Decompression of acute megacolon or sigmoid volvulus
Balloon dilation of stenotic lesions (e.g., anastomotic strictures)
Palliative treatment of stenosing or bleeding neoplasms (e.g., laser, electrocoagulation, stenting)
Marking a neoplasm for localization

Adapted from the ASGE/ACG Task Force on Quality in Endoscopy, 2015, with permission from the American College of Gastroenterology [3]

patients can be referred by non-GI providers and may arrive with limited information. Historically, the recommendation has been for colon cancer screening in average-risk individuals to begin at age 50, although in recent years the United States Preventive Services Task Force and American Cancer Society have recommended that average-risk individuals should screen patients beginning at age 45 up to the age of 75 [2, 5]. This has been supported by guidelines from the major GI societies, although the benefit of screening remains greater in average-risk patients aged >50 compared to those aged 45–49 [6]. For patients aged 76–85, selective screening is recommended based on the patient's health, prior screening history, and personal preferences.

Certain factors increase the risk of colon cancer and warrant earlier or more frequent screening. Patients with a first-degree relative who was diagnosed with colon cancer or advanced polyps under age 60 or patients with two first-degree relatives with CRC or advanced polyps of any age are considered to have increased risk. Colorectal cancer screening is recommended to begin at age 40 or 10 years before the youngest affected relative and to continue at minimum of 5-year intervals [6]. One study of first-degree relatives of patients with CRC indicated that only 28% were aware of their increased risk for cancer and only 22% were aware of the correct age to start screening [7]. This suggests that we are likely under-screening these high-risk patient populations, and the endoscopist should ask and document the family history for every patient arriving for screening colonoscopy.

In addition, women with a personal history of uterine or ovarian cancer before age 50 are also considered to have an increased risk of colorectal cancer, and colonoscopy is recommended at 5-year intervals. Patients with known hereditary colon cancer syndromes such as Lynch syndrome or familial adenomatous polyposis require stringent screening and surveillance which is beyond the scope of this chapter.

There has not been adequate time to measure the adherence to the updated guidelines recommending an earlier age for colon cancer screening, but as of 2019, 67.1% of adults aged 50–75 had received some form of colorectal cancer screening [8]. Undoubtedly extending the age range to include patients aged 45–75 would lead to a lower adherence rate. While there is no available data on how many patients may be getting screening colonoscopies at too early of an age, it has been shown that patients are receiving repeat colonoscopies after a negative screening colonoscopy much more frequently than recommended [9].

Appropriate post-polypectomy surveillance intervals will be covered later in this chapter. The goal is that >90% of patients will undergo appropriate colorectal screening and post-polypectomy surveillance. However, we are likely overutilizing surveillance in low-risk individuals and underutilizing surveillance in high-risk individuals. A systemic review of 16 studies showed that less than 50% of surveillance colonoscopies followed guidelines on recommended intervals [10]. Surveys of endoscopists suggest that this may be due to a combination of not knowing the guidelines, disagreement with published guidelines, concerns about legal risk, or reimbursement factors [11, 12]. Lack of adherence with guidelines is more common among surgeons, nonacademic physicians, and low-volume colonoscopists [13, 14]. But even among endoscopists that knew the guidelines, some may disagree and perform surveillance sooner than recommended [12]. The endoscopist should properly document the indication for each colonoscopy, and if the timing differs from established guidelines, an accompanying explanation is warranted. Proper adherence to recommended colorectal screening and post-polypectomy surveillance intervals must be identified during the referral/triage process, before the patient has undergone bowel prep and has arrived for the procedure.

Surveillance colonoscopy is recommended for patients with ulcerative colitis or Crohn's colitis with a minimum of 8 years of disease and at least 30% of colon disease involvement and continued every 1–3 years, due to the increased long-term risk of colorectal cancer [15, 16]. An exception to this rule is patients with concomitant primary sclerosing cholangitis (PSC) who have a significantly increased risk of colorectal cancer and thus require annual surveillance beginning at the time of diagnosis of ulcerative colitis. Multiple studies support the survival benefit of a surveillance colonoscopy program in ulcerative colitis and Crohn's colitis patients [17, 18]. Patients with active inflammation, endoscopic scarring, post-inflammatory polyp formation, personal history of stricture/dysplasia, or a family history of cancer may require more frequent surveillance. Notably European guidelines suggest that in select endoscopically normal patients without intermediate- or high-risk features, surveillance may be extended out to every 5 years [19]. Given the wide variance of surveillance guidelines, there is significant variability in surveillance frequency in clinical practice as well. However, one study at a tertiary Canadian center showed that patients were getting surveillance colonoscopies at an appropriate frequency up to 75% of the time. One exception to this was patients with PSC, who were adherent to the recommended annual colonoscopy only between one-third and one-half of the time [20]. Regardless, the gastrointestinal community is likely falling short of the target of >90% of surveillance colonoscopies following appropriate surveillance intervals.

Precautions in Colonoscopy

A careful review of the medical history is necessary to determine the risks of colonoscopy for the patient. There are a few situations when colonoscopy is strictly contraindicated, such as known/suspected perforation, toxic megacolon/fulminant colitis, and acute diverticulitis. It is also important to consider factors which may increase risk of perforation during colonoscopy, including but not limited to patient age, multiple comorbidities, poor nutritional status, critical illness, and ischemic colitis [21]. Other factors to consider prior to the colonoscopy include anatomic issues (such as prior abdominal surgeries or presence of hernias) which may complicate the colonoscopy itself or the ability to safely provide abdominal pressure, comorbidities that may increase risks of sedation and/or safety of airway intubation, chronic use of medications that may affect patient's tolerance to anesthesia, and the presence of implanted cardiac defibrillator or pacemaker which may need to be turned off when using electrocautery. Use of the Mallampati classification can predict difficulty with airway management and potential endotracheal intubation. The American Society of Anesthesiologists Physical Status Classification System (ASA) can help guide the proper choice of anesthesia (moderate vs deep vs general) and the proper location for the procedure to be performed (ambulatory vs hospital). The ASGE recommends that anesthesia provider assistance be considered if anticipate any of the following: a prolonged or therapeutic endoscopic procedure, intolerance to standard sedation, increased risk for airway obstruction due to anatomy, or increased risk for adverse event due to comorbidities (ASA class 4 or 5) [22].

The optimal management of the patient's anticoagulation should also be addressed prior to colonoscopy. This requires balancing the procedural risk of bleeding (low vs high) with the risk of a thromboembolic event (low vs high) for the patient if the anticoagulation is stopped. Diagnostic colonoscopy with biopsy is considered low risk, while polypectomy or dilation is considered high risk. The risk of thromboembolic events depends on the indications, but high-risk patients include those with $CHAD_2S_2$-VASC ≥ 2 in atrial fibrillation, drug-eluting coronary stents placed $\leq$12 months prior or bare metal coronary stents placed $\leq$ 1 month prior, history of prior stent occlusion, prior venous thromboembolism within 3 months or severe thrombophilia, any mitral valve prosthesis or caged-ball/tilting disc aortic valve prosthesis, and CVA/TIA $\leq$6 months prior. The ASGE guidelines on this subject are summarized in Table 2.3 [23].

Consenting for Colonoscopy

Prior to undergoing colonoscopy, the patient must appropriately understand the risks and benefits and be able to consent for the procedure. The patient should understand the present medical diagnosis, nature of the proposed procedure, reason for the procedure, benefits of the procedure, risks and complications of the procedure, reasonable alternatives, and prognosis if the procedure is declined [24]. ASGE guidelines recommend that endoscopists learn the specific standard of informed consent in the locale where they are practicing. Informed consent may be obtained by any member of the GI team who is thoroughly knowledgeable of and able to communicate the indications, risks, benefits, and alternatives of the procedure [25]. A third-party witness to the consent process is recommended. The consent form should be written and communicated in simple lay language. In multilingual settings, the use of consent forms in foreign languages and certified translators can ensure the patient fully understands what is being consented to. Family members should not be used as translators, as this has inherent bias and creates uncertainty about the nature of what is being communicated.

Consent must be completed prior to beginning the procedure and prior to any sedation. The increase in open access endoscopy creates a more challenging environment for informed consent, as there is less time for the patient to consider and review information provided. Studies suggest that patients undergoing open access endoscopy felt less informed about their endoscopic procedure and were less likely to understand the indication for the procedure compared with patients that had previously been seen in an office visit [26, 27]. However, patient satisfaction appears to

Table 2.3 Management of antithrombotic agents in elective endoscopy

	Endoscopy-induced bleeding risk				
Cardiovascular risk		Low risk		High risk	
	Low risk	AC	1. Continue warfarin and NOAC	AC	1. Discontinue AC 2. Restart warfarin on same day of procedure 3. Delay reinitiating NOACs until adequate hemostasis is achieved
		APA	1. Continue standard doses of ASA/NSAIDs 2. Continue thienopyridines	APA	1. Continue standard doses of ASA/NSAIDs[a] 2. Discontinue thienopyridines at least 5 days before switching to ASA[b] 3. Dual APA; hold thienopyridines for at least 5 days, and continue ASA[b]
	High risk	AC	1. Continue warfarin and NOAC	AC	1. Discontinue AC 2. Bridge therapy 3. Restart warfarin on same day of procedure 4. Delay reinitiating NOACs until adequate hemostasis is achieved
		APA	1. Continue standard doses of ASA/NSAIDs 2. Continue thienopyridines	APA	1. Continue standard doses of ASA/NSAIDs 2. Discontinue thienopyridines at least 5 days before endoscopy or switch to ASA[b] 3. Dual APA; hold thienopyridines for at least 5 days, and continue ASA[b]

Adapted from the ASGE Standards of Practice Committee statement on the management of antithrombotic agents for patients undergoing GI endoscopy [23]
AC anticoagulants, *APA* antiplatelet agent, *NOAC* novel oral anticoagulant, *ASA* acetylsalicylic acid, or aspirin, *NSAID* nonsteroidal anti-inflammatory drug
[a] There is evidence to hold APA in patients undergoing ESD and EMR who have a low risk for a thromboembolic event
[b] Ticagrelor should be held for 3–5 days, and all other thienopyridines should be held for 5–7 days

be similar, and there is strong desire for patients and providers to continue to offer open access endoscopy [28]. Strategies such as mailing consent forms or pre-procedural educational information may improve the ability to adequately provide consent and patient adherence to instructions in the open access endoscopy setting [29, 30]. The informed consent process is a common area to be involved in medical legal action, and while there is little literature on how often informed consent is documented, the more critical legal question often regards the adequacy of the informed consent. The use of templates can facilitate proper documentation and remind the endoscopist of important details to be included in the discussion. As patient recall of the written or verbal consent process is poor even in healthy volunteers, the use of pie graphs or pictograms can also help improve patient understanding about risks and benefits of colonoscopy [31, 32].

Intra-procedure Metrics

The main goal for most colonoscopy procedures is to detect and remove precancerous and cancerous lesions. To achieve this goal, the bowel must be adequately clean so that the mucosa can be well inspected, the cecum should be reached so that the colon can be examined in its entirety, the withdrawal time should be adequate to allow for a thorough inspection of the colon, and the endoscopist should be able to detect precancerous lesions (adenomas).

Bowel Preparation

A key procedure factor for a high-quality colonoscopy exam is bowel preparation for the colonoscopy. Adequate bowel preparation as defined by the ability to detect polyps smaller than 5 mm is essential for achieving a high-quality examination during colonoscopy. More than 85% of colonoscopies for all indications and ≥90% of screening colonoscopies should be scored adequate or better to meet the ASGE/ACG colonoscopy quality indicator goals. Inadequate preparation can cause failure to detect all types of lesions: neoplastic, adenomatous, or serrated [33]. Poor bowel preparation results in repeat procedures which lead to increased health-care costs and burden on the health-care system. The three most commonly used classifications to grade the quality of preparation are the Aronchick, Ottawa, and Boston scales. The Aronchick scale grades preparation prior to any rinsing maneuvers on a scale of 1 (excellent) to 5 (inadequate with repeat procedure needed). The Ottawa scale grades each of three colon segments prior to cleansing on a scale of 0 (excellent) to 4 (inadequate), as well as the amount of fluid in the colon from 0 (small amount) to 2 (large amount). The scores are then summed for a composite score ranging from 0 (excellent) to 14 (very poor) [33]. The Boston Bowel Preparation

Scale is the most favored scale based on high reliability and ease of use. Each of three colon segments is rated after cleansing maneuvers have been performed from 0 (unprepared with solid stool) to 3 (entire mucosa well visualized). These scores are then summed for a range from 0 (very poor) to 9 (excellent) [34]. Choksi et al. showed that patients with bowel preparation classified as poor or inadequate/unsatisfactory result in an adenoma miss rate of 47.9% with the majority (64.8%) of those missed in the proximal colon [35]. The ADR with poor prep was calculated as 25.7% in the study's participants. Of the participants who underwent repeat colonoscopy, 33.8% had at least one new adenoma found that was not initially detected [35]. Thus, poor bowel preparation is one of the factors contributing to missed advanced polyps or malignancies, and it may be prudent to abort a procedure with poor preparation rather than attempt to complete it. Patients with an inadequate bowel prep should be scheduled for a repeat procedure within a year with a different or 2-day bowel preparation. Lieberman et al. showed that among patients who had a repeat examination within 1 year (nearly three quarters of whom because their original examination had inadequate bowel preparation or was incomplete), 6.5% had large polyps [36].

Inadequate bowel preparation can also impair detection of nonpolypoid colorectal lesions [37], which are innately more difficult to detect visually due to being nearly flat (protruding 2.5 mm or less into the colon lumen) or depressed and have been shown to have more advanced pathology than polypoid neoplasms. The estimated risk of missing a nonpolypoid colorectal neoplasm due to poor preparation was calculated as 45–51%. Fair-quality bowel preparation has been shown to significantly lower the detection of nonpolypoid colorectal neoplasms from 12.9% to 8.5%, suggesting that fair preparation should prompt shortening of surveillance intervals.

Many experts discourage the use of the term "fair" to describe bowel preparation quality. The impact of fair-quality preparation on colonoscopy has been the subject of several studies attempting to determine the best surveillance interval in patients with fair preparation as well as its effect on ADR. Anderson et al. showed the overall ADR as well as the proximal colon ADR in colonoscopies with fair preparation was similar to those with an optimal (good or excellent) preparation [38]. A meta-analysis showed that patients with intermediate- or fair-quality preparation do not have a significantly different ADR from patients with high-quality bowel preparation nor a significant difference between preparations classified as good and excellent [39]. The authors suggested that patients with fair or intermediate bowel preparation should be given standard surveillance intervals and perhaps there is no clinical necessity to distinguishing between good and excellent bowel preparation. Patient education regarding appropriate preparation prior to a colonoscopy is important to achieve adequate bowel preparation. Detailed written or audiovisual prep instructions and split-dose bowel preparation have been shown to improve bowel preparation for colonoscopy [40].

It is now known that bowel preparation quality decreases as the interval from preparation completion to start of the procedure increases. This is particularly true for the right side of the colon. A split-dose preparation with one-half of the preparation taken the day before and the other taken the day of the procedure is now considered the standard of care to achieve a high-quality bowel preparation, resulting in both better preparation quality and better patient acceptance [41]. For procedures scheduled in the afternoon, it is acceptable to have the entire bowel preparation the same morning.

With increased emphasis on making health care more affordable in the United States, bundled payment arrangements have been proposed. According to the American Gastroenterological Association Institute, a colonoscopy bundled payment would include one payment for a pre-procedure visit, the preparation medication, the procedure itself, and any post-procedural complications for a defined period. As most bundled payment plans also include repeat colonoscopies done due to poor bowel preparation, the physician performing the procedure would receive no reimbursement for the repeat procedure and would hence affect the physician's bottom line. It is recommended that the percentage of repeat colonoscopies in less than a year due to inadequate bowel prep should not exceed 15%. This data must be tracked, and endoscopists with >15% of examinations with inadequate bowel prep should re-examine their bowel preparation protocols, patient instructions, choice of purgatives, and split-dose protocol. Thus, it is imperative that every effort be made by gastroenterology practices to provide the patient comprehensive pre-procedure instructions which are reinforced prior to the procedure to ensure that the bowel preparation quality is adequate.

Cecal Intubation

Cecal intubation is defined as the passage of the colonoscope proximal to the ileocecal valve until the cecal caput, medial cecal wall, and appendiceal orifice are visualized. Cecal intubation is an important measure of quality and signifies that the colon was visualized in its entirety. The present performance target for cecal intubation is ≥90% for all colonoscopies and ≥95% for screening examinations. Higher cecal intubation rates are associated with better ADR and lower incidence of interval colon cancer particularly from the proximal (right) colon [42]. There must be both photographic (Fig. 2.1) and written documentation within the procedure note that cecal intubation was achieved.

A retrospective study using the Clinical Outcomes Research Initiative (CORI) database found that bleeding and other nonspecific indications for colonoscopy had the highest risk of incomplete examination, while screening exams had the highest chance of a complete examination [43]. The study also found that males had higher completion rates than females, community settings had higher completion than academic or Veterans Affairs centers, and increasing age resulted in lower rates of complete examinations. Other reported predictors of incomplete colonoscopy include low body mass index, history of hysterectomy, history of diverticular disease, inflammation, anatomy, and bowel preparation quality [44].

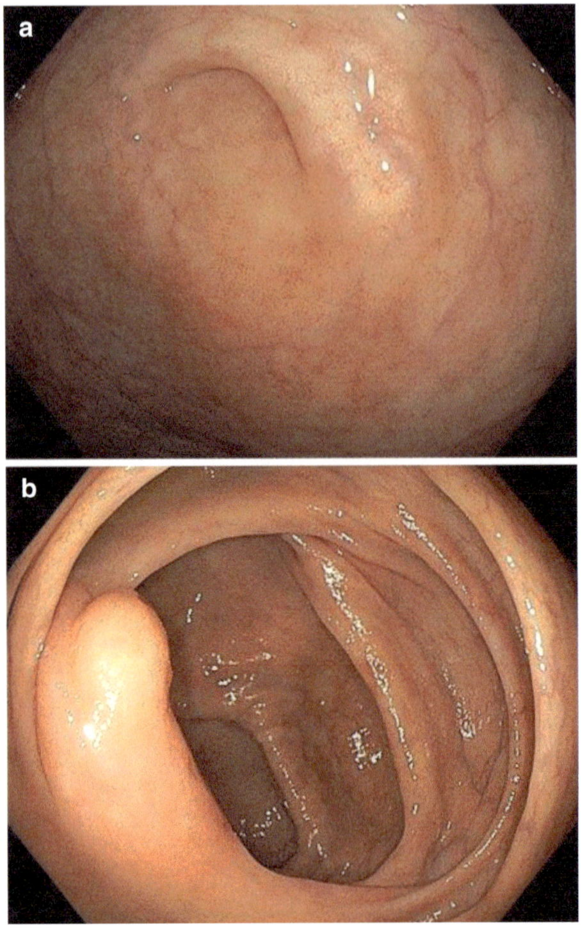

Fig. 2.1 Photographic documentation of cecal intubation showing the appendiceal orifice (**a**) and ileocecal valve (**b**)

Several techniques have been proposed to increase cecal intubation rate, including water infusion, carbon dioxide insufflation, the use of an ultrathin (9.2 mm) colonoscope, magnetic endoscopic imaging, device-assisted colonoscopy (single-balloon colonoscopy), and sedation [45]. Understanding the reason for failure to achieve cecal intubation should guide which approach to use in subsequent colonoscopy attempts.

Withdrawal Time

Withdrawal time is the time spent during endoscopy when the colonic mucosa is carefully inspected for lesions as the instrument is withdrawn from the cecum to the rectum. Present quality measures indicated that the withdrawal time should be ≥6 min in patients with intact colons (after subtracting time used to perform polypectomy or other interventions). Studies have shown that longer withdrawal time is associated with higher ADR [46]. Studies have challenged whether 6 min is long enough to ensure high-quality colonoscopy. Shaukat et al. found that the incidence of interval colorectal cancer was lowest with a mean withdrawal time of ≥8 min. They also found that ADR increased by 3.6% with every minute of increased withdrawal time [47]. A British study found that in colonoscopies with a mean withdrawal time of <7 min, the mean ADR was 42.5%, while those with a mean withdrawal time of ≥11 min had an ADR of 47.1%. The extra lesions detected with longer withdrawal times were mainly small or right-sided adenomas; detection of advanced adenomas did not increase. Their data showed that a withdrawal time of more than 10 min resulted in a minimal increase in ADR [48]. Butterly et al. evaluated withdrawal time and adenoma detection rate, as well as clinically significant serrated polyp rate (defined as serrated polyps and hyperplastic polyps proximal to the sigmoid colon). They found that a withdrawal time of 9 min was associated with a 13% increase in the detection of overall polyps, a 14% increase in the detection of adenomas, and a 30% increase in the detection of clinically significant serrated polyps [49]. Thus, based on these studies, the suggested guideline of ≥6 min of withdrawal time should be re-evaluated in light of new evidence. In addition to monitoring adherence to withdrawal time, proper technique when withdrawing the scope such as washing the mucosa, suctioning fluid, distending the colon adequately, and inspecting behind folds will increase ADR.

Adenoma Detection Rate

Adenoma detection rate (ADR) is defined by the proportion of average-risk individuals undergoing screening colonoscopy in whom an adenoma or colon cancer is found.

ADR is the sine qua non of quality measures for colonoscopy due to a landmark study by Kaminski et al. showing that a patient receiving a colonoscopy from a physician with an ADR below 20% had a tenfold higher chance of developing interval colorectal cancer than a colonoscopy performed by a physician with an ADR of greater than 20% [50]. Corley et al. found that with every 1% increase in adenoma detection rate, there was a 3% decrease in the risk of subsequent colon cancer [51]. A prospective study of individuals who underwent screening colonoscopy within a national colorectal cancer screening program showed increased ADR with a reduced risk of interval colorectal cancer and death [52]. The present benchmark metrics for ADR are 20% for women, 30% for men, and a combined ADR rate of 25% with both sexes combined. However, sessile serrated lesions are not considered when calculating ADR at this time due to inconsistencies in detecting these lesions and variability in pathologist's reporting of these lesions.

There is a high variability of ADR among endoscopists and across practices [53]. The maximum threshold of ADR beyond which there may be no added benefit of a high ADR is presently unknown. Although ADR is calculated using colonoscopies performed for screening only, it has been suggested that the metric should be changed to include adenomas detected during a colonoscopy performed for any reason, called the adenoma per colonoscopy rate. Two major limitations of ADR are a "one and done" practice pattern and inability to capture complete polyp resection. Further refinement in ADR has been proposed, since ADR does not capture the total number of adenomas removed during a procedure [54]. Studies that examine proximal versus distal ADR are underway and may be incorporated as a quality metric in the future.

Additionally, ADR does not distinguish between advanced (high-risk) adenomas and non-advanced (low-risk) adenomas. This is a major limitation since the biology of the lesion also matters as shown in a systematic review and meta-analysis that demonstrated that the risk of metachronous CRC and mortality is significantly higher for patients with high-risk adenomas (HRAs), defined as an advanced adenoma (villous histology, high-grade dysplasia, or ≥10 mm) or ≥3 adenomas), versus patients with low-risk adenomas (LRAs), defined as one to two tubular adenomas <10 mm with low-grade dysplasia, who have a risk profile comparable to patients with no adenomas. This has implications for surveillance colonoscopy intervals as follow-up of patients with LRAs detected at index colonoscopy should be the same as for persons with no adenomas [55]. Multiple studies have shown that interval colorectal cancer (iCRC) is inversely correlated with provider ADR [56, 57]. In a study of over 700,000 Kaiser patients, there was a hazard ratio of 0.97 for every 1% increase in ADR, across ADR groups from <20% to >50%. When comparing results by physicians above and below the median ADR in the study (>28.3% vs <28.3%), the hazard ratio was 0.26 [56]. Lam et al. showed that a quality improvement program focused on split-dose bowel preparation, quality metric measurement, provider education, and feedback led to increased ADRs and decreased iCRC rates over time [57]. iCRC rate measurement should be considered a feasible, outcomes-driven institutional metric of colonoscopy quality.

New data proposes that serrated lesion detection rate (SDR) should get calculated similarly to ADR as the number of screening colonoscopies with one or more sessile serrated lesion (SSL) divided by the total number of screening colonoscopies for a given period of time. The goal SDR for an endoscopist is recommended to be ≥7%. There is a wide variability of SDR among colonoscopists, just as there is variability of ADR [58, 59]. There is a definite association between withdrawal time and SDR suggesting careful inspection on withdrawal impacts SDR [49]. Since SDR is dependent on the pathologists' interpretation more so than ADR, any remediation to improve SDR should involve both the endoscopist and the reading pathologist [60].

Several interventions have been proposed to improve ADR. Two studies showed that the use of a physician "report card" with individual quality metrics results in increased ADR [61, 62]. A study at the Mayo Clinic showed that the implementation of an educational intervention for staff endoscopists (termed endoscopic quality improvement program, or EQUIP) improved adenoma detection rates. EQUIP training consisted of two sessions lasting approximately 1 h each. Those in the trial arm of the study also received monthly feedback on their ADR. After the intervention, the ADR of "trained" physicians increased from 35% to 47%, where the control group's adenoma detection rate remained steady at 35% [63]. Critics of this study point out that the endoscopists involved had a higher ADR than the average endoscopist in practice and that there is no way to determine whether it was the educational intervention, the monthly report of ADR, or a combination of the two which resulted in the improvement. In addition, serrated polyps were not separately reported in the study [64]. Abdul-Baki et al. showed that public reporting of ADR as a part of a quality improvement initiative increased ADR for all types of colonoscopies from 34.3% to 39.2% [65]. Proposed endoscopic techniques to improve ADR are water-aided colonoscopy, retroflexion in the cecum, and change in patient position during the procedure [66–68]. Several endoscopic technological advances may aid the endoscopist in achieving a higher ADR by exposing more mucosa during inspection and improving visibility and polyp detection [69]. High-definition white light endoscopy gives more detailed images than standard white light [70]. Some studies have shown that it increases ADR and decreases polyp miss rates compared to standard white light [71]. Several new technologies have been proposed to aid in viewing parts of the colon that have traditionally been difficult to see, such as flexures, behind large haustral folds, and the proximal edges of mucosal folds [72]. Full-spectrum endoscopy (FUSE) allows a 330-degree view of the colon using three separate video monitors. A small study showed a significantly lower adenoma miss rate with this technology versus standard forward viewing endoscopes, with 70% of the adenomas missed with the standard endoscope and then detected with FUSE in the right colon [73]. The third eye retroscope uses an additional scope introduced through the working channel of the main endoscope to allow a backward view of the colon. A study showed that this technology has a 41.5% additional adenoma detection rate [74]. However, it has been criticized because the third eye is expensive and gives a 50% reduction in suction during colonoscopy, and the retroscope must be removed from the working channel if another accessory device is needed, such a biopsy forceps.

Narrowband imaging and chromoendoscopy are other suggested interventions to improve ADR [75]. The use of distal attachment devices such as the Endocuff, Endocap, and Endoring that flatten large mucosal folds has been shown to increase polyp detection rate by 14% particularly for polyps of the cecum and sigmoid colon [76–78]. The use of artificial intelligence (AI) software with colonoscopy has been shown to improve polyp detection and ADR [79, 80]. However, cost of the system limits its widespread use and is not substitute for good colonoscopy technique.

The process of calculating ADR can be tedious and time-consuming, as pathology reports and procedure reports must often be compared and entered manually. Natural language processing (NLP) has been proposed as a potential solution. NLP is a computer program that uses artificial intelligence to identify and extract information from free text notes, such as procedure reports, which it then links to other data sources, such as pathology reports [81–83]. It has been shown to be comparable to manual review in calculation of ADR [82].

Index Colonoscopy

Performing a high-quality index colonoscopy has long-lasting implications on risk stratification and prognosis for patients. A negative index colonoscopy has a prolonged protective effect with associated reductions in colorectal cancer risk for at least the first 10 years and potentially even beyond 20 years [84, 85]. One study of patients with a negative index colonoscopy who underwent colonoscopy 5 years later found no colorectal cancer and extremely low rates of advanced adenomas (1.3%) [86]. A recent study of 165,887 patients in the Polish colon cancer screening program showed that a high-quality colonoscopy (defined as a complete examination to the cecum, with adequate bowel prep, performed by endoscopists with an ADR >20%) resulted in a significantly lower incidence of colorectal cancer (0.16–0.32) and mortality (0.10 vs 0.32) compared to patients that received an index low-quality colonoscopy. These differences in colorectal cancer incidence persisted for 0–5 years, 5–10 years, and 10–17 years of follow-up [87]. When polyps are found, it has been well described that polyp pathology is predictive of future colon cancer risk. This risk is reflected in the guidelines on polyp surveillance requiring more frequent follow-up for findings of high-risk adenomas compared to low-risk adenomas or no adenomas [88]. However, one factor that has yet to be incorporated into guidelines is that the quality of the endoscopist performing the screening exam also has significant impact on the prognostic power of the index colonoscopy. Another study using the Polish and Austrian colon cancer screening programs showed that exams done by high-performing endoscopists (ADR >20%) were more protective compared to exams done by low-performing endoscopists (ADR <20%), regardless of the findings on the index exam. At 10 years of follow-up, the colorectal cancer incidence for exams performed by high-quality vs low-quality endoscopist based on findings at index exam was as follows: no adenomas (0.15% vs 0.30%), low-risk adenomas (0.22% vs 0.55%), and high-risk adenomas (0.43% vs 1.14%). So having a high-quality endoscopist find a high-risk adenoma was actually more protective than having a low-quality endoscopist find a low-risk adenoma [89]! This discrepancy may be due to multiple factors including a missed lesion developing into colon cancer, misclassification of future cancer risk due to missed lesions, or patients with an index colonoscopy by high-performing endoscopists who end up undergoing more surveillance colonoscopies. Regardless, this clarifies the importance of having a high-quality index colonoscopy to adequately provide colorectal cancer risk stratification for patients.

Endoscopic Removal of Polyps <20 mm

With advances in colonoscopy and polypectomy techniques, many polyps that were previously being sent for surgery can and should be removed endoscopically. However, referral of nonmalignant colorectal polyps to surgery remains common and seems to be increasing in recent years [90]. In particular, polyps <20 mm in size should be considered routine polypectomy and generally be resected by the initial endoscopist. In instances where the polypectomy is technically difficult, referral to an expert endoscopist for an endoscopic resection should be done rather than referring to surgery. One study showed that half of all patients (for any size of polyp) referred for surgery were candidates for attempted endoscopic resection, with complete resection achieved in 87% of these patients and no association between size of polyps and modality of resection [91]. Compared with surgical resection, endoscopic resection is safer for the patient and more cost-effective [92]. If the initial endoscopist anticipates referral for resection, any incomplete intervention such as partial resection, biopsy, or injection should be avoided to avoid creating scarring which can make subsequent endoscopic resection more difficult [5].

Completeness of Adenoma Removal

Missed lesions and incomplete polyp resection are the major contributors to interval colorectal cancer [93–95]. It is estimated that incomplete resection may be responsible for up to 30% of interval colorectal cancer [96]. Adenomas and neoplasia have a proclivity to recur in regions with prior adenomas, which may represent either a "field effect" or recurrence due to incomplete resections [97]. A systemic review of 32 studies, comprising 9282 polyps, provided a comprehensive look at incomplete resection rates (IRR). Snare removal of polyps 1–10 mm had an IRR of 15.9%, and snare removal of polyps 10–20 mm had an IRR of 20.8% [98]. There was a much higher IRR for sessile serrated adenomas (28.5%) compared to adenomas (13.3%).

There has been tremendous interest in whether different techniques or modalities can improve completeness of polyp resection. Guidelines recommend cold snare polypectomy be used for polyps 3–9 mm and only using forceps for polyps <2 mm [99]. In the aforementioned systemic review, cold snare for polyps <5 mm was found to have a lower IRR compared to use of cold forceps (4.4% vs 9.9%) [98]. There was also no significant difference in IRR for hot snare vs cold snare and for use or nonuse of submucosal injection for polyps under 10 mm. There was no data available to compare the use or nonuse of submucosal injection for polyps >10 mm [98]. Cold snare polypectomy has similar efficacy to hot snare polypectomy but is preferred for polyps <10 mm given the lower rates of delayed post-polypectomy bleeding, avoiding the risk of thermal injury, and likely reduced risk of perforation [99–101]. Polypectomy should aim for a 2–3 mm border around the lesion. With cold snare polypectomy, the snare should be pushed into the mucosa on resection to maintain a wide resection area and improve likelihood of complete resection. In contrast, with hot snare polypectomy, the polyp must be tented up to avoid cauterization, which may result in a less wide resection border [102].

One area of ongoing discussion is whether piecemeal cold snare polypectomy or attempted en bloc endoscopic mucosal resection with a submucosal injection lift is preferred for polyps >10 mm. While no guidelines have explicitly endorsed a specific approach, systemic reviews suggest that cold snare polypectomy may be able to provide complete resection with low rates of residual polypectomy (4.1%) and low rates of post-procedural bleeding (0.5%) [103]. Studies focused on polyps >20 mm have shown equal efficacy of piecemeal cold snare polypectomy to conventional EMR while virtually eliminating the risk of delayed bleeding and perforation [104]. Underwater endoscopic mucosal resection, which relaxes the bowel wall and does not utilize submucosal injection, was initially developed for en bloc resection of large polyps but has also shown promise as a technique to also increase the likelihood of R0 resection (en bloc resection with negative margins) for polyps sized 10–20 mm, compared to conventional EMR (69% vs 50%) [105]. Resection of pedunculated polyps has historically been the domain of hot snares given the higher risk of bleeding, but this may be evolving as well. For pedunculated polyps <10 mm in size, a technique to "choke" the polyp base for >10 s may be used, which decreases the likelihood of immediate bleeding by 97% [106].

The European Society of Gastrointestinal Endoscopy guidelines recommend that at least 80% of polyps should be completely resected, although no guidance is given on how to measure this. Measurements could include visual assessment (least reliable), margin biopsy, or histologic assessment of the polyp margin [107].

Colonoscopy for Chronic Diarrhea

In the workup of chronic diarrhea, it is recommended that random biopsies are taken in every patient, in order to rule out microscopic colitis. There is a higher prevalence in females and patients aged >60 [108]. Colonoscopy and biopsy lead to a diagnosis in over 15% of patients with chronic diarrhea, with lymphocytic or collagenous colitis diagnosed in over 8% of patients [109, 110]. Distribution of microscopic colitis can be isolated to the right or left colon, or throughout the entire colonic mucosa. Given the varied distribution, biopsies should ideally be taken from each segment of the colon to improve the yield [111, 112]. There are no clear guidelines on the optimal number of biopsies but a minimum of eight biopsies throughout the colon recommended—four biopsies in both the right and the left colon [5, 112]. Historically, less than 80% of patients undergoing colonoscopy for chronic diarrhea have gotten biopsies [113, 114].

Colonoscopy for Inflammatory Bowel Disease

In patients with inflammatory bowel disease, a more extensive exam and reporting are required. A complete colonoscopy in the workup of inflammatory bowel disease should include intubation of the ileum and biopsies of both affected and unaffected areas of the colon. Histologic disease can be seen even in endoscopically normal colonic mucosa, and it is important to define the extent of disease. There is mixed data on whether biopsy of a normal-appearing ileum is strictly required, although this is often done in clinical practice [115–117]. A RAND appropriateness panel identified 48 elements across themes of "disease background," "findings and interventions," "Crohn's disease with an ileocolonic anastomosis," and "pouchoscopy" which should be included in the colonoscopy report, as detailed in Table 2.4 [119].

Table 2.4 Colonoscopy reporting in inflammatory bowel disease

Disease background elements
General description of disease type and extent
Specific indication for procedure
Specific IBD therapy at time of procedure
Description of symptoms at time of present evaluation
Reporting elements
Description of whether DRE performed at the time of examination
Description of pertinent positives/negatives regarding stigmata of perianal CD (fissures, fistulas, skin tags) in CD
Maximal extent of examination
Ileal intubation? (Y/N)
Rational for failure to intubate terminal ileum
Description of maximal extent of endoscopically visible disease (for UC only)
Adequate description of degree of endoscopic disease activity in UC using Mayo endoscopy score [118]
Adequate description of degree of endoscopic disease activity in CD using the Simple Endoscopic Score for Crohn's Disease (SES-CD) [118]
Description of morphology and location of raised lesion (diminutive, sessile, pedunculated, flat, laterally spreading)
Description of whether lesion is in endoscopically colitic or non-colitic mucosa
Description of completeness of endoscopic removal of polypoid lesion
Description of technique of endoscopic removal of polypoid lesion (biopsy forceps, jumbo forceps, snare cautery, snare cautery with submucosal lifting, cold snare)
Description of whether biopsies obtained adjacent to polypoid lesions
Description of any special techniques for visualization (NBI, iScan, dye spray chromoendoscopy, endomicroscopy)
Description of segmental location of biopsies obtained
Description of the approximate number of biopsies obtained overall
A summary of findings is provided
Summary should specifically address the stated indication for the procedure
Explicit instructions should be provided on when and how to arrange a follow-up appointment
Exam with an ileocolonic anastomosis
Maximal extent of examination
Intubation of neoterminal ileum? (Y/N)
Maximal distance of neoterminal ileal insertion
Rationale for failure to intubate the neoterminal ileum

(continued)

Table 2.4 (continued)

Description of degree of anastomotic and neoterminal ileal inflammation using Rutgeerts score or findings 2 and 3 (below)
Adequate description of anastomotic inflammation using general descriptors
Adequate description of neoterminal ileal inflammation using general descriptors
Segmental description of colonic/rectal inflammation if present
With a pouch exam
Indication for procedure
Specific IBD therapy at the time of procedure
Symptoms at the time of evaluation
Description of whether DRE performed at the time of examination
Description of pertinent positives/negatives regarding stigmata of perianal CD (fissures, fistulas, skin tags)
Maximal pouch insertion (cm)
Intubation of prepouch ileum (Y/N)
Maximal distance of prepouch ileal intubation (cm)
Rationale for failure of intubation of prepouch ileum
Description of distribution and nature of pouch inflammation
Description of whether cuff is present
Description of cuff mucosa
Description of pouch inlet
Description of prepouch ileum
Description of proximal prepouch ileum (.5 cm into prepouch ileum)
Description of location of biopsies
Description of whether cuff surveillance biopsies obtained

Adapted from Recommendations for Quality Colonoscopy Reporting for Patients with Inflammatory Bowel Disease: Results from a RAND Appropriateness Panel [119]

As detailed earlier in this chapter, surveillance colonoscopy is recommended for patients with ulcerative colitis or Crohn's colitis with a minimum of 8 years of disease and at least 30% of colon disease involvement [15, 16]. These should be conducted during disease remission, and during the exam, the endoscopist should focus on identifying raised lesions and abnormal pit patterns and perform targeted biopsies. The use of high-definition white light (HDWL) colonoscopes is strongly preferred and can be used with chromoendoscopy (CE) or narrowband imaging (NBI) to identify dysplasia. Studies suggest that NBI has similar dysplasia detection capabilities as CE while allowing for a shorter procedural time [120, 121]. If only standard definition colonoscopies are available, then use of CE with methylene blue or indigo carmine is recommended. While it adds time to the duration of procedure, which is likely the main barrier to widespread adoption, there appears to be a minimal learning curve and similar dysplasia detection between expert and nonexpert endoscopists [122]. Previous guidelines had recommended biopsies in four quadrants every 10 cm of the colon for a minimum of 32 biopsies. However, it is unclear if these segmental random biopsies are actually beneficial, as many studies have demonstrated only a 0.1–0.2% rate of dysplasia detection with non-targeted biopsies [16]. One randomized controlled trial comparing targeted biopsies alone to targeted biopsies + random biopsies showed similar proportions of neoplasia detection despite decreased procedural time and less pathology samples required in the group with targeted biopsies alone [123]. Previous studies had shown poor adherence to guidelines on random biopsies, and a recent study including the options of virtual or dye-based CE still had a low percentage of patients receiving an adequate endoscopic surveillance [124, 125]. Data is conflicting on if HDWL alone may provide similar dysplasia detection compared to the use of NBI and CE [121, 126–128]. At present, if HDWL is used alone, then non-targeted biopsies are still recommended [129]. If HDWL with targeted biopsies alone becomes a recommended surveillance technique, then we will need new methods to track completion of an appropriate surveillance colonoscopy, such as an IBD-specific dysplasia detection rate or recommended withdrawal time.

There is no perfect method to endoscopically differentiate colitis-associated dysplasia and sporadic dysplasia. Dysplastic lesions should be described as either polypoid (>2.5 mm tall), nonpolypoid (<2.5 mm), or invisible (detected on non-targeted biopsy) [129]. Colitis-associated dysplasia tends to be flat or spreading rather than sessile or pedunculated. Dysplasia that is found on non-targeted biopsies or in areas of prior active disease is also thought to be more likely to be colitis-associated. It is important to describe the size, shape, pit pattern, clarity of borders, presence of ulceration, location, presence within area of past/present colitis, perceived completeness of resection, and whether any special techniques were used for visualization in the colonoscopy report [16, 129]. If invisible dysplasia is found, then repeat examination by an experienced endoscopist using HDWL with dye spray CE under optimal viewing conditions is recommended.

For patients with pseudopolyps, targeted biopsies of representative or concerning pseudopolyps are appropriate. Dye spray CE is not recommended for use within a field of pseudopolyps [95]. In cases of extensive pseudopolyposis where it may not be feasible to have adequate surveillance with colonoscopy, there should be individualized decision-making. This may include more frequent colonoscopy surveillance, increased non-targeted biopsies of involved areas, or discussion with a surgeon about resection depending on the individual patient goals and clinical situation.

For patients with a pouch, surveillance is recommended annually in those with prior colorectal cancer or dysplasia, a diagnosis of PSC, or moderate-severe pouchitis/ileitis.

Post-procedure Quality Metrics

Post-procedural quality indicators monitor complications of colonoscopy such as bleeding and perforation and selection of an appropriate surveillance interval, based on guidelines and exam quality and histology. Although perforation is a rare complication, the consequences may be serious. The expected perforation rate should be less than 0.2% for all colonoscopies and less than 0.1% for screening examinations. Post-polypectomy bleeding is another potentially serious complication and should be less than 1%, of which less than 10% should require surgical intervention [130]. Although the rate of adverse events of colonoscopy is low, they are frequently underestimated. As more colonoscopies are performed, the number of interventions such as polypectomies will also increase which will increase the probability of complications. While intra-procedure complications are frequently captured, post-procedure complications that occur after the patient leaves the endoscopy unit are rarely captured. This is due to the fact that patient may end up seeking care elsewhere and the records pertaining to the management of these complications may not reach the endoscopist in order to be documented in the endoscopy report. Endoscopy units should routinely provide contact information for the practice with instructions to call the practice or seek urgent medical care should they experience a complication related to their procedure. Serious adverse events such as perforation, death, or interval CRC should be reviewed for quality improvement purposes.

The key post-procedure quality indicator is the selection of an appropriate surveillance interval, based on present guidelines, histopathology of the polyp, and exam quality. Multiple studies have shown that the suggested surveillance interval for colonoscopies is often not consistent with national guidelines set forth by the US Multi-Society Task Force on Colorectal Cancer. The Task Force's most recent update was published in 2020 and *assumes a high-quality baseline* colonoscopy, defined as complete examination to the cecum, adequate bowel preparation, performance by an endoscopist with a good ADR, and attention to complete polyp excision [131]. Based on the updated guidelines, the recommended surveillance intervals are shown in Table 2.5.

Table 2.5 US Multi-Society Task Force recommendations for post-colonoscopy follow-up in average-risk patients based on baseline colonoscopy findings

Baseline colonoscopy finding	Recommended colonoscopy surveillance interval
Normal colonoscopy, or <20 hyperplastic polyps <10 mm	10 years
1–2 adenomas <10 mm	7–10 years
5–10 adenomas, adenoma ≥10 mm, or adenoma with villous component or high-grade dysplasia	3 years
>10 adenomas	1 year[a]
Piecemeal resection of adenoma ≥20 mm	6 months, then 1 year later, then 3 years after the second examination
1–2 sessile serrated polyps (SSPs) <10 mm	5–10 years
3–4 SSPs <10 mm or hyperplastic polyp ≥10 mm	3–5 years
5–10 SSPs, SSP ≥10 mm, SSP with dysplasia, or traditional serrated adenoma	3 years

Adapted from recommendations for follow-up after colonoscopy and polypectomy: a consensus update by the US Multi-Society Task Force on Colorectal Cancer [131]

[a] Consider genetic testing based on age, adenoma burden, or family history

Based on present data, there is stronger evidence for the recommended 10-year surveillance interval for average-risk individuals with a negative high-quality baseline examination [132]. Emerging evidence also shows that finding one to two diminutive adenomas (<6 mm) is not significantly associated with a significant risk of interval colon cancer which prompted the change from 5–10 years to 7–10 years for patients with these findings. Although it is anticipated that many endoscopists will err on the side of caution when selecting these new intervals, the updated recommendations are nevertheless a step in the right direction for gastroenterologists who perform high-quality colonoscopies.

Underutilization of colonoscopy risks a potential interval cancer, while overutilization of colonoscopy exposes patients to unnecessary risk from the procedure and drains health-care resources [133]. Schoen et al. showed that in community practice there is substantial overuse of surveillance colonoscopy in low-risk patients and underuse in patients with advanced adenomas [13]. An analysis of 25 Veterans Health Administration facilities found that 16% of patients without adenomas received a follow-up colonoscopy too early, 26.4% of patients with low-risk adenomas (defined as one to two adenomas <1 cm in size) received a follow-up colonoscopy too early, and 54.1% of patients with high-risk adenomas (defined as size measuring $\geq$1 cm, high-grade dysplasia, or $\geq$ three adenomas) received a follow-up colonoscopy too late. Non-gastroenterologists performing colonoscopies were more likely to recommend a follow-up colonoscopy too early in this data [134]. Another study by Kruse et al. also found that average-risk patients were more likely to receive a follow-up exam earlier than national guidelines, while 25% of patients with adenomas detected did not receive appropriate surveillance intervals according to guidelines suggesting that endoscopist recommendations are the key factor behind overuse [135]. Similarly, a study of Medicare patients who are colorectal cancer survivors found that they frequently receive colonoscopies sooner than guidelines recommend and that patients over the age of 80 and those with significant medical comorbidities had a higher likelihood of receiving surveillance sooner than recommended [136]. Following national practice guidelines for colonoscopy, surveillance intervals can be challenging because it often requires clinical records from other providers or health-care systems apart from knowledge of the present recommended surveillance intervals. Natural language processing is promising technology to link findings from procedure and pathology reports but is limited by variation in endoscopy reporting software and electronic health record platforms [83]. We recommend strict adherence to national colonoscopy surveillance guidelines unless there is a documented reason that the national guideline is not being followed (e.g., poor preparation). Perhaps future versions of endoscopy reporting software will incorporate the appropriate surveillance interval in the procedure report if no polyps are found or once polyp histopathology has been reviewed by the endoscopist. Auditing an endoscopist's indication for procedure and suggested surveillance interval may help improve appropriate use and surveillance interval for colonoscopies and prevent overuse.

Patient Satisfaction

Patient satisfaction with the colonoscopy is a topic that requires further study, as it could determine whether patients are willing to undergo repeat examinations. Sharing a poor experience, particularly with the widespread use of social media, could negatively influence other patients against screening. There are conflicting data regarding whether there is a correlation between patient satisfaction scores and measurement of procedural quality. Yadlapati et al. and colleagues found weak or no correlation between known quality metrics and patient satisfaction scores [137]. Ekkelenkamp et al. found that endoscopists with a higher cecal intubation rate caused less patient discomfort, found more precancerous lesions, and used less sedation [138]. It has been suggested that patient comfort should be deemed an "auditable outcome" that should be measured, reviewed, and acted upon, although a concrete performance guideline cannot be defined. We agree that patient satisfaction should be considered an independent quality goal secondary to high-quality colonoscopy.

Conclusion

Colonoscopy quality measures are widely available for providers and institutions to implement and monitor. It is essential that both individual providers and practices commit to performing high-quality colonoscopies and monitor quality metrics. Pre-procedure documentation should always include consent, an appropriate indication, and notation of relevant precautions including anesthesia and procedural risk factors. Key intra-procedure quality metrics must include bowel preparation quality, cecal intubation rate, ADR, and completeness of polyp resection. Post-procedure follow-up recommendations must follow national practice guidelines, and adverse events must be documented. Promising new technology that aids low performers improve their quality metrics will similarly help skilled endoscopists who are already performing high-quality examinations. Measuring colonoscopy quality is important because quality cannot be improved if it is not measured.

References

1. Siegel RL, Miller KD, Fuchs HE, Jemal A. Cancer statistics, 2022. CA Cancer J Clin. 2022;72(1):7–33.
2. Force USPST, Davidson KW, Barry MJ, Mangione CM, Cabana M, Caughey AB, et al. Screening for colorectal cancer: US Preventive Services Task Force Recommendation Statement. JAMA. 2021;325(19):1965–77.
3. Rex DK, Schoenfeld PS, Cohen J, Pike IM, Adler DG, Fennerty MB, et al. Quality indicators for colonoscopy. Gastrointest Endosc. 2015;81(1):31–53.

4. Hassan C, Di Giulio E, Marmo R, Zullo A, Annibale B. Appropriateness of the indication for colonoscopy: systematic review and meta-analysis. J Gastrointestin Liver Dis. 2011;20(3):279–86.
5. Early DS, Ben-Menachem T, Decker GA, Evans JA, Fanelli RD, et al. Appropriate use of GI endoscopy. Gastrointest Endosc. 2012;75(6):1127–31.
6. Shaukat A, Kahi CJ, Burke CA, Rabeneck L, Sauer BG, Rex DK. ACG clinical guidelines: colorectal cancer screening 2021. Am J Gastroenterol. 2021;116(3):458–79.
7. Salimzadeh H, Bishehsari F, Delavari A, Barzin G, Amani M, Majidi A, et al. Cancer risk awareness and screening uptake in individuals at higher risk for colon cancer: a cross-sectional study. BMJ Open. 2016;6(12):e013833.
8. Colorectal Cancer Screening: National Cancer Institute. Available from: https://progress-report.cancer.gov/detection/colorectal_cancer#:~:text=In%202019%2C%2067.1%25%20of%20adults,on%20the%20most%20recent%20guidelines.
9. Goodwin JS, Singh A, Reddy N, Riall TS, Kuo YF. Overuse of screening colonoscopy in the Medicare population. Arch Intern Med. 2011;171(15):1335–43.
10. Djinbachian R, Dube AJ, Durand M, Camara LR, Panzini B, Bouchard S, et al. Adherence to post-polypectomy surveillance guidelines: a systematic review and meta-analysis. Endoscopy. 2019;51(7):673–83.
11. Shah TU, Voils CI, McNeil R, Wu R, Fisher DA. Understanding gastroenterologist adherence to polyp surveillance guidelines. Am J Gastroenterol. 2012;107(9):1283–7.
12. Saini SD, Nayak RS, Kuhn L, Schoenfeld P. Why don't gastroenterologists follow colon polyp surveillance guidelines: results of a national survey. J Clin Gastroenterol. 2009;43(6):554–8.
13. Schoen RE, Pinsky PF, Weissfeld JL, Yokochi LA, Reding DJ, Hayes RB, et al. Utilization of surveillance colonoscopy in community practice. Gastroenterology. 2010;138(1):73–81.
14. Iskandar H, Yan Y, Elwing J, Early D, Colditz GA, Wang JS. Predictors of poor adherence of US Gastroenterologists with colonoscopy screening and surveillance guidelines. Dig Dis Sci. 2015;60(4):971–8.
15. Lichtenstein GR, Loftus EV, Isaacs KL, Regueiro MD, Gerson LB, Sands BE. ACG clinical guideline: management of Crohn's disease in adults. Am J Gastroenterol. 2018;113(4):481–517.
16. Rubin DT, Ananthakrishnan AN, Siegel CA, Sauer BG, Long MD. ACG clinical guideline: ulcerative colitis in adults. Am J Gastroenterol. 2019;114(3):384–413.
17. Hata K, Anzai H, Ikeuchi H, Futami K, Fukushima K, Sugita A, et al. Surveillance colonoscopy for ulcerative colitis-associated colorectal cancer offers better overall survival in real-world surgically resected cases. Am J Gastroenterol. 2019;114(3):483–9.
18. Basseri RJ, Basseri B, Vassilaki ME, Melmed GY, Ippoliti A, Vasiliauskas EA, et al. Colorectal cancer screening and surveillance in Crohn's colitis. J Crohns Colitis. 2012;6(8):824–9.
19. Magro F, Gionchetti P, Eliakim R, Ardizzone S, Armuzzi A, Barreiro-de Acosta M, et al. Third European Evidence-based consensus on diagnosis and management of ulcerative colitis. Part 1: definitions, diagnosis, extra-intestinal manifestations, pregnancy, cancer surveillance, surgery, and ileo-anal pouch disorders. J Crohns Colitis. 2017;11(6):649–70.
20. Singh K, Al Khoury A, Kurti Z, Gonczi L, Reinglas J, Verdon C, et al. High adherence to surveillance guidelines in inflammatory bowel disease patients results in low colorectal cancer and dysplasia rates, while rates of dysplasia are low before the suggested onset of surveillance. J Crohns Colitis. 2019;13(10):1343–50.
21. Jigar Bhagatwala AS, Aldrugh S, Sherid M, Sifuentes H, Sridhar S. Colonoscopy – indications and contraindications. Screening for Colorectal Cancer with Colonoscopy. 2015.
22. Early DS, Lightdale JR, Vargo JJ, Acosta RD, Chandrasekhara V, et al. Guidelines for sedation and anesthesia in GI endoscopy. Gastrointest Endosc. 2018;87(2):327–37.
23. Acosta RD, Abraham NS, Chandrasekhara V, Chathadi KV, Early DS, et al. The management of antithrombotic agents for patients undergoing GI endoscopy. Gastrointest Endosc. 2016;83(1):3–16.

24. Zuckerman MJ, Shen B, Harrison ME, Baron TH, Adler DG, et al. Informed consent for GI endoscopy. Gastrointest Endosc. 2007;66(2):213–8.
25. Storm AC, Fishman DS, Buxbaum JL, Coelho-Prabhu N, Al-Haddad MA, et al. American Society for Gastrointestinal Endoscopy guideline on informed consent for GI endoscopic procedures. Gastrointest Endosc. 2022;95(2):207–15.
26. David M, Staff KS, Rochling F, et al. Does open access endoscopy close the door to an adequately informed patient? Gastrointest Endosc. 2000;52(2):212–7.
27. Radha Menon AS, Miller E, et al. Open access endoscopy is a barrier to effective colonoscopy. Gastrointest Endosc. 2007;65:5.
28. Chandrasekhara V, Eloubeidi MA, Bruining DH, Chathadi K, Faulx AL, et al. Open-access endoscopy. Gastrointest Endosc. 2015;81(6):1326–9.
29. Denberg TD, Coombes JM, Byers TE, Marcus AC, Feinberg LE, Steiner JF, et al. Effect of a mailed brochure on appointment-keeping for screening colonoscopy: a randomized trial. Ann Intern Med. 2006;145(12):895–900.
30. Hanson M, Pitt D. Informed consent for surgery: risk discussion and documentation. Can J Surg. 2017;60(1):69–70.
31. Gett RM, Cooray AR, Gold D, Danta M. Evaluating informed consent for colonoscopy. Surg Laparosc Endosc Percutan Tech. 2014;24(4):345–52.
32. Fortun P, West J, Chalkley L, Shonde A, Hawkey C. Recall of informed consent information by healthy volunteers in clinical trials. QJM. 2008;101(8):625–9.
33. Saltzman JR, Cash BD, Pasha SF, Early DS, Muthusamy VR, et al. Bowel preparation before colonoscopy. Gastrointest Endosc. 2015;81(4):781–94.
34. Calderwood AH, Jacobson BC. Comprehensive validation of the Boston Bowel Preparation Scale. Gastrointest Endosc. 2010;72(4):686–92.
35. Chokshi RV, Hovis CE, Hollander T, Early DS, Wang JS. Prevalence of missed adenomas in patients with inadequate bowel preparation on screening colonoscopy. Gastrointest Endosc. 2012;75(6):1197–203.
36. Lieberman DA, Holub JL, Morris CD, Logan J, Williams JL, Carney P. Low rate of large polyps (>9 mm) within 10 years after an adequate baseline colonoscopy with no polyps. Gastroenterology. 2014;147(2):343–50.
37. Oh CH, Lee CK, Kim JW, Shim JJ, Jang JY. Suboptimal bowel preparation significantly impairs colonoscopic detection of non-polypoid colorectal neoplasms. Dig Dis Sci. 2015;60(8):2294–303.
38. Anderson JC, Butterly LF, Robinson CM, Goodrich M, Weiss JE. Impact of fair bowel preparation quality on adenoma and serrated polyp detection: data from the New Hampshire colonoscopy registry by using a standardized preparation-quality rating. Gastrointest Endosc. 2014;80(3):463–70.
39. Clark BT, Rustagi T, Laine L. What level of bowel prep quality requires early repeat colonoscopy: systematic review and meta-analysis of the impact of preparation quality on adenoma detection rate. Am J Gastroenterol. 2014;109(11):1714–23; quiz 24.
40. Guo X, Yang Z, Zhao L, Leung F, Luo H, Kang X, et al. Enhanced instructions improve the quality of bowel preparation for colonoscopy: a meta-analysis of randomized controlled trials. Gastrointest Endosc. 2017;85(1):90–7.
41. Enestvedt BK, Tofani C, Laine LA, Tierney A, Fennerty MB. 4-Liter split-dose polyethylene glycol is superior to other bowel preparations, based on systematic review and meta-analysis. Clin Gastroenterol Hepatol. 2012;10(11):1225–31.
42. Lund M, Trads M, Njor SH, Erichsen R, Andersen B. Quality indicators for screening colonoscopy and colonoscopist performance and the subsequent risk of interval colorectal cancer: a systematic review. JBI Database System Rev Implement Rep. 2019;17(11):2265–300.
43. Gupta M, Holub JL, Eisen G. Do indication and demographics for colonoscopy affect completion? A large national database evaluation. Eur J Gastroenterol Hepatol. 2010;22(5):620–7.
44. Pullens HJ, Siersema PD. Quality indicators for colonoscopy: current insights and caveats. World J Gastrointest Endosc. 2014;6(12):571–83.

45. Committee AT, Trindade AJ, Lichtenstein DR, Aslanian HR, Bhutani MS, Goodman A, et al. Devices and methods to improve colonoscopy completion (with videos). Gastrointest Endosc. 2018;87(3):625–34.
46. Barclay RL, Vicari JJ, Doughty AS, Johanson JF, Greenlaw RL. Colonoscopic withdrawal times and adenoma detection during screening colonoscopy. N Engl J Med. 2006;355(24):2533–41.
47. Shaukat A, Rector TS, Church TR, Lederle FA, Kim AS, Rank JM, et al. Longer withdrawal time is associated with a reduced incidence of interval cancer after screening colonoscopy. Gastroenterology. 2015;149(4):952–7.
48. Lee TJ, Blanks RG, Rees CJ, Wright KC, Nickerson C, Moss SM, et al. Longer mean colonoscopy withdrawal time is associated with increased adenoma detection: evidence from the Bowel Cancer Screening Programme in England. Endoscopy. 2013;45(1):20–6.
49. Butterly L, Robinson CM, Anderson JC, Weiss JE, Goodrich M, Onega TL, et al. Serrated and adenomatous polyp detection increases with longer withdrawal time: results from the New Hampshire Colonoscopy Registry. Am J Gastroenterol. 2014;109(3):417–26.
50. Kaminski MF, Regula J, Kraszewska E, Polkowski M, Wojciechowska U, Didkowska J, et al. Quality indicators for colonoscopy and the risk of interval cancer. N Engl J Med. 2010;362(19):1795–803.
51. Corley DA, Jensen CD, Marks AR, Zhao WK, Lee JK, Doubeni CA, et al. Adenoma detection rate and risk of colorectal cancer and death. N Engl J Med. 2014;370(14):1298–306.
52. Kaminski MF, Wieszczy P, Rupinski M, Wojciechowska U, Didkowska J, Kraszewska E, et al. Increased rate of adenoma detection associates with reduced risk of colorectal cancer and death. Gastroenterology. 2017;153(1):98–105.
53. Corley DA, Jensen CD, Marks AR, Zhao WK, de Boer J, Levin TR, et al. Variation of adenoma prevalence by age, sex, race, and colon location in a large population: implications for screening and quality programs. Clin Gastroenterol Hepatol. 2013;11(2):172–80.
54. Wang HS, Pisegna J, Modi R, Liang LJ, Atia M, Nguyen M, et al. Adenoma detection rate is necessary but insufficient for distinguishing high versus low endoscopist performance. Gastrointest Endosc. 2013;77(1):71–8.
55. Duvvuri A, Chandrasekar VT, Srinivasan S, Narimiti A, Dasari C, Nutalapati V, et al. Risk of colorectal cancer and cancer related mortality after detection of low-risk or high-risk adenomas, compared with no adenoma, at index colonoscopy: a systematic review and meta-analysis. Gastroenterology. 2021;160(6):1986–96.
56. Schottinger JE, Jensen CD, Ghai NR, Chubak J, Lee JK, Kamineni A, et al. Association of Physician Adenoma detection rates with postcolonoscopy colorectal cancer. JAMA. 2022;327(21):2114–22.
57. Lam AY, Li Y, Gregory DL, Prinz J, O'Reilly J, Manka M, et al. Association between improved adenoma detection rates and interval colorectal cancer rates after a quality improvement program. Gastrointest Endosc. 2020;92(2):355–64.
58. Crockett SD, Gourevitch RA, Morris M, Carrell DS, Rose S, Shi Z, et al. Endoscopist factors that influence serrated polyp detection: a multicenter study. Endoscopy. 2018;50(10):984–92.
59. Je IJ, de Wit K, van der Vlugt M, Bastiaansen BA, Fockens P, Dekker E. Prevalence, distribution and risk of sessile serrated adenomas/polyps at a center with a high adenoma detection rate and experienced pathologists. Endoscopy. 2016;48(8):740–6.
60. Gourevitch RA, Rose S, Crockett SD, Morris M, Carrell DS, Greer JB, et al. Variation in pathologist classification of colorectal adenomas and serrated polyps. Am J Gastroenterol. 2018;113(3):431–9.
61. Kahi CJ, Ballard D, Shah AS, Mears R, Johnson CS. Impact of a quarterly report card on colonoscopy quality measures. Gastrointest Endosc. 2013;77(6):925–31.
62. Keswani RN, Yadlapati R, Gleason KM, Ciolino JD, Manka M, O'Leary KJ, et al. Physician report cards and implementing standards of practice are both significantly associated with improved screening colonoscopy quality. Am J Gastroenterol. 2015;110(8):1134–9.

63. Coe SG, Crook JE, Diehl NN, Wallace MB. An endoscopic quality improvement program improves detection of colorectal adenomas. Am J Gastroenterol. 2013;108(2):219–26; quiz 27.
64. Robertson DJ. EQUIPping ourselves for future quality improvements in colonoscopy. Am J Gastroenterol. 2013;108(2):228–30.
65. Abdul-Baki H, Schoen RE, Dean K, Rose S, Leffler DA, Kuganeswaran E, et al. Public reporting of colonoscopy quality is associated with an increase in endoscopist adenoma detection rate. Gastrointest Endosc. 2015;82(4):676–82.
66. Fuccio L, Frazzoni L, Hassan C, La Marca M, Paci V, Smania V, et al. Water exchange colonoscopy increases adenoma detection rate: a systematic review with network meta-analysis of randomized controlled studies. Gastrointest Endosc. 2018;88(4):589–97.
67. Hewett DG, Rex DK. Miss rate of right-sided colon examination during colonoscopy defined by retroflexion: an observational study. Gastrointest Endosc. 2011;74(2):246–52.
68. Zhao SB, Wan H, Fu HY, Liu ZX, Wang QS, Ji L, et al. Quantitative assessment of the effect of position changes during colonoscopy withdrawal. J Dig Dis. 2016;17(6):357–65.
69. Facciorusso A, Triantafyllou K, Murad MH, Prokop LJ, Tziatzios G, Muscatiello N, et al. Compared abilities of endoscopic techniques to increase colon adenoma detection rates: a network meta-analysis. Clin Gastroenterol Hepatol. 2019;17(12):2439–54.
70. Gomez V, Wallace MB. Advances in diagnostic and therapeutic colonoscopy. Curr Opin Gastroenterol. 2014;30(1):63–8.
71. Gomez V, Racho RG, Heckman MG, Diehl NN, Wallace MB. High-definition white-light (HDWL) colonoscopy and higher adenoma detection rate and the potential for paradoxical over surveillance. Dig Dis Sci. 2014;59(11):2749–56.
72. Committee AT, Konda V, Chauhan SS, Abu Dayyeh BK, Hwang JH, Komanduri S, et al. Endoscopes and devices to improve colon polyp detection. Gastrointest Endosc. 2015;81(5):1122–9.
73. Gralnek IM, Siersema PD, Halpern Z, Segol O, Melhem A, Suissa A, et al. Standard forward-viewing colonoscopy versus full-spectrum endoscopy: an international, multicentre, randomised, tandem colonoscopy trial. Lancet Oncol. 2014;15(3):353–60.
74. Leufkens AM, DeMarco DC, Rastogi A, Akerman PA, Azzouzi K, Rothstein RI, et al. Effect of a retrograde-viewing device on adenoma detection rate during colonoscopy: the TERRACE study. Gastrointest Endosc. 2011;73(3):480–9.
75. Matsuda T, Ono A, Sekiguchi M, Fujii T, Saito Y. Advances in image enhancement in colonoscopy for detection of adenomas. Nat Rev Gastroenterol Hepatol. 2017;14(5):305–14.
76. Biecker E, Floer M, Heinecke A, Strobel P, Bohme R, Schepke M, et al. Novel endocuff-assisted colonoscopy significantly increases the polyp detection rate: a randomized controlled trial. J Clin Gastroenterol. 2015;49(5):413–8.
77. Dik VK, Gralnek IM, Segol O, Suissa A, Belderbos TD, Moons LM, et al. Multicenter, randomized, tandem evaluation of EndoRings colonoscopy–results of the CLEVER study. Endoscopy. 2015;47(12):1151–8.
78. Gkolfakis P, Tziatzios G, Facciorusso A, Muscatiello N, Triantafyllou K. Meta-analysis indicates that add-on devices and new endoscopes reduce colonoscopy adenoma miss rate. Eur J Gastroenterol Hepatol. 2018;30(12):1482–90.
79. Kudo SE, Misawa M, Mori Y, Hotta K, Ohtsuka K, Ikematsu H, et al. Artificial intelligence-assisted system improves endoscopic identification of colorectal neoplasms. Clin Gastroenterol Hepatol. 2020;18(8):1874–81.
80. Wang P, Berzin TM, Glissen Brown JR, Bharadwaj S, Becq A, Xiao X, et al. Real-time automatic detection system increases colonoscopic polyp and adenoma detection rates: a prospective randomised controlled study. Gut. 2019;68(10):1813–9.
81. Hou JK, Imler TD, Imperiale TF. Current and future applications of natural language processing in the field of digestive diseases. Clin Gastroenterol Hepatol. 2014;12(8):1257–61.
82. Raju GS, Lum PJ, Slack RS, Thirumurthi S, Lynch PM, Miller E, et al. Natural language processing as an alternative to manual reporting of colonoscopy quality metrics. Gastrointest Endosc. 2015;82(3):512–9.

83. Imler TD, Morea J, Kahi C, Sherer EA, Cardwell J, Johnson CS, et al. Multi-center colonoscopy quality measurement utilizing natural language processing. Am J Gastroenterol. 2015;110(4):543–52.
84. Lee JK, Jensen CD, Levin TR, Zauber AG, Schottinger JE, Quinn VP, et al. Long-term risk of colorectal cancer and related deaths after a colonoscopy with normal findings. JAMA Intern Med. 2019;179(2):153–60.
85. Brenner H, Chang-Claude J, Seiler CM, Hoffmeister M. Long-term risk of colorectal cancer after negative colonoscopy. J Clin Oncol. 2011;29(28):3761–7.
86. Imperiale TF, Glowinski EA, Lin-Cooper C, Larkin GN, Rogge JD, Ransohoff DF. Five-year risk of colorectal neoplasia after negative screening colonoscopy. N Engl J Med. 2008;359(12):1218–24.
87. Pilonis ND, Bugajski M, Wieszczy P, Franczyk R, Didkowska J, Wojciechowska U, et al. Long-term colorectal cancer incidence and mortality after a single negative screening colonoscopy. Ann Intern Med. 2020;173(2):81–91.
88. Gupta S, Lieberman D, Anderson JC, Burke CA, Dominitz JA, Kaltenbach T, et al. Recommendations for follow-up after colonoscopy and polypectomy: a consensus update by the US Multi-Society Task Force on colorectal cancer. Gastrointest Endosc. 2020;91(3):463–85.
89. Wieszczy P, Waldmann E, Loberg M, Regula J, Rupinski M, Bugajski M, et al. Colonoscopist performance and colorectal cancer risk after adenoma removal to stratify surveillance: two nationwide observational studies. Gastroenterology. 2021;160(4):1067–74.
90. Peery AF, Cools KS, Strassle PD, McGill SK, Crockett SD, Barker A, et al. Increasing rates of surgery for patients with nonmalignant colorectal polyps in the United States. Gastroenterology. 2018;154(5):1352–60.
91. Moon N, Aryan M, Khan W, Jiang P, Madhok I, Wilson J, et al. Effect of referral pattern and histopathology grade on surgery for nonmalignant colorectal polyps. Gastrointest Endosc. 2020;92(3):702–11.
92. Onken JE, Friedman JY, Subramanian S, Weinfurt KP, Reed SD, Malenbaum JH, et al. Treatment patterns and costs associated with sessile colorectal polyps. Am J Gastroenterol. 2002;97(11):2896–901.
93. David A, Johnson M, Wallace MB, Kaul V, Kaltenbach T. Incomplete resection rates in polyps smaller than 2 centimeters. Gastroenterol Hepatol. 2018;14:5.
94. Lieberman DA, Rex DK, Winawer SJ, Giardiello FM, Johnson DA, Levin TR. Guidelines for colonoscopy surveillance after screening and polypectomy: a consensus update by the US Multi-Society Task Force on Colorectal Cancer. Gastroenterology. 2012;143(3):844–57.
95. Pohl H, Srivastava A, Bensen SP, Anderson P, Rothstein RI, Gordon SR, et al. Incomplete polyp resection during colonoscopy-results of the complete adenoma resection (CARE) study. Gastroenterology. 2013;144(1):74–80 e1.
96. Adler J, Robertson DJ. Interval colorectal cancer after colonoscopy: exploring explanations and solutions. Am J Gastroenterol. 2015;110(12):1657–64; quiz 65.
97. Pohl H, Robertson DJ, Mott LA, Ahnen DJ, Burke CA, Barry EL, et al. Association between adenoma location and risk of recurrence. Gastrointest Endosc. 2016;84(4):709–16.
98. Djinbachian R, Iratni R, Durand M, Marques P, von Renteln D. Rates of incomplete resection of 1- to 20-mm colorectal polyps: a systematic review and meta-analysis. Gastroenterology. 2020;159(3):904–14.
99. Keswani RN, Crockett SD, Calderwood AH. AGA clinical practice update on strategies to improve quality of screening and surveillance colonoscopy: expert review. Gastroenterology. 2021;161(2):701–11.
100. Shinozaki S, Kobayashi Y, Hayashi Y, Sakamoto H, Lefor AK, Yamamoto H. Efficacy and safety of cold versus hot snare polypectomy for resecting small colorectal polyps: systematic review and meta-analysis. Dig Endosc. 2018;30(5):592–9.
101. Jegadeesan R, Aziz M, Desai M, Sundararajan T, Gorrepati VS, Chandrasekar VT, et al. Hot snare vs. cold snare polypectomy for endoscopic removal of 4–10 mm colorectal polyps dur-

ing colonoscopy: a systematic review and meta-analysis of randomized controlled studies. Endosc Int Open. 2019;7(5):E708–16.
102. Anderson JC. Techniques for detection and complete resection of sessile serrated polyps. Gastroenterol Hepatol. 2021;17(8):384–6.
103. Thoguluva Chandrasekar V, Spadaccini M, Aziz M, Maselli R, Hassan S, Fuccio L, et al. Cold snare endoscopic resection of nonpedunculated colorectal polyps larger than 10 mm: a systematic review and pooled-analysis. Gastrointest Endosc. 2019;89(5):929–36.
104. van Hattem WA, Shahidi N, Vosko S, Hartley I, Britto K, Sidhu M, et al. Piecemeal cold snare polypectomy versus conventional endoscopic mucosal resection for large sessile serrated lesions: a retrospective comparison across two successive periods. Gut. 2021;70(9):1691–7.
105. Yamashina T, Uedo N, Akasaka T, Iwatsubo T, Nakatani Y, Akamatsu T, et al. Comparison of underwater vs conventional endoscopic mucosal resection of intermediate-size colorectal polyps. Gastroenterology. 2019;157(2):451–61.
106. Fatima HM, Tooba MD, Gilmore A, Kim HN, Tang J, Ghabril M, Abdeljawad K. Bleeding risk with cold snare polypectomy of ≤10 mm pedunculated colon polyps. J Clin Gastroenterol. 2022;57(3):294–9.
107. Kaminski MF, Thomas-Gibson S, Bugajski M, Bretthauer M, Rees CJ, Dekker E, et al. Performance measures for lower gastrointestinal endoscopy: a European Society of Gastrointestinal Endoscopy (ESGE) quality improvement initiative. United European Gastroenterol J. 2017;5(3):309–34.
108. Nguyen GC, Smalley WE, Vege SS, Carrasco-Labra A, Clinical Guidelines C. American Gastroenterological Association Institute guideline on the medical management of microscopic colitis. Gastroenterology. 2016;150(1):242–6; quiz e17-8.
109. Genta RM, Sonnenberg A. The yield of colonic biopsy in the evaluation of chronic unexplained diarrhea. Eur J Gastroenterol Hepatol. 2015;27(8):963–7.
110. Shah RJ, Fenoglio-Preiser C, Bleau BL, Giannella RA. Usefulness of colonoscopy with biopsy in the evaluation of patients with chronic diarrhea. Am J Gastroenterol. 2001;96(4):1091–5.
111. Thijs WJ, van Baarlen J, Kleibeuker JH, Kolkman JJ. Microscopic colitis: prevalence and distribution throughout the colon in patients with chronic diarrhoea. Neth J Med. 2005;63(4):137–40.
112. Peixoto A, Silva M, Pereira P, Macedo G. Biopsies in gastrointestinal endoscopy: when and how. GE Port J Gastroenterol. 2016;23(1):19–27.
113. Harewood GC, Olson JS, Mattek NC, Holub JL, Lieberman DA. Colonic biopsy practice for evaluation of diarrhea in patients with normal endoscopic findings: results from a national endoscopic database. Gastrointest Endosc. 2005;61(3):371–5.
114. Villafuerte-Galvez J, Sotelo-Olivera MI, Cok J, Piscoya-Rivera A, Huerta-Mercado J. Colonoscopic findings in Peruvian patients with chronic diarrhea. PLoS One. 2012;7(10):e46690.
115. Neilson LJ, Bevan R, Panter S, Thomas-Gibson S, Rees CJ. Terminal ileal intubation and biopsy in routine colonoscopy practice. Expert Rev Gastroenterol Hepatol. 2015;9(5):567–74.
116. Velidedeoglu M, Enes Arikan A, Kagan ZA. Diagnostic value of terminal ileum biopsies in patients with abnormal terminal ileum mucosal appearance. Ulus Cerrahi Derg. 2015;31(3):152–6.
117. Koksal AR, Boga S, Alkim H, Ergun M, Bayram M, Sakiz D, et al. How does a biopsy of endoscopically normal terminal ileum contribute to the diagnosis? Which patients should undergo biopsy? Libyan J Med. 2014;9:23441.
118. Schroeder KW, Tremaine WJ, Ilstrup DM. Coated oral 5-aminosalicylic acid therapy for mildly to moderately active ulcerative colitis. A randomized study. N Engl J Med. 1987;317(26):1625–9.
119. Devlin SM, Melmed GY, Irving PM, Rubin DT, Kornbluth A, Kozuch PL, et al. Recommendations for quality colonoscopy reporting for patients with inflammatory bowel disease: results from a RAND appropriateness panel. Inflamm Bowel Dis. 2016;22(6):1418–24.

120. Bisschops R, Bessissow T, Joseph JA, Baert F, Ferrante M, Ballet V, et al. Chromoendoscopy versus narrow band imaging in UC: a prospective randomised controlled trial. Gut. 2018;67(6):1087–94.
121. Ignjatovic A, East JE, Subramanian V, Suzuki N, Guenther T, Palmer N, et al. Narrow band imaging for detection of dysplasia in colitis: a randomized controlled trial. Am J Gastroenterol. 2012;107(6):885–90.
122. Carballal S, Maisterra S, Lopez-Serrano A, Gimeno-Garcia AZ, Vera MI, Marin-Garbriel JC, et al. Real-life chromoendoscopy for neoplasia detection and characterisation in long-standing IBD. Gut. 2018;67(1):70–8.
123. Watanabe T, Ajioka Y, Mitsuyama K, Watanabe K, Hanai H, Nakase H, et al. Comparison of targeted vs random biopsies for surveillance of ulcerative colitis-associated colorectal cancer. Gastroenterology. 2016;151(6):1122–30.
124. Santi G, Michetti P, Froehlich F, Rossel JB, Pittet V, Maillard MH. Adherence to recommendations and quality of endoscopic colorectal cancer surveillance in long-standing ulcerative colitis. Inflamm Intest Dis. 2021;6(1):25–31.
125. Kaltz B, Bokemeyer B, Hoffmann J, Porschen R, Rogler G, Schmiegel W. Surveillance colonoscopy in ulcerative colitis patients in Germany. Z Gastroenterol. 2007;45(4):325–31.
126. Iannone A, Ruospo M, Wong G, Principi M, Barone M, Strippoli GFM, et al. Chromoendoscopy for surveillance in ulcerative colitis and Crohn's disease: a systematic review of randomized trials. Clin Gastroenterol Hepatol. 2017;15(11):1684–97.
127. Mooiweer E, van der Meulen-de Jong AE, Ponsioen CY, Fidder HH, Siersema PD, Dekker E, et al. Chromoendoscopy for surveillance in inflammatory bowel disease does not increase neoplasia detection compared with conventional colonoscopy with random biopsies: results from a large retrospective study. Am J Gastroenterol. 2015;110(7):1014–21.
128. van den Broek FJ, Fockens P, van Eeden S, Stokkers PC, Ponsioen CY, Reitsma JB, et al. Narrow-band imaging versus high-definition endoscopy for the diagnosis of neoplasia in ulcerative colitis. Endoscopy. 2011;43(2):108–15.
129. Murthy SK, Feuerstein JD, Nguyen GC, Velayos FS. AGA clinical practice update on endoscopic surveillance and management of colorectal dysplasia in inflammatory bowel diseases: expert review. Gastroenterology. 2021;161(3):1043–51.
130. Kothari ST, Huang RJ, Shaukat A, Agrawal D, Buxbaum JL, Abbas Fehmi SM, et al. ASGE review of adverse events in colonoscopy. Gastrointest Endosc. 2019;90(6):863–76.
131. Gupta S, Lieberman D, Anderson JC, Burke CA, Dominitz JA, Kaltenbach T, et al. Recommendations for follow-up after colonoscopy and polypectomy: a consensus update by the US Multi-Society Task Force on colorectal cancer. Gastroenterology. 2020;158(4):1131–53.
132. Lieberman D, Sullivan BA, Hauser ER, Qin X, Musselwhite LW, O'Leary MC, et al. Baseline colonoscopy findings associated with 10-year outcomes in a screening cohort undergoing colonoscopy surveillance. Gastroenterology. 2020;158(4):862–74.
133. Murphy CC, Lewis CL, Golin CE, Sandler RS. Underuse of surveillance colonoscopy in patients at increased risk of colorectal cancer. Am J Gastroenterol. 2015;110(5):633–41.
134. Murphy CC, Sandler RS, Grubber JM, Johnson MR, Fisher DA. Underuse and overuse of colonoscopy for repeat screening and surveillance in the Veterans Health Administration. Clin Gastroenterol Hepatol. 2016;14(3):436–44.
135. Kruse GR, Khan SM, Zaslavsky AM, Ayanian JZ, Sequist TD. Overuse of colonoscopy for colorectal cancer screening and surveillance. J Gen Intern Med. 2015;30(3):277–83.
136. Singh A, Kuo YF, Goodwin JS. Many patients who undergo surgery for colorectal cancer receive surveillance colonoscopies earlier than recommended by guidelines. Clin Gastroenterol Hepatol. 2013;11(1):65–72.
137. Yadlapati R, Gawron A, Keswani RN. Patient satisfaction does not correlate with established colonoscopy quality metrics. Am J Gastroenterol. 2014;109(7):1089–91.
138. Ekkelenkamp VE, Dowler K, Valori RM, Dunckley P. Patient comfort and quality in colonoscopy. World J Gastroenterol. 2013;19(15):2355–61.

Chapter 3
Quality in Upper Endoscopy

Thomas J. Wang and Hiroyuki Aihara

Table of Quality Measures/Metrics

T. J. Wang
Division of Gastroenterology Hepatology and Endoscopy, Brigham and Women's Hospital, Boston, MA, USA
e-mail: twang16@partners.org

H. Aihara (✉)
Division of Gastroenterology Hepatology and Endoscopy, Brigham and Women's Hospital, Boston, MA, USA

Department of Medicine, Harvard Medical School, Boston, MA, USA
e-mail: haihara@bwh.harvard.edu

J. D. Feuerstein, D. J. Stein (eds.), *Quality in Gastroenterology*,
https://doi.org/10.1007/978-3-031-58492-3_3

Key Points

- A detailed discussion on the indication, appropriateness, risk/benefits of the procedure, and alternative options should occur well before the procedure date to ensure proper patient understanding.
- Attention to ergonomics and judicious use of insufflation can reduce the risk of musculoskeletal injuries and improve the quality of endoscopy.
- For urgent endoscopies, their indications, timings, and periprocedural recommendations should be reviewed and discussed in advance with the care team.
- The chromoendoscopy and image-enhanced endoscopy are essential tools in enhancing the quality and diagnostic yield of upper endoscopy, particularly in gastric cancer screening.
- Gastric polyp diagnosis should be performed based on the endoscopic findings as well as biopsies to determine the treatment plan and endoscopic surveillance intervals.

Pre/Post-procedure Management

Consent Process

Informed consent is the cornerstone of GI endoscopy and, from a medicolegal and moral perspective, must be provided to the patient before performing endoscopy. Failing to provide informed consent can put an endoscopist under legal liability for negligence and, at the same time, protect providers from claims of medical injury due to the procedure [1]. There are, however, no specific guidelines on the exact timing [2]. In the ideal setting, there should be a thorough discussion about the procedure when the upper endoscopy is proposed to the patient, which often could be months in advance. Any discussion should be paired with appropriate documentation of that conversation and include the rationale/indication behind performing the procedure, benefits, risks, procedural description, and alternatives to performing the procedure [3]. In particular, a discussion of risks should include any heightened risks based on patients' known medical comorbidities and possible additional interventions (e.g., biopsy, polyp removal, hemostasis, and dilation). Supplemental reading or video material is highly encouraged and can substantially improve information recall on the contents of the informed consent [4].

Consent obtained the same day as the procedure should ideally reinforce any prior discussion and formally review standard risks and benefits that may have been missed in prior discussions or forgotten by the patient. However, same-day consent should not formally substitute prior, more detailed discussions, as the demanding workflow and high time pressure setting during endoscopy setup can make it very challenging for patients to properly comprehend the information provided and make an informed decision on the spot [5].

Ideally, consent should be provided by the clinician performing the procedure. However, it is also reasonable for consent to be provided by a nurse, trainee, or advanced practice provider, with the caveat that the provider obtaining consent is highly knowledgeable and able to effectively communicate the indication, benefits, risks, and descriptions of the procedure [3]. An alternate consenting provider allows the primary endoscopist to practice at the top of their license and more effectively juggle an often very busy clinical workflow. Moreover, it frequently gives more time to the patient to ask questions and more effectively process information provided by the consenting provider.

Appropriate Indications

It is important that, before performing an upper endoscopy, patients are properly screened for the appropriate indication. In one large study of more than 2000 patients referred for diagnostic endoscopy, 39% of referred patients were considered to have an inappropriate indication, and patients who had appropriate or uncertain (i.e., borderline appropriate) indications had an odds ratio (OR) of 2.6 in increased yield of finding significant diagnoses on endoscopy (60 vs. 37%, OR 2.6, 95% confidence interval (CI) 2.2–3.2) [6]. The majority of patients with inappropriate indications were those referred for dyspepsia symptoms, with 68% considered inappropriate. Those patients had not been given an adequate trial of therapy for their dyspepsia symptoms prior to consideration of endoscopy [7]. More urgent indications, such as hematemesis, melena, iron deficiency anemia, dysphagia, and odynophagia, were almost all considered appropriate and should be prioritized urgently, as their diagnostic yield and risks from delayed endoscopy are much higher in comparison [6].

A full list of appropriate indications for upper endoscopy can be found in the ASGE 2012 guidelines "appropriate use of GI endoscopy" [8]. A summary of indications is outlined in Table 3.1.

Choice of Sedation

Sedation choices for upper endoscopy can be classified into three major categories: unsedated, moderate conscious sedation, and deep sedation [9].

Unsedated upper endoscopy is rare in the United States but is more common in other countries in Asia and Europe [10]. When they do occur, they are often performed with sufficient topical anesthesia to minimize patient discomfort.

Moderate sedation typically involves a combination of a benzodiazepine and narcotic to manage anxiety and pain during the endoscopy and is administered per

Table 3.1 Summary of indications appropriate for upper endoscopy

Category	Details
Upper GI symptoms	Odynophagia, dysphagia, or those refractory to the appropriate initial therapy for nausea/vomiting, gastroesophageal reflux disease, and dyspepsia. Patients with alarm features (older than age 50, family history of cancers in the upper GI tract, unintentional weight loss, smoking history) should be more urgently evaluated and should not be delayed in the evaluation of therapy response
Bleeding or concern for bleeding	Hematemesis, melena, iron deficiency anemia (along with colonoscopy), variceal screening in patients with suspected portal hypertension
Ingestion	Removal of impacted foreign body, assessment of acute injury after caustic ingestion
Diarrhea	Only if small bowel disease is suspected (e.g., celiac)
Malignancy screening	High-risk individuals (e.g., those with a family history of esophageal or gastric cancer, Barrett's esophagus, familial adenomatous polyposis (FAP) syndrome)
Radiographic findings (e.g., CT, barium swallow)	Suspected malignancy, esophageal or gastric ulcers, obstruction, stricture. Upper endoscopy should not be performed for patients found to have sliding hiatal hernia or uncomplicated duodenal ulcer
Therapeutic treatment of a known condition	Placement of feeding tube, dilation, stenting, botulinum toxin injection (for achalasia)

instructions from the endoscopist [11]. At our center, we favor midazolam and fentanyl due to their fast onset of action and short duration, though other centers may be more familiar with other alternative agents (e.g., diazepam, meperidine). Patients who are difficult to sedate but do not meet criteria for monitored anesthesia due to lack of indication or availability may also be trialed on adjunct agents such as diphenhydramine (i.e., Benadryl), though this carries the risk of longer recovery times [9].

Deep sedation typically involves propofol and must be administered with the aid of an anesthesia provider. For some patients, deep sedation may be preferred due to anxiety, discomfort with the procedure with moderate sedation, patients' comorbidities, shorter sedation and recovery period, or adverse events from moderate sedation agents [9]. Deep sedation can be further categorized into monitored anesthesia care (MAC) or general anesthesia. General anesthesia requires intubation, often for airway protection in patients with an increased risk of pulmonary aspiration (e.g., food impaction, vomiting in the past 24 h, history of aspiration pneumonia) [11]. These criteria should be carefully weighed by the provider ordering the endoscopy and discussed with the patient prior to scheduling to maximize patient satisfaction and minimize the risk of procedure failure from the inability to tolerate the selected sedation.

One large retrospective, observational cohort study comparing moderate and deep sedation, including 508,000 upper endoscopies, demonstrated an increased risk of serious adverse events in patients with deep sedation over moderate sedation (OR 1.33, 95% CI 1.18–1.5) [12]. As such, the choice of deep sedation versus moderate sedation should be carefully weighed, striking a balance between patient comfort/satisfaction, patient safety, and expectations of ability to complete the upper endoscopy without deep sedation.

Regarding the topical anesthesia for upper endoscopy with deep sedation, two randomized controlled trials (RCT) demonstrated no effect on patient discomfort, the necessary dose of propofol, or anesthesia/endoscopist's satisfaction intra-procedure [13, 14]. Topical anesthesia makes little difference in patients who undergo deep sedation. It likely only adds to increased time pre-procedure and results in temporary but unnecessary patient discomfort during the application, which should be reserved for unsedated or moderate sedated procedures [15].

Diet Protocol

Prior to endoscopy, clear instructions on diet restriction should be provided for the patient. At a minimum, before any upper endoscopy, regardless of anesthesia choice, patients should not drink any clear liquid at least 2 h before scheduled upper endoscopy, not drink or eat full liquid or light meals at least 6 h prior, and not eat heavier foods (fried, fatty, or meat) at least 8 h prior [16]. For convenience, a cutoff of nothing by mouth after midnight is often easy to remember for patients but not necessary. For patients who did not follow the diet protocol prior to endoscopy, the endoscopy should be delayed until at least the minimum time restriction cutoff is met unless the procedure is emergent (e.g., food impaction). In rare emergent cases, general anesthesia with intubation for airway protection would likely have to be considered to reduce the risk of pulmonary aspiration.

Best Practices During Upper Endoscopy

Ergonomics

A proper understanding of ergonomics is essential to prevent musculoskeletal injury for endoscopists. In one study, more than half of endoscopists (53%) reported a musculoskeletal injury either certainly or likely related to endoscopy. The frequency of injury was associated with higher procedure volume, longer work hours, and the cumulative number of years worked [17].

Endoscopists should ensure that before starting a procedure, they should place themselves in a neutral body position with minimal strain on their upper body muscles [18]. One should adjust or request the monitor to be adjusted so that the center of the screen is 15° below resting eye positioning to reduce neck strain. The hospital bed should be adjusted 0–10 cm below elbow height in a resting position while holding the scope. A finger grip (i.e., "cigar-rolling" technique) over the gastroscope is preferred over a fist grip to allow for more precise control of the endoscope. The scopes should always be adjusted before the procedure to be in a neutral position. Both the finger grip and neutral position can help reduce excessive manipulation and turning of the scope.

Insufflation

Proper visualization of the upper GI tract is essential in upper endoscopies. The stomach should be appropriately distended to avoid missing small gastric lesions or key findings (e.g., dysplasias, ulcers, and arteriovenous malformations) hidden behind the gastric folds [19]. However, once the stomach lining begins to blanch in color, air should be taken out to reduce post-procedural abdominal discomfort. Unlike colonoscopies [20], no randomized studies for upper endoscopies have compared the use of air or CO_2 in terms of patient comfort, so there exists no general consensus on whether there is an advantage to using either for insufflation purposes.

Use of Simethicone

Simethicone is an essential tool that can be deployed by endoscopists to enhance mucosal assessment and lesion detection in the upper gastrointestinal tract [21]. Simethicone is a defoaming agent in clearing bubbles that, when present, can impair adequate visualization of the mucosa, leading to longer procedural times or reducing the detection rate of potential notable findings [22]. Unfortunately, there is no other alternative agent commercially available that achieves similar goals. Simethicone can either be applied directly through the scope channel or added to lavage fluid, with a suggested concentration of 2–3 mL of 120 mg/mL added to 1 L of sterile water, though the evidence of an optimal concentration or dose is lacking.

Specific Scenarios

In this section, we describe more specific best practices and quality metrics for upper endoscopies for certain indications. For best practices in endoscopic ultrasound (EUS), endoscopic retrograde cholangiopancreatography (ERCP), and esophageal cancer screening, refer to the other chapters for more information.

Upper Endoscopy in an Urgent Setting

In this section, we overview best practices for upper endoscopy in urgent situations. This almost exclusively occurs in the emergency or inpatient setting, with the most common indications being suspected acute upper gastrointestinal bleeding (e.g., hematemesis or melena), foreign body ingestion and food impaction, and caustic injury requiring urgent evaluation and treatment.

For suspected acute upper gastrointestinal bleeding, in general, upper endoscopy should be performed within 24 h [23]. However, the establishment of adequate intravenous (IV) access (at least two 18 gauge peripheral IVs or equivalent) followed by resuscitation with intravenous fluids and packed red blood cell transfusion should be prioritized. Hemoglobin goal should be aimed at >7 (or >21 if using hematocrit) for patients who are hemodynamically stable [24], while for patients with hemodynamic instability with concern for active gastrointestinal hemorrhage, resuscitation should be based on hemodynamics and less so on a specific hemoglobin goal. For patients who have active hematemesis or with concerns for impending or ongoing respiratory failure, intubation for airway protection should also occur in parallel. Patients who exhibit hemodynamic instability should be transferred to an intensive care unit for close monitoring prior to bedside endoscopy. Lastly, one should consider a reversal of anticoagulant agents when possible and initiation of IV proton pump inhibitor therapy.

There is no mortality benefit in scoping more urgently within 12 h versus scoping within 24 h for patients with acute GI bleeding [25]. The exception to this rule is patients with suspicion for variceal bleeding (e.g., history or imaging/lab findings of cirrhosis and portal hypertension), of which, although no strong evidence exists, general consensus per Baveno VII guidelines is to perform endoscopy in less than 12 h when able [26].

For foreign body ingestion and food impaction, urgent endoscopies should be subdivided into patients who may require emergent endoscopy versus those who may need urgent endoscopy [27]. Emergent endoscopy (within 6 h of ingestion) should be reserved for patients with evidence of complete esophageal obstruction (i.e., cannot manage secretions) or those with disk batteries or sharp-pointed objects in the esophagus, as either type of object would be at high risk of perforation. For patients with ingestion of a disk battery or sharp object, an emergent chest X-ray should be performed to stratify the patient between the emergent or urgent categories. For patients with emergent indications, general anesthesia with elective intubation is preferred, given the high risk of aspiration and airway damage while pursuing foreign body removal.

If sharp objects have already passed into the stomach or duodenum, then endoscopy is recommended within 24 h of ingestion (i.e., urgent) [27]. The same strategy applies to patients with food impaction with incomplete obstruction. Disk and cylindrical batteries that have passed into the stomach without suspicious findings of gastric injury or GI symptoms can be observed for as long as 48 h, though if the battery continues to be retained, then endoscopic removal should be pursued.

For food impactions, once the acute impaction is resolved, careful inspection of the esophagus should be performed to look for areas of ulceration and endoscopic findings that may be consistent with eosinophilic esophagitis (EoE). EoE is highly prevalent (up to 50%) in patients who present with acute food impaction, especially in younger patients [28].

Table 3.2 Zargar classification system for caustic injury

Caustic injury grade	Description
0	Normal
1	Mucosal edema and erythema
2A	Superficial ulceration and exudates
2B	Deep focal or circumferential ulcers
3A	Focal necrosis with numerous or deep ulcerations
3B	Extensive necrosis

Lastly, patients with caustic ingestion, regardless of an acidic or alkali source, should undergo urgent endoscopy within 24 h of ingestion. The primary purpose of the upper endoscopy is diagnostic, with documentation of the severity of mural injury based on the Zargar classification system as outlined in Table 3.2 [29]. If there is a concern for deep mural damage (grade 2B or higher), then a computed tomography (CT) scan would be performed to better characterize the extent of the damage. Higher grades are also predictive of the development of adverse events (e.g., bleeding, fistula formation, and stricture), so follow-up endoscopy may also be warranted depending on the severity of the injury.

Gastric Cancer Screening

Gastric cancer screening should be considered for patients who are at high risk of developing gastric adenocarcinoma. A systematic review and meta-analysis demonstrated that endoscopic screening was linked to a 40% relative risk reduction in mortality from gastric cancer [30]. High-risk populations include patients with evidence on prior biopsy of chronic atrophic gastritis (AG) or intestinal metaplasia (IM), those with a family history of gastric cancer in a first-degree relative, or those who originated from high-risk regions, such as countries in Eastern Europe, East Asia, and South America [31]. High-risk patients are often referred for upper endoscopies for gastric cancer screening, either at age 50 or 10 years before the age of diagnosis for a first-degree relative [32, 33]. Regarding these patients, they should undergo systematic endoscopic examination and biopsies under the Sydney protocol, which entails five different sites of biopsies in two different bottles [34]. Three of the sites are in the distal stomach, with biopsies all collected into one bottle from locations in the A1 (3 cm from the pylorus in the antral lesser curvature), A2 (3 cm from the pylorus in the antral greater curvature), and IA (incisura angularis) regions. The second bottle should consist of biopsies from two additional sites in the B1 (middle of the gastric body, lesser curvature) and B2 (middle of the gastric body, greater curvature) regions. Endoscopic findings concerning for atrophic gastritis or intestinal metaplasia should be clearly documented and differentiated based on location, in particular, whether the involvement is primarily in the distal stomach (i.e., antrum and incisura), in the proximal stomach (i.e., gastric body), or both, as more proximal involvement does increase the risk of progression to gastric adenocarcinoma.

Any additional targeted biopsies should be obtained from any sites of concern (e.g., changes in color [red or white areas] and shape [depressed or elevated areas]) detected on white light endoscopy (WLE). These sites should also be evaluated by chromoendoscopy and image-enhanced endoscopies (IEE), such as narrowband imaging (NBI) and blue light imaging (BLI). A minimum examination time of 7 min should be performed to find small dysplastic lesions during a gastric cancer screening [34].

If *H. pylori* are present, but there is no evidence of AG or IM, then the patient should be prescribed eradication therapy and scheduled for follow-up endoscopy in 3–5 years. If AG/IM is present or there is strong family history in a first-degree relative, then patients should be scheduled for surveillance endoscopy for a shorter duration of 1–2 years. The 1-year interval should be considered if an adenomatous polyp is resected [32], and it should be shortened to 6 months in case of high-grade dysplasia [35]. If there is neither a family history nor the presence of AG/IM/*H. pylori*, then no further follow-up is required [36, 37].

Polyp Evaluation in the Stomach

Gastric polyps are often incidentally discovered during routine upper endoscopies, and it can be challenging to know how best to manage (e.g., biopsy vs. resection) at the time of endoscopy. We outline below common gastric polyps that endoscopists may encounter, how to distinguish types of polyps, and how to manage them based on endoscopic appearance, size, and the biopsy results.

Fundic gland polyps are the most commonly encountered polyps in the stomach, making up 47% of all polyps seen [38]. These polyps are often seen in the gastric body and fundus, with the surface color often appearing identical to that of surrounding gastric mucosa. These polyps also characteristically do not have a stalk. Although fundic gland polyps can often be differentiated reliably on endoscopy, biopsy sampling of likely fundic gland polyps should be performed to exonerate dysplasia or adenocarcinoma [39]. Polyps >1 cm should be completely resected to reduce the risk of sampling error. If numerous fundic gland polyps are seen, then familial adenomatous polyposis (FAP) should be suspected, especially if the patient is young, and lower endoscopy may be warranted.

Hyperplastic polyps, on the other hand, are often sessile or pedunculated in appearance. They can occur anywhere in the stomach but typically reside in the antrum [35]. These polyps are often associated with *H. pylori* and/or chronic gastritis. If hyperplastic polyps are suspected, gastric biopsies in the body and antrum for *H. pylori* screening should also be performed, with eradication treatment if present since these polyps often regress with *H. pylori* eradication [40]. Guidelines on whether these polyps should be resected or biopsied are lacking; hyperplastic polyps often have a low potential for dysplasia but sometimes may be difficult to differentiate from gastric adenomas. Recommendations for size cutoff resection vary from 0.5 cm to 2 cm.

Gastric adenomas, unlike fundic gland polyps and hyperplastic polyps, are often more flat or sessile in appearance. All suspected gastric adenomas, regardless of size, should be completely resected due to their potential to develop into high-grade dysplasia and gastric cancer [35].

Acknowledgments None.

Disclosures Thomas Wang has nothing to disclose.
Hiroyuki Aihara is a consultant for Olympus America, Fujifilm Medical Systems, Boston Scientific, ConMed, Medtronic, and 3D-Matrix.

Funding Support No funding to declare.

References

1. Gerstenberger PD, Plumeri PA. Malpractice claims in gastrointestinal endoscopy: analysis of an insurance industry database. Gastrointest Endosc. 1993;39(2):132–8.
2. Proctor DD, Price J, Minhas BS, Gumber SC, Christie EM. Patient recall and appropriate timing for obtaining informed consent for endoscopic procedures. Am J Gastroenterol. 1999;94(4):967–71.
3. Storm AC, Fishman DS, Buxbaum JL, Coelho-Prabhu N, Al-Haddad MA, Amateau SK, et al. American Society for Gastrointestinal Endoscopy guideline on informed consent for GI endoscopic procedures. Gastrointest Endosc. 2022;95(2):207–15.
4. Farrell EH, Whistance RN, Phillips K, Morgan B, Savage K, Lewis V, et al. Systematic review and meta-analysis of audio-visual information aids for informed consent for invasive healthcare procedures in clinical practice. Patient Educ Couns. 2014;94(1):20–32.
5. Woodrow SR, Jenkins AP. How thorough is the process of informed consent prior to outpatient gastroscopy? Digestion. 2006;73(2–3):189–97.
6. Froehlich F, Repond C, Müllhaupt B, Vader JP, Burnand B, Schneider C, et al. Is the diagnostic yield of upper GI endoscopy improved by the use of explicit panel-based appropriateness criteria? Gastrointest Endosc. 2000;52(3):333–41.
7. Shaukat A, Wang A, Acosta RD, Bruining DH, Chandrasekhara V, Chathadi KV, et al. The role of endoscopy in dyspepsia. Gastrointest Endosc. 2015;82(2):227–32.
8. Early DS, Ben-Menachem T, Decker GA, Evans JA, Fanelli RD, Fisher DA, et al. Appropriate use of GI endoscopy. Gastrointest Endosc. 2012;75(6):1127–31.
9. Early DS, Lightdale JR, Vargo JJ, Acosta RD, Chandrasekhara V, Chathadi KV, et al. Guidelines for sedation and anesthesia in GI endoscopy. Gastrointest Endosc. 2018;87(2):327–37.
10. Aljebreen A. Unsedated endoscopy: is it feasible? Saudi J Gastroenterol. 2010;16(4):243.
11. Vargo JJ, DeLegge MH, Feld AD, Gerstenberger PD, Kwo PY, Lightdale JR, et al. Multisociety sedation curriculum for gastrointestinal endoscopy. Gastrointest Endosc. 2012;76(1):e1–25.
12. Vargo JJ, Niklewski PJ, Williams JL, Martin JF, Faigel DO. Patient safety during sedation by anesthesia professionals during routine upper endoscopy and colonoscopy: an analysis of 1.38 million procedures. Gastrointest Endosc. 2017;85(1):101–8.
13. de la Morena F, Santander C, Esteban C, de Cuenca B, García JA, Sánchez J, et al. Usefulness of applying lidocaine in esophagogastroduodenoscopy performed under sedation with propofol. World J Gastrointest Endosc. 2013;5(5):231–9.

14. Sun X, Xu Y, Zhang X, Li A, Zhang H, Yang T, et al. Topical pharyngeal anesthesia provides no additional benefit to propofol sedation for esophagogastroduodenoscopy: a randomized controlled double-blinded clinical trial. Sci Rep. 2018;8(1):6682.
15. Tsai HI, Tsai YF, Liou SC, Su MY, Lin CC, Chang CJ, et al. The questionable efficacy of topical pharyngeal anesthesia in combination with propofol sedation in gastroscopy. Dig Dis Sci. 2012;57(10):2519–26.
16. ASA. Practice guidelines for preoperative fasting and the use of pharmacologic agents to reduce the risk of pulmonary aspiration: application to healthy patients undergoing elective procedures: an updated report by the American Society of Anesthesiologists Task Force on preoperative fasting and the use of pharmacologic agents to reduce the risk of pulmonary aspiration. Anesthesiology. 2017;126(3):376–93.
17. Ridtitid W, Coté GA, Leung W, Buschbacher R, Lynch S, Fogel EL, et al. Prevalence and risk factors for musculoskeletal injuries related to endoscopy. Gastrointest Endosc. 2015;81(2):294–302.
18. Walsh CM, Qayed E, Aihara H, Anand GS, Byrne K, Chahal P, et al. Core curriculum for ergonomics in endoscopy. Gastrointest Endosc. 2021;93(6):1222–7.
19. Lee SH, Park YK, Cho SM, Kang JK, Lee DJ. Technical skills and training of upper gastrointestinal endoscopy for new beginners. World J Gastroenterol. 2015;21(3):759.
20. Wu J, Hu B. The role of carbon dioxide insufflation in colonoscopy: a systematic review and meta-analysis. Endoscopy. 2012;44(2):128–36.
21. Manfredi G, Bertè R, Iiritano E, Alicante S, Londoni C, Brambilla G, et al. Premedication with simethicone and N-acetylcysteine for improving mucosal visibility during upper gastrointestinal endoscopy in a Western population. Endosc Int Open. 2021;9(2):E190–4.
22. Devereaux BM, Taylor AC, Athan E, Wallis DJ, Brown RR, Greig SM, et al. Simethicone use during gastrointestinal endoscopy: Position statement of the Gastroenterological Society of Australia. J Gastroenterol Hepatol. 2019;34(12):2086–9.
23. Laine L, Barkun AN, Saltzman JR, Martel M, Leontiadis GI. ACG clinical guideline: upper gastrointestinal and ulcer bleeding. ACG. 2021;116(5):899–917.
24. Villanueva C, Colomo A, Bosch A, Concepción M, Hernandez-Gea V, Aracil C, et al. Transfusion strategies for acute upper gastrointestinal bleeding. N Engl J Med. 2013;368(1):11–21.
25. Jairath V, Kahan BC, Logan RFA, Hearnshaw SA, Doré CJ, Travis SPL, et al. Outcomes following acute nonvariceal upper gastrointestinal bleeding in relation to time to endoscopy: results from a nationwide study. Endoscopy. 2012;44(8):723–30.
26. De Franchis R, Bosch J, Garcia-Tsao G, Reiberger T, Ripoll C, Abraldes JG, et al. Baveno VII–renewing consensus in portal hypertension. J Hepatol. 2022;76(4):959–74.
27. Ikenberry SO, Jue TL, Anderson MA, Appalaneni V, Banerjee S, Ben-Menachem T, et al. Management of ingested foreign bodies and food impactions. Gastrointest Endosc. 2011;73(6):1085–91.
28. Lucendo AJ, Molina-Infante J, Arias Á, von Arnim U, Bredenoord AJ, Bussmann C, et al. Guidelines on eosinophilic esophagitis: evidence-based statements and recommendations for diagnosis and management in children and adults. UEG J. 2017;5(3):335–58.
29. Zargar SA, Kochhar R, Mehta S, Mehta SK. The role of fiberoptic endoscopy in the management of corrosive ingestion and modified endoscopic classification of burns. Gastrointest Endosc. 1991;37(2):165–9.
30. Zhang X, Li M, Chen S, Hu J, Guo Q, Liu R, et al. Endoscopic screening in Asian countries is associated with reduced gastric cancer mortality: a meta-analysis and systematic review. Gastroenterology. 2018;155(2):347–54.
31. Karimi P, Islami F, Anandasabapathy S, Freedman ND, Kamangar F. Gastric cancer: descriptive epidemiology, risk factors, screening, and prevention gastric cancer. Cancer Epidemiol Biomarkers Prev. 2014;23(5):700–13.
32. Evans JA, Chandrasekhara V, Chathadi KV, Decker GA, Early DS, Fisher DA, et al. The role of endoscopy in the management of premalignant and malignant conditions of the stomach. Gastrointest Endosc. 2015;82(1):1–8.

33. Kim GH, Liang PS, Bang SJ, Hwang JH. Screening and surveillance for gastric cancer in the United States: is it needed? Gastrointest Endosc. 2016;84(1):18–28.
34. Banks M, Graham D, Jansen M, Gotoda T, Coda S, Di Pietro M, et al. British Society of Gastroenterology guidelines on the diagnosis and management of patients at risk of gastric adenocarcinoma. Gut. 2019;68(9):1545–75.
35. Islam RS, Patel NC, Lam-Himlin D, Nguyen CC. Gastric polyps: a review of clinical, endoscopic, and histopathologic features and management decisions. Gastroenterol Hepatol. 2013;9(10):640–51.
36. Yamaguchi D, Kodashima S, Fujishiro M, Ono S, Niimi K, Mochizuki S, et al. Evaluation of image-enhanced endoscopic technology using advanced diagnostic endoscopy for the detection of early gastric cancer: a pilot study. Endosc Int Open. 2017;5(9):E825–33.
37. Choi HJ, Lee YN. Focused review series: image enhanced endoscopy: open access; advanced imaging technology in biliary tract diseases: narrow-band imaging of the bile duct. Clin Endosc. 2015;48(6):498–502.
38. Stolte M, Sticht T, Eidt S, Ebert D, Finkenzeller G. Frequency, location, and age and sex distribution of various types of gastric polyp. Endoscopy. 1994;26(8):659–65.
39. Goddard AF, Badreldin R, Pritchard DM, Walker MM, Warren B. The management of gastric polyps. Gut. 2010;59(9):1270–6.
40. Ohkusa T, Takashimizu I, Fujiki K, Suzuki S, Shimoi K, Horiuchi T, et al. Disappearance of hyperplastic polyps in the stomach after eradication of Helicobacter pylori: a randomized, controlled trial. Ann Intern Med. 1998;129(9):712–5.

Chapter 4
Quality in ERCP

Lawrence Jun Leung, Ryan B. Perumpail, and Mandeep S. Sawhney

Table of Quality Measures/Metrics

Key Points

- Prioritized measures for ERCP quality include ERCP indication, cannulation success rate, stone extraction success rate, stent placement success rate, and rate of post-ERCP pancreatitis.
- Other quality metrics encompass aspects of documentation and follow-up, appropriate antibiotic use, fluoroscopy duration, and adverse events.
- Quality metrics to mitigate post-ERCP pancreatitis include pharmacologic prophylaxis and endoscopic techniques.

Since the first endoscopic access of the ampulla of Vater in 1968 [1], endoscopic retrograde cholangiopancreatography (ERCP) has evolved over the decades from a solely diagnostic procedure into a predominantly therapeutic [2]. It has increasingly

L. J. Leung
Kaiser Permanente San Francisco, San Francisco, CA, USA
e-mail: Lawrence.j.leung@kp.org

R. B. Perumpail
Genesis Health Group, Gastroenterology Associates, Bettendorf, IA, USA
e-mail: perumpailr@genesishealth.com

M. S. Sawhney (✉)
Beth Israel Deaconess Medical Center, Boston, MA, USA
e-mail: msawhney@bidmc.harvard.edu

J. D. Feuerstein, D. J. Stein (eds.), *Quality in Gastroenterology*,
https://doi.org/10.1007/978-3-031-58492-3_4

Table 4.1 Priority ERCP quality indicators

Priority ERCP quality indicators
ERCP indication
Cannulation success rate
Stone extraction success rate
Stent placement success rate
Rate of post-ERCP pancreatitis

become the first treatment option for pancreatic and biliary disease management [2]. ERCP patient outcomes can vary significantly [3], and procedure-related complications can be significant [3–6].

ERCP procedures have relatively high rates of adverse events and can be associated with a high rate of morbidity and mortality [7, 8]. The most common serious complication is post-ERCP pancreatitis (PEP) [8]. Other adverse events include infection, including cholangitis, cholecystitis, and duodenoscope-related transmission; bleeding; perforation, which is classified based on location; cardiopulmonary complications; and reaction to contrast material and medications [8].

In order to maximize success and minimize complications, the American Society for Gastrointestinal Endoscopy (ASGE) and the American College of Gastroenterology (ACG) have emphasized training factors and metrics to maximize quality and decrease the high adverse events rate in ERCP [9]. Different quality indicators have been described to allow for a successful ERCP [9–11]; however, certain indicators have been deemed priority indicators [9]. **Priority quality indicators** are summarized in Table 4.1 [9–11].

Priority Quality Indicators

ERCP indication refers to the frequency in which an ERCP is performed for an appropriate indication [9]. Pre-procedural patient selection is key and prevents unnecessary exposure to the potential procedural complications. It is recommended that an appropriate indication should be at a target rate of 90% or higher due to the high risk of adverse events [9, 12]. This is compared to other endoscopic procedures where appropriate indications have a target rate of 80% or higher [9]. Indications that have previously been published are summarized in Table 4.2 [9, 12–14]. Most appropriate indications are for patients with objective data requiring therapeutic purposes, such as objective evidence of obstructive jaundice [12, 15]. One listed indication includes the need to perform a sphincterotomy. Appropriate indications to perform a sphincterotomy include: choledocholithiasis, papillary stenosis or sphincter of Oddi dysfunction, to facilitate biliary stent placement or dilation of biliary strictures, bile leak, Sump syndrome, choledochocele involving the major papilla, ampullary carcinoma in patients who are not candidates for surgery, and to facilitate access to the pancreatic duct [9]. Additionally, although ERCP and sphincterotomy can be indicated for sphincter of Oddi dysfunction, this does not

Table 4.2 ERCP indications

ERCP indications
Jaundiced, suspect biliary obstruction
No jaundice but labs or imaging suggesting pancreatic or biliary tract disease
Evaluation of pancreatic malignancy when direct imaging is equivocal or normal
Evaluation of pancreatitis of unknown etiology
Preoperative evaluation of chronic pancreatitis and/or pseudocyst
Empirical biliary sphincterotomy is not recommended in type III sphincter of Oddi dysfunction
Sphincterotomy indications
Stent placement across strictures, fistulae, postoperative bile leak, or in high-risk patients with large unremovable common duct stones
Dilation of ductal strictures
Balloon dilation of the papilla
Pancreatic pseudocyst drainage in appropriate cases
Tissue sampling from pancreatic or bile ducts
Ampullectomy of adenomatous neoplasms of the major papilla
Therapy of disorders of the biliary and pancreatic ducts
Facilitation of cholangioscopy and/or pancreatoscopy

hold true in type III when there is no objective evidence of pancreatic or biliary pathology [16].

Another priority indicator is the **rate of deep cannulation in native papillae without surgically altered anatomies** [9]. One of the key steps that allows access to the pancreatic and biliary system involves cannulation into the duct of interest. This allows visualization with contrast injection and the ability for instrumentation to achieve the intended purpose. High rates of deep cannulation allow for a successful ERCP and minimize the need for a potential repeat procedure—whether another ERCP, interventional radiology procedure, or surgical intervention. Prior reports have demonstrated varying rates of successful cannulation depending on user experience and prior papillae alterations [17, 18]. Verma et al. showed that successful cannulation rates increased with further training and experience and proposed this metric to be a standard for ERCP training [19]. DeBenedet et al. demonstrated in a meta-analysis comparing ERCP performance that cannulation success rate was approximately 89.3% for a bile duct and 85% for a pancreatic duct [20]. Additionally, a prior analysis showed that almost 25% of independently practicing endoscopists did not reach 90% for their rate of deep cannulation [5]. Regardless, this intra-procedural quality indicator is recommended to have a target rate of 90% or higher [6, 9].

A priority indicator for ERCP procedures involving stone extraction is the **success rate of common duct stone removal that is less than 1 cm in size in patients with normal bile duct anatomy** [9]. Stone extraction is a common indication for ERCP [12, 15], and successful removal of small to medium stones in unaltered anatomy is a marker of a trained and competent ERCP endoscopist [13, 21]. This intra-procedural quality indicator is recommended to have a target success rate of 90% or higher [9]. Unlike the prior rate of deep cannulation metric, a success rate of 90% or higher for successful small to medium stone removal is more prevalent. Cotton et al. demonstrated that approximately 3% of ERCP endoscopists did not meet the 90% threshold for successful stone removal [5].

A priority indicator for ERCP procedures involving stents is the **success rate of stent placement for non-hilar biliary obstruction in patients with normal anatomy** [9]. In addition to stone extraction, biliary stent placement is a common indication for ERCP [12, 15]. Biliary stents can help relieve obstruction, including from malignancy, strictures, or stones [12, 13]. Stents in non-hilar biliary obstruction are used as a metric because obstructions involving the hilum and above the bifurcation are more technically challenging and may require further experience or training [5, 9]. The recommended threshold for successful stent placement is 90% or higher [9].

The last priority quality indicator and only post-procedure priority metric is the **rate of post-ERCP pancreatitis** [9]. PEP is defined as pancreatitis after an ERCP, and rates can range from 3% to 10% if the indication is appropriate [7, 8, 22–26]. Traditional criteria for pancreatitis diagnosis include abdominal pain with concurrent lipase elevation to three or more times the upper limit of normal or radiographic evidence [9]. A performance target is not recommended for PEP because many factors, including type of ERCP, indication, and skill level of the endoscopists, contribute to the development of PEP [9]. Quality metrics to decrease PEP, such as rectal indomethacin [27–29], will be discussed later in the chapter.

Other Quality Metrics

Additional quality metrics to maximize ERCP quality are summarized in Table 4.3 [9].

Table 4.3 Other quality metrics

Other quality metrics
Informed consent obtained
Pre-procedure antibiotics when appropriate
Volume of ERCPs performed per year
Fluoroscopy time and radiation dose
Complete ERCP report
Acute adverse events and hospital transfers
Rate and type of perforation
Rate of clinically significant hemorrhage after sphincterotomy or sphincteroplasty
Frequency with which patients are contacted ≥14 days

Obtaining **informed consent** pre-procedure at a frequency of over 98% is a recommended quality metric [9]. ERCP procedures carry significantly higher risk than most endoscopic procedures, and patients should be informed of the potential complications before agreeing to proceed [7, 9, 23]. This includes PEP, infection, bleeding, cardiopulmonary compromise, perforation, and reactions to contrast and medications [7, 23].

Frequency for pre-procedure **antibiotics prior to ERCP when appropriate** is recommended to be over 98% [9]. Some appropriate indications for antibiotics include ongoing biliary obstruction, immunosuppressed patients, and active infections (including cholangitis) [30].

Frequency with which the **volume of ERCPs performed per year** is recorded per endoscopist is recommended to be over 98% [9]. Case volume has been shown to be associated with higher success rates [31–33]. Although the volume may not similarly predict success compared to the actual success rate, it does provide a useful tool to track an endoscopist's continued practice of the procedure [33].

Frequency with which **fluoroscopy time and radiation dose are measured** and documented is recommended to be above 98% [9]. ERCP requires radiation exposure to the patient, endoscopists, and intra-procedural staff and thus should be minimized as much as possible. More experienced ERCP endoscopists have been shown to use less fluoroscopy time, whereas those less experienced have been shown to use more fluoroscopy time [34]. There are other factors affecting radiation dose beyond fluoroscopy time, including radiation equipment and ERCP indications and complexity; however, overall radiation exposure should be minimized [9].

Frequency with which a **complete ERCP report** that details the specific techniques performed, particular accessories used, and all intended outcomes is prepared is recommended to be above 98% [9]. As with all procedure reports, the ERCP report serves to communicate pertinent findings, events, outcomes, and the impressions [35]. Additional key details that ERCP reports should include are whether the deep cannulation of the desired duct was achieved, frequency of unintended cannulation and injection of the pancreatic duct, fluoroscopic images, and photo documentation of key endoscopic findings [9].

Frequency with which **acute adverse events and hospital transfers** are documented is recommended to be above 98% [9]. This includes the aforementioned priority metric of post-ERCP pancreatitis, the **rate and type of perforation** (recommended less than 0.2%), and the **rate of clinically significant hemorrhage after sphincterotomy or sphincteroplasty** (recommended less than 1%) [9]. ERCP perforation rates can range and can be up to 0.6% or more [23, 25]. ERCP perforations are classified based on location, as summarized by Table 4.4 [36, 37]. ERCP-related hemorrhage is usually mild and self-resolves but can occur in up to

Table 4.4 Post-ERCP perforation types

Post-ERCP perforation types
Type I: Free duodenal wall perforation
Type II: Retroperitoneal duodenal perforation secondary to periampullary injury
Type III: Perforation of the pancreatic or bile duct
Type IV: Retroperitoneal air alone

1–2% of cases [25, 32]. Most ERCP-related hemorrhage is related to post-sphincterotomy, thus the necessity to track post-sphincterotomy bleeding as a metric [9, 25, 32]. Post-sphincterotomy hemorrhage is generally defined as objective evidence of bleeding (drop in hemoglobin or overt signs of bleeding) within 10 days after an ERCP [38].

Frequency with which **patients are contacted at or greater than 14 days to detect and record the occurrence of delayed adverse events** after ERCP is recommended to be above 90% [9]. Most places have some form of follow-up. This is essential to monitoring patient outcomes and ensuring quality patient care post-ERCP.

Quality Metrics to Prevent Post-ERCP Pancreatitis

Post-ERCP pancreatitis is one of the most common complications from the procedure and can occur in up to 10% of cases [7, 8, 25, 26]. Given the significant morbidity and mortality of this complication [7], strategies to mitigate the risk of PEP have been recommended in the appropriate context. General principles for maximizing ERCP quality as described prior, including proper patient selection, are essential [9].

Pharmacological prophylaxis with rectal nonsteroidal anti-inflammatory drugs pre-procedure has been proven to be effective in preventing PEP in those without contraindications [39, 40], typically indomethacin suppository 100 mg or diclofenac suppository 100 mg [27–29, 39–41]. Additionally, aggressive hydration peri-procedure with lactated Ringer's solution has been shown to be effective in minimizing PEP [42, 43].

Emphasizing quality **endoscopic techniques** can help to prevent PEP. Limiting cannulation attempts and duration [44, 45], using a guidewire to assist initial cannulation [46], and pancreatic stenting for higher-risk patients [47] can help minimize the risk for PEP. The use of a pancreatic stent may assist with pressure reduction by supporting drainage and can be helpful in cases with repeat unintentional manipulation of the pancreatic duct and pancreatic sphincterotomy [48].

References

1. McCune WS, Shorb PE, Moscovitz H. Endoscopic cannulation of the ampulla of vater: a preliminary report. Ann Surg. 1968;167:752–6.
2. Huang RJ, Thosani NC, Barakat MT, et al. Evolution in the utilization of biliary interventions in the United States: results of a nationwide longitudinal study from 1998 to 2013. Gastrointest Endosc. 2017;86:319–26.
3. Keswani RN, Qumseya BJ, O'Dwyer LC, et al. Association between endoscopist and center endoscopic retrograde cholangiopancreatography volume with procedure success and adverse outcomes: a systematic review and meta-analysis. Clin Gastroenterol Hepatol. 2017;15:1866–75.
4. Huang RJ, Barakat MT, Girotra M, et al. Unplanned hospital encounters after endoscopic retrograde cholangiopancreatography in 3 large North American States. Gastroenterology. 2019;156:119–29.
5. Cotton PB, Romagnuolo J, Faigel DO, et al. The ERCP quality network: a pilot study of benchmarking practice and performance. Am J Med Qual. 2013;28:256–60.
6. Cotton PB. Income and outcome metrics for the objective evaluation of ERCP and alternative methods. Gastrointest Endosc. 2002;56:283–90.
7. Mallery J, Baron T, Dominitz J, et al. Complications of ERCP. Gastrointest Endosc. 2003;57:633–8.
8. Chandrasekhara V, Khashab MA, Muthusamy VR, et al. Adverse events associated with ERCP. Gastrointest Endosc. 2017;85:32–47.
9. Adler DG, Lieb JG, Cohen J, et al. Quality indicators for ERCP. Gastrointest Endosc. 2015;81:54–66.
10. Jorgensen J, Kubiliun N, Law JK, et al. Endoscopic retrograde cholangiopancreatography (ERCP): core curriculum. Gastrointest Endosc. 2016;83:279–89.
11. Faulx AL, Lightdale JR, Acosta RD, et al. Guidelines for privileging, credentialing, and proctoring to perform GI endoscopy. Gastrointest Endosc. 2017;85:273–81.
12. Adler DG, Baron TH, Davila RE, et al. ASGE guideline: the role of ERCP in diseases of the biliary tract and the pancreas. Gastrointest Endosc. 2005;62:1–8.
13. Carr-Locke DL. Therapeutic role of ERCP in the management of suspected common bile duct stones. Gastrointest Endosc. 2002;56:S170–4.
14. Hawes RH. Diagnostic and therapeutic uses of ERCP in pancreatic and biliary tract malignancies. Gastrointest Endosc. 2002;56:201–5.
15. Johanson JF, Cooper G, Eisen GM, et al. Quality assessment of ERCP. Endoscopic retrograde cholangiopancreatography. Gastrointest Endosc. 2002;56:165–9.
16. Brawman-Mintzer O, Durkalski V, Wu Q, et al. Psychosocial characteristics and pain burden of patients with suspected sphincter of Oddi dysfunction in the EPISOD multicenter trial. Am J Gastroenterol. 2014;109:436–42.
17. Schlup MMT, Williams SM, Barbezat GO. ERCP: a review of technical competency and workload in a small unit. Gastrointest Endosc. 1997;46:48–52.
18. Jewell PS. Endoscopic retrograde cholangiopancreatography: toward a better understanding of competence. Endoscopy. 1999;31:755–7.
19. Verma D, Gostout CJ, Petersen BT, et al. Establishing a true assessment of endoscopic competence in ERCP during training and beyond: a single-operator learning curve for deep biliary cannulation in patients with native papillary anatomy. Gastrointest Endosc. 2007;65:394–400.
20. Debenedet AT, Elmunzer BJ, McCarthy ST, et al. Intraprocedural quality in endoscopic retrograde cholangiopancreatography: a meta-analysis. Am J Gastroenterol. 2013;108:1696–704.
21. Lauri A, Horton RC, Davidson BR, et al. Endoscopic extraction of bile duct stones: management related to stone size. Gut. 1993;34:1718–21.
22. Cotton PB, Lehman G, Vennes J, et al. Endoscopic sphincterotomy complications and their management: an attempt at consensus. Gastrointest Endosc. 1991;37:383–93.

23. Cotton PB, Garrow DA, Gallagher J, et al. Risk factors for complications after ERCP: a multivariate analysis of 11,497 procedures over 12 years. Gastrointest Endosc. 2009;70:80–8.
24. Adler DG, Verma D, Hilden K, et al. Dye-free wire-guided cannulation of the biliary tree during ERCP is associated with high success and low complication rates: outcomes in a single operator experience of 822 cases. J Clin Gastroenterol. 2010;44:e57–62.
25. Andriulli A, Loperfido S, Napolitano G, et al. Incidence rates of post-ERCP complications: a systematic survey of prospective studies. Am J Gastroenterol. 2007;102:1781–8.
26. Kochar B, Akshintala VS, Afghani E, et al. Incidence, severity, and mortality of post-ERCP pancreatitis: a systematic review by using randomized, controlled trials. Gastrointest Endosc. 2015;81:143–9.
27. Smith ZL, Elmunzer BJ, Cooper GS, et al. Real-world practice patterns in the era of rectal indomethacin for prophylaxis against post-ERCP pancreatitis in a high-risk cohort. Am J Gastroenterol. 2020;115:934–40.
28. Elmunzer BJ, Scheiman JM, Lehman GA, et al. A randomized trial of rectal indomethacin to prevent post-ERCP pancreatitis. N Engl J Med. 2012;366:1414–22.
29. Elmunzer BJ, Higgins PDR, Saini SD, et al. Does rectal indomethacin eliminate the need for prophylactic pancreatic stent placement in patients undergoing high-risk ERCP? Post hoc efficacy and cost-benefit analyses using prospective clinical trial data. Am J Gastroenterol. 2013;108:410–5.
30. Khashab MA, Chithadi KV, Acosta RD, et al. Antibiotic prophylaxis for GI endoscopy. Gastrointest Endosc. 2015;81:81–9.
31. Kapral C, Duller C, Wewalka F, et al. Case volume and outcome of endoscopic retrograde cholangiopancreatography: results of a nationwide Austrian benchmarking project. Endoscopy. 2008;40:625–30.
32. Freeman ML, Nelson DB, Sherman S, et al. Complications of endoscopic biliary sphincterotomy. N Engl J Med. 1996;335:909–19.
33. Coté GA, Imler TD, Xu H, et al. Lower provider volume is associated with higher failure rates for endoscopic retrograde cholangiopancreatography. Med Care. 2013;51:1040–7.
34. Jorgensen JE, Rubenstein JH, Goodsitt MM, et al. Radiation doses to ERCP patients are significantly lower with experienced endoscopists. Gastrointest Endosc. 2010;72:58–65.
35. Rizk MK, Sawhney MS, Cohen J, et al. Quality indicators common to all GI endoscopic procedures. Gastrointest Endosc. 2015;81:3–16.
36. Howard TJ, Tzujen T, Lehman GA, et al. Classification and management of perforations complicating endoscopic sphincterotomy. Surgery. 1999;126:658–65.
37. Stapfer M, Selby RR, Stain SC, et al. Management of duodenal perforation after endoscopic retrograde cholangiopancreatography and sphincterotomy. Ann Surg. 2000;232:191–8.
38. Tenca A, Pugliese D, Consonni D, et al. Bleeding after sphincterotomy in liver transplanted patients with biliary complications. Eur J Gastroenterol Hepatol. 2011;23:778–81.
39. Kubiliun NM, Adams MA, Akshintala VS, et al. Evaluation of pharmacologic prevention of pancreatitis after endoscopic retrograde cholangiopancreatography: a systematic review. Clin Gastroenterol Hepatol. 2015;13:1231–9.
40. Luo H, Zhao L, Leung J, et al. Routine pre-procedural rectal indometacin versus selective post-procedural rectal indometacin to prevent pancreatitis in patients undergoing endoscopic retrograde cholangiopancreatography: a multicentre, single-blinded, randomised controlled trial. Lancet. 2016;387:2293.
41. Akshintala VS, Husain SZ, Brenner TA, et al. Rectal INdomethacin, oral TacROlimus, or their combination for the prevention of post-ERCP pancreatitis (INTRO Trial): protocol for a randomized, controlled, double-blinded trial. Pancreatology. 2022;22:887–93.
42. Buxbaum J, Yan A, Yeh K, et al. Aggressive hydration with lactated Ringer's solution reduces pancreatitis following endoscopic retrograde cholangiopancreatography. Clin Gastroenterol Hepatol. 2014;12:303.

43. Talukdar R, Kamal A, Akshintala VS, et al. Fluid type and volume reduce risk of post-ERCP pancreatitis and length of hospital stay in high-risk patients: a secondary analysis of the INDIEH trial. Endosc Int Open. 2020;8:E834.
44. Wang P, Li ZS, Liu F, et al. Risk factors for ERCP-related complications: a prospective multicenter study. Am J Gastroenterol. 2009;104:31–40.
45. Testoni PA, Mariani A, Giussani A, et al. Risk factors for post-ERCP pancreatitis in high- and low-volume centers and among expert and non-expert operators: a prospective multicenter study. Am J Gastroenterol. 2010;105:1753–61.
46. Testoni PA, Mariani A, Aabakken L, et al. Papillary cannulation and sphincterotomy techniques at ERCP: European Society of Gastrointestinal Endoscopy (ESGE) clinical guideline. Endoscopy. 2016;48:657–83.
47. Hanna MS, Portal AJ, Dhanda AD, et al. UK wide survey on the prevention of post-ERCP pancreatitis. Frontline Gastroenterol. 2014;5:103–10.
48. Freeman ML. Pancreatic stents for prevention of post-endoscopic retrograde cholangiopancreatography pancreatitis. Clin Gastroenterol Hepatol. 2007;5:1354–65.

Chapter 5
Quality in Endoscopic Ultrasound

Daniel S. Strand and Andrew Y. Wang

Table of Quality Measures/Metrics

D. S. Strand (✉) · A. Y. Wang
Division of Gastroenterology and Hepatology, University of Virginia, Charlottesville, VA, USA
e-mail: dss7a@virginia.edu; ayw7d@virginia.edu

J. D. Feuerstein, D. J. Stein (eds.), *Quality in Gastroenterology*, https://doi.org/10.1007/978-3-031-58492-3_5

Abbreviations

ACG	American College of Gastroenterology
AE	Adverse event
ASGE	American Society for Gastrointestinal Endoscopy
CME	Continuing medical education
CT	Computed tomography
ESGE	European Society of Gastrointestinal Endoscopy
EUS	Endoscopic ultrasound
EUS-FNA	EUS-directed fine needle aspiration
FNB	Fine needle biopsy
GI	Gastrointestinal
GRADE	Grading of recommendations, assessment, development, and evaluations
MRI	Magnetic resonance imaging
ROSE	Rapid on-site evaluation
TEESAT	The EUS and ERCP Skills Assessment Tool
TUS	Transabdominal ultrasound
U.S.	United States

Key Points

- Proposed quality indicators (QIs) for endoscopic ultrasound have been developed with the support of multiple professional GI societies.
- Although several priority QIs are supported by evidence, extensive validation of these proposed metrics remains elusive.
- Barriers to further progress include the significant heterogeneity of EUS procedures and indications, intra- and interobserver variability, and differences in documentation and data reporting practices.

Introduction

First pioneered in the late 1970s, radial [1] and curvilinear [2] endoscopic ultrasound (EUS) has become indispensable in assessing malignant and nonmalignant conditions of the gastrointestinal (GI) tract and adjacent structures. Although EUS in the United States (U.S.) had historically been centralized at tertiary care or academic medical centers, recent data suggest a rapidly increasing number of endosonographic procedures performed by a steadily growing number of endoscopists in a variety of clinical settings [3]. This American diaspora of EUS procedures outside of traditional referral centers is witnessed in the context of increasingly available endosonographic training. Although such instruction has been present for decades via a conventional apprenticeship in therapeutic endoscopy [4, 5], the number of these programs has expanded over time. Additionally, there are now opportunities to obtain EUS skills by continuing medical education (CME) curricula, offered in didactic and hands-on format by GI professional societies [6]. Due to the complex and operator-dependent nature of EUS, it is frequently regarded by interventional endoscopists to be among the most challenging procedural skills to acquire, refine, and perfect [7].

Despite the known degree of difficulty, an ever-expanding panoply of EUS-based procedures, and a national focus on the delivery of high-quality health care [8, 9], the milieu of quality assessment in endosonography is nascent when compared to parallel endoscopic procedures. This is especially true when considered through the lens of colorectal cancer screening, where a robust assortment of quality indicators (QIs) exists that is tied to important clinical outcomes, such as the incidence of interval colon cancer or cancer-associated mortality [10–13]. Although evidence-based QIs for EUS have been previously published [14], there remains a paucity of data regarding the reporting and validation of these proposed metrics [15]. In this chapter, we will review the present state of quality in endosonography and outline the potential components of a high-quality EUS examination. For each component of a typical EUS exam, we will review the individual challenges of quality assessment.

The State of Quality Assessment in Endoscopic Ultrasound

The ability to provide high-quality medical care to patients is a crucial responsibility of physicians, nurses, and other medical professionals. Despite a long-held ethical principle of "doing no harm," awareness of potentially avoidable medical errors in the early 2000s [8, 9] prompted broad reassessment of the US health-care delivery system and an increased focus on quality. Conceptually speaking, health-care quality can be objectively measured by directly comparing the performance of an individual or group with a benchmark tied to a desired patient outcome [16]. The relative performance of the physician, surgeon, or provider may then be objectively presented as a "scorecard" for quality, to be judged programmatically. The assessments of performance on objective quality metrics may be internal (e.g., individual review) or external (by stakeholders). The latter form may have significant real-world consequences for the subject, including through guarantor initiatives such as "pay for performance" [17] or "value-based care" [18]. Given the overall importance of quality in medicine and the high-stakes nature of procedures, serious attention to outcome-based quality is in the interest of patients and physicians. Accordingly, the development and validation of evidence-based quality indicators (QIs) in endoscopic care is a paramount responsibility of GI professional societies and federal governing agencies, such as the Centers for Medicare and Medicaid Services.

In 2006, the American Society for Gastrointestinal Endoscopy (ASGE) and the American College of Gastroenterology (ACG) published the first joint practice

Table 5.1 Proposed quality indicators specific to EUS. Adapted from Joint-Society Guideline (used with permission) [14]

Quality indicator	Priority indicator	Performance target (%)
Pre-procedure QIs		
EUS is performed for an appropriate indication		≥98
Informed consent is obtained after discussion of specific risks and alternatives		≥98
Medication management: appropriate plan for periprocedural antibiotics		n/a
Medication management: appropriate plan for anticoagulants		n/a
Intra-procedural QIs		
Documented appearance of relevant structures, specific to the indication for EUS		≥98
Use of AJCC TNM staging to describe gastrointestinal cancers at EUS	√	≥98
• Measurement of pancreatic mass along with vascular involvement, lymphadenopathy, and distant metastases		≥98
• Documentation of EUS wall layers involved in subepithelial lesions		≥98
Diagnostic rate of adequate sample for solid lesions undergoing EUS-FNA		≥85
• Frequency of EUS-directed tissue sampling of distant metastases and primary lesion, when it would change management		≥98
• Diagnostic rate and sensitivity for malignancy in patients with solid pancreatic tumors	√	≥70, ≥85
Post-procedural QIs		
Frequency of documentation of adverse events after EUS-directed tissue sampling		≥98
Incidence of adverse events following EUS-directed tissue sampling (varies by complication)	√	<2

guideline on quality for endoscopic ultrasonography. That manuscript, the product of a multi-society quality task force, outlined a series of indicators (Table 5.1) to "aid in the recognition of high-quality EUS examinations" [19]. Given the available data at the time of publication, many of these proposed QIs were based solely upon expert opinion, and evidence in support of them was considered weak by traditional grading of recommendations, assessment, development, and evaluations (GRADE) methodology [20, 21]. This guideline was revisited and updated in 2015 to highlight the incorporation of substantive interval data and to prioritize QIs that had "wide-ranging clinical application, were associated with variation in practice and outcomes and were validated in clinical studies" [14]. The freshly revised guideline included a total of 13 EUS-specific proposed QIs, classified as either *process* (those which assess performance during delivery of care) or *outcome* measures (those which assess the results of the care provided). Additional QIs, common to all endoscopic procedures, were also summarized in the manuscript. Process-related indicators were further subdivided by the associated phase of care: *pre-procedure, intra-procedure, and post-procedure* [14].

Notably, and despite the 9-year interval between first publication and subsequent guideline revision, the summation of evidence for eight of the 13 QIs remained compatible with expert opinion alone. As such, evidence-based benchmark performance targets could not be readily established for nine of the measures, though several were conscientiously deemed to be "never events" and assigned a compliance target of >98% (one was given no recommendation at all). Additionally, it is essential to note that several of the proposed EUS QIs are measured entirely by the completeness of post-procedural documentation. For example, if a normal pancreas is visualized during EUS examination for choledocholithiasis, and this unremarkable appearance is not described in the report, the endosonographer would be considered deficient with regard to the associated QI. Failure to establish compliance with proposed benchmarks, then, may accurately be judged as a deficiency of comprehensive documentation in the medical record rather than a failure of endoscopist performance [22]. In this context, it would be easy to demonstrate how methodologic differences in the generation of a procedure report (e.g., dictation, typographical template use, or specialized endoscopy reporting software) could produce highly disparate results in QI compliance representative of the same physician or the same endosonographic exam. Furthermore, data that would provide validation for many of the proposed process EUS QIs remains lacking [15]. These limitations were not inapparent to the guideline authors, who acknowledged the implicit flaw of using measures of *process*, rather than *outcome*, as a surrogate for quality. This weakness is especially true in settings where there is no clear or implied thread which ties process to a clinically meaningful result (as is seen in the previous example of withdrawal time in colorectal cancer screening) [14]. If the endoscopist does not ritually document an anticipated normal finding, does this truly affect a patient and represent suboptimal quality of care? Perhaps, or perhaps not. This is acknowledged by the joint-society authors, who note that proposed EUS QIs did "not necessarily reflect the standard of care." This observation is particularly incisive and appropriate, given previously mentioned evidentiary limitations. Despite this critique, meaningful progress has been made by simply establishing potential targets for quality assessment in EUS—and the task of further refining and validating these targets remains a critical priority for practicing endosonographers.

Training and Competency in EUS

As with many medical disciplines, traditional training in EUS has been structured according to an apprenticeship model. This training is typified by graduated responsibility, beginning with observation and concluding with independent performance of endosonography—ideally carried out under the supervision of a motivated, expert proctor [23]. A collaborative environment appears to be essential, as unsupervised self-directed learning of EUS has been shown to be ineffective [24, 25]. In the past, the components of an EUS training curriculum had been left to the sole discretion of individual instructors and the institution which was offering training [26]. In addition, no formal tool existed to help assess learners during EUS training with regard to competency or define their individual learning curve [27]. Thus, training was a variation of the old adage "see *one*, do *one*, teach *one*" where *one* is substituted by an integer deemed appropriate by the mentor.

Fortunately, recent efforts have provided valuable data regarding skill acquisition in advanced endoscopy procedures, including EUS. As such, there have been efforts to standardize the approach to education by both the ASGE and European Society of Gastrointestinal Endoscopy (ESGE) [23, 26, 28]. Both societies now recommended the adoption of formal in-training assessment tools, such as the EUS and ERCP Skills Assessment Tool (TEESAT). This validated instrument, which relies on cumulative sum analysis, should be used regularly throughout leaning to track trainee performance and assess individual learning curve.

Data from prospective incorporation of TEESAT into ASGE accredited training programs has also implied what degree of trainee experience can predict competency in an "average" learner [29–32]. In the setting of primarily diagnostic pancreatobiliary EUS (70%), most trainees achieve competence at approximately 225 cases [29]. To ensure adequacy, the ESGE has recently recommended a training experience of at least 250 EUS cases (including >75 fine needle aspirations) prior to independent practice. This assessment appears to be a reasonable minimum threshold, as graduates from training programs that employ TEESAT routinely achieve compliance with EUS-specific QIs by the end of their first year in practice [32]. The degree of experience necessary to achieve competence in more complex tasks, such as EUS-guided therapeutics, is likely to be significantly more extensive—though specific data are lacking. It is our recommendation that these procedures continue to be consolidated at referral centers which possess broad institutional expertise in interventional endoscopy.

Quality in EUS: Before the Endoscopy

> "Give me 6 hours to chop down a tree and I will spend the first four sharpening the ax."
> —Abraham Lincoln

Providing high-quality care in a procedural specialty does not begin with the procedure itself; rather, it begins with preparation. Historically, preparation by the proceduralist was initiated during consultation with the patient in either an office or hospital setting. In the world of endoscopy, direct referral of patients to the GI lab rather than for clinical consultation is commonplace practice [33, 34]. This approach, now standard in many settings for colorectal cancer screening, has become increasingly prevalent for EUS due to perceived costs and time advantages. Given this trend, it is imperative that the endosonographer carefully consider each referral to ensure the delivery of high-quality care.

Indication and Clinical Context

The indication for EUS is the first fundamental issue to be considered by the endoscopist. Indeed, the first QI considered in the ASGE/ACG guideline is defined as the "frequency with which EUS is performed for an indication that is included in a

Table 5.2 Appropriate indications for EUS

Diagnostic indications for EUS
Staging of localized tumors of the GI tract or adjacent structures (including pancreas, bile duct, or mediastinum)
Evaluation of biliary tree abnormalities (dilation, lithiasis, obstruction, or stricture)
Evaluation of pancreatic abnormalities (masses, cystic lesions, and pancreatitis)
Evaluation of subepithelial lesions of the GI tract
Evaluation of perianal or perirectal lesions
Screening for patient at high risk for pancreatic carcinoma (PRSS-1, BRCA, Peutz-Jeghers)
Direct measurement of portal pressure gradient for selected patients with suspected portal hypertension
Therapeutic indications for EUS
Drainage of symptomatic pancreatic fluid collections (pseudocysts and walled off necrosis)
Guiding access to biliary and/or pancreatic ducts
Placement of radiologic fiducial markers into an EUS accessible mass lesion
Celiac plexus block or neurolysis
Establishing trans-gastric or entero-enteric access for endoscopy or relief of obstruction
Drainage of luminal-adjacent structures as an alternative to surgery (gallbladder, abscess)
Directed ablative treatment of luminal adjacent cysts or mass lesions
Transluminal vascular interventions (e.g., vascular coil placement, variceal gluing, or pressure measurement)

published standard list of appropriate indications and the indication is documented." Acceptable indications for EUS have been published [35, 36], though the value of EUS often depends upon context (Table 5.2). For example, abdominal magnetic resonance imaging (MRI) and EUS are acceptable diagnostic modalities to determine the etiology for presumed idiopathic acute pancreatitis [37, 38]. Although EUS may offer an overall advantage in determining an etiology (driven by occult biliary lithiasis), MRI may be more sensitive in cases of anomalous pancreatic ductal anatomy [39]. In cases of a cancer diagnosis, formal endosonographic TNM staging is generally not beneficial for patients with metastasis already confirmed by other means. While EUS may still be useful for tissue acquisition or some other therapeutic purpose (placement of a fiducial, etc.), the indication for staging is not appropriate. These examples, along with many others, reflect circumstances where there is no substitute for clinical judgment in determining whether or not to pursue EUS over an alternative study for an individual patient.

A clear understanding of context at EUS also assists the focus of the endosonographer to maximize the value of the exam to the patient. This effect is clearly shown by blinding expert endosonographers to clinical history, laboratory results, and prior imaging in the case of esophageal, gastric, and pancreatic malignancy [40]. When missing clinical context and reviewing EUS video alone, the accuracy of T-staging for 101 patients decreased from 73% to 52% compared to routine analysis [40]. Context also provides the basis for sound judgment, not just accurate image interpretation. For example, the significance and differential diagnosis for incidentally discovered bile duct dilation (without an obvious obstruction) depends entirely on the patient's symptoms and liver biochemistries [41]. While some experts argue for a universal comprehensive exam [42, 43], limiting the scope of EUS in the face of a clear indication may also help mitigate the potential for adverse events [14]. For example, EUS interrogation of the pancreaticobiliary axis in cases of esophageal cancer staging is time-consuming and may be unnecessary. Furthermore, in patients where dilation of a malignant esophageal stricture is required, gastroduodenal intubation with an echoendoscope may be dangerous [44, 45]. The additional incremental risk may be justifiable to pursue information that is critical to subsequent oncologic care, but it is less justifiable for the purposes of completing a systematic EUS examination.

Informed Consent

Informed consent is an ethical responsibility of medical practitioners for *any* intervention beyond those with trivial risk. As such, all endoscopic procedures (including EUS) should be preceded by a detailed discussion between the patient and physician. This process should include explaining the indication for the procedure, a comprehensive accounting of the procedure itself, a review of the potential benefit derived from intervention, and a description of suitable alternative(s). Of critical importance, the patient should be advised (in terms that are understandable to them) of the potential for harm or adverse outcomes which may accompany the intended procedure. This process should be free of duress, and the patient should be encouraged to ask questions and relay understanding [46, 47]. If the patient determines to move forward with endoscopy, a decision which may be withdrawn at any time, documentation of this decision should be recorded using an informed consent form in at least 98% of cases [14].

The details of informed consent should be tailored to EUS rather than simply inclusive of any generic provisions included with esophagogastroduodenoscopy [42]. This is significant as the incidence of adverse events (AEs) following diagnostic EUS is reported to be higher than that observed for general upper endoscopy. [48]. Completing an EUS exam requires the passage of a radial or curvilinear echoendoscope, typified by the presence of a relatively rigid (4–5 cm) transducer on the distal end. This difference in mechanics and impaired forward visibility account for an increased luminal perforation rate estimated to be between 0.03% and 0.09% [49]. The perforation risk of diagnostic EUS may be higher in patients with esophageal carcinoma, particularly in the elderly, patients with a stricture, or those with a proximal mass lesion [14].

In cases where EUS-directed tissue sampling is indicated (by fine needle aspiration (FNA) or biopsy (FNB)), the risk of an AE increases further. Given the very low absolute rate of complications seen during routine diagnostic EUS, this increase in risk for FNA/FNB is estimated to be tenfold compared to an imaging-only procedure. The overall rate of complication(s) secondary to EUS-directed tissue sampling is estimated to be 1%, though analysis of prospective studies suggests this may be as high as 2.44% [50]. The majority of complications following FNA/FNB include post-procedure pain (34%) and pancreatitis (34%), though infection and bleeding are also notable (13–16%). Targeting pancreatic or mediastinal cystic lesions is generally thought to be more dangerous than solid ones by EUS. Thankfully, other immediate complications such as perforation or bile leaks remain rare [50]. Tumor seeding following EUS-guided sampling is a devastating potential complication, though it is reported infrequently [51–54]. In cases of hilar cholangiocarcinoma, avoidance of EUS-directed lesion sampling has been previously recommended [14, 55], though more recent data suggests that EUS-based tissue sampling may not affect patient outcomes [56, 57] outside of exceptional circumstances such as a liver transplant protocol.

As therapeutic endoscopy has matured, a panoply of novel therapeutic EUS-based interventions has emerged. This suite of radically disparate procedures includes EUS-directed biliary or pancreatic duct access, drainage of pancreatic fluid collections, celiac plexus neurolysis, and ablative therapies for cysts and mass lesions. In some instances, interventional EUS has supplanted traditional surgical interventions, such as direct pancreatic necrosectomy, EUS-directed gastrojejunostomy, or gastric access for temporary endoscopy (GATE). Direct EUS-guided portal pressure measurement has recently emerged as an alternative to traditional catheter-derived hepatic vein wedge pressure(s) to assess portal hypertensive complications. Each of these interventions is inherently unique and is accompanied by its own profile of associated risks, ranging from those with a long track record of safety (celiac plexus neurolysis) to those with overall complication rates that can approach 10–20% [58, 59]. Given these differences, informed consent for therapeutic EUS procedures should be comprehensive and individualized to a specific patient and circumstance.

A wide variety of variables have been demonstrated to influence the rate of AEs in association with EUS, including the operator's experience. This observation prompted the inclusion of a QI in the joint-society guideline stating that >98% of EUS exams should be performed by a "trained endosonographer." This represents a formally trained physician who has gained the necessary technical and cognitive skills to perform EUS. Until recently, there were no established data to indicate a minimum standard benchmark for EUS competency [29, 30], though most graduating interventional endoscopy trainees successfully meet QI thresholds from published guidelines by the end of their first year of independent practice [32].

Medication Management: Anticoagulants and Antibiotics

As mentioned previously, in the past, most patients were often seen in consultation before scheduling and performing an EUS. This provided the opportunity to obtain a comprehensive history and afforded ample time to consider preoperative testing and develop a plan for ancillary care surrounding EUS. Open-access endosonography compresses this process, but it does not prevent it. Among all of the various considerations required of a physician, two elements are frequently relevant with respect to EUS: perioperative anticoagulation management and prophylactic antimicrobials [14, 42].

Bleeding at the time of EUS, even in the face of fine needle aspiration or tissue biopsy, is not common. Although many professional GI societies classify EUS-directed fine needle aspiration (EUS-FNA) to be among a category of "high-risk endoscopic procedures" [35, 59–62], bleeding associated with EUS or EUS-FNA occurs in less than 1% of cases [49, 50]. The rationale often provided for this classification is the observation that bleeding, when it occurs, can be serious. In addition, contrary to bleeding from intraluminal sources, bleeding for EUS-FNA/B may occur in locations inaccessible to immediate endoscopic treatment [42]. In a prospective trial that included 85 patients who underwent EUS-FNA of solid lesions without interruption of anticoagulation, two (2.4%) developed bleeding events. One patient developed melena after 8 days; the other developed immediate hemothorax and required surgical intervention [63]. Additionally, this incident risk may be lower for some patients (such as those with subepithelial lesions [64]) and higher for others (such as cystic lesions [65]). To make matters more complicated: aspirin, non-aspirin antiplatelet agents, warfarin, heparin, and direct-acting oral anticoagulants (DOACs) all demonstrate differential risk when patients are exposed to EUS tissue sampling [63, 66, 67].

Nearly all present guidelines suggest careful consideration of the balance between the risk of interruption of anticoagulation and the risk of bleeding accompanied by the intended procedure [60–62]. In general, the existing consensus recommendations suggest interruption of anticoagulation (apart from aspirin) for procedures that are appreciated to be high risk and for individuals whose indication for anticoagulation is understood to be of low thromboembolic risk [60–62]. A full vetting of this context is often not straightforward as the patient background (e.g., uncomplicated atrial fibrillation vs. mechanical mitral valve), medication used (warfarin, DOAC, aspirin), and procedure target for FNA (e.g., mediastinum, pancreatic cystic lesion, subepithelial lesion) come with myriad variation. The most recent ACG-CAG guideline highlighted the limitations in the existing literature and overall poor quality of data regarding the interruption of anticoagulation. Although they recommended the continuation of warfarin for elective GI procedures, the authors note that the "absence of studies in advanced endoscopic procedures (with higher baseline bleeding risk), and differences in clinical consequences of luminal and extraluminal bleeding associated with such endoscopic GI procedures, limits our ability to comment on the safety of proceeding without interrupting warfarin" [61]. In practice, aspirin monotherapy appears safe [66] to continue prior to EUS, but other anticoagulants should be assessed and temporarily interrupted if tissue acquisition may be performed during the exam [59–63, 65].

Historically, antibiotic prophylaxis was often recommended during EUS-guided aspiration of cystic lesions [68]. The rationale for antibiotic administration was the observation that the instrumentation of cystic lesions was associated with a much higher rate of infection than solid lesions (0.5% vs. 14%) [69]. Despite the persistence of this recommendation over time, high-quality data on the effectiveness of antibiotic prophylaxis in FNA of cystic lesions are lacking. Recently, a multicenter, prospective, randomized controlled trial that included 226 patients was conducted in Spain comparing perioperative prophylaxis with ciprofloxacin to placebo. During this trial, only one patient developed an infection, and no statistically significant difference was observed between groups. This result, consistent with more contemporary retrospective data [70, 71], suggests that antibiotic prophylaxis is unnecessary for EUS-directed FNA.

Quality in EUS: During the Endoscopy

EUS examination is an integrated task of image acquisition and interpretation. This fact is apparent when one considers places like Great Britain, where EUS is performed not only by gastroenterologists but also by radiologists. However, unlike typical imaging exams, EUS involves the invasive components of upper diagnostic endoscopy. From the time of patient sedation through endoscope removal, the endoscopist performs all of the technical aspects of EUS [72]. For this reason, the proposed QIs which pertain to the intra-procedural portion of EUS is focused on discrete components such as successful imaging of intended structures, appropriate oncologic staging, and successful tissue sampling by FNA [14].

Image Acquisition and Interpretation

The first proposed intra-procedural QI is the frequency with which the appearance of relevant structures specific to the indication for EUS is documented [14]. Despite straightforward and innocuous language, this statement actually represents performance of a complex task with a significant learning curve [7, 30]. Success requires the endosonographer to understand the indication and anatomical basis for the procedure and demonstrate the technical motor ability to position the echoendoscope to visualize the target. Depending upon circumstance, this may require comprehensive visualization of the pancreatobiliary organs or a detailed inspection of specific luminal wall layers (as with epithelial or subepithelial GI malignancy) [72]. Beyond the endoscopist, selecting either a radial or curvilinear echoendoscope probe may suggest how successful imaging of a desired structure will be [73]. Further, modern ultrasound equipment is extremely complicated, and acquiring high-quality images often requires the operator to adjust transducer frequency and ultrasound gain, apply tissue harmonic imaging, and manipulate various Doppler settings [74].

Although visualization of incidental or unexpected findings at EUS is not considered a QI, for reasons of safety and efficiency discussed previously, identification of these anomalies can be important [43]. Incidental findings at EUS are not uncommon when a comprehensive examination is performed (approximately 10%) [75], and sometimes they can have significant clinical ramifications. Perhaps the most overt example would be identifying previously unknown metastases that could alter downstream oncologic management. While a proposed QI represents this circumstance, others are not: the identification of incidental bile duct stones, a cystic pancreatic lesion, a renal or adrenal mass, features of cirrhosis, and so on. Given that incidental findings are not rare, providing a high-quality EUS should include thoughtful assessment by the endoscopist to determine under what circumstances a focused exam is warranted and when a systematic and thorough exam is more appropriate [43].

Inter-operator variation is another factor that complicates ideal compliance with the goal of providing accurate image assessment and description. Such variation is not uncommon in EUS for a variety of disease states, which affects the likelihood that two endoscopists would “see (a particular finding) the same way.” Note the QI associated with this portion of EUS includes only a requirement to *document* the “appearance of relevant structures” [14] without qualification regarding accuracy. As supporting evidence: EUS-based diagnosis of chronic pancreatitis [76], cystic pancreatic lesions [76], some subepithelial lesions [77], MALT lymphoma [78], and even biliary sludge [79] have all been shown to have suboptimal interobserver reliability, even among experienced endoscopists.

Universal conformity with standard AJCC/TNM staging is also considered to be a high-priority QI for EUS diagnosis of malignancy. EUS is a particularly useful tool for assessment of the “T” (tumor) and “N” (lymph node) component of this system, though the “M” (distant metastases) is often more accurately assessed by other means [80, 81]. In this setting, EUS may have an intrinsic tendency to systematically over- or under-stage some lesions in some circumstances (such as T2 rectal cancer) [82]. As an illustration, EUS assessment of vascular invasion in the case of pancreatic carcinoma appears to be consistently less accurate when compared with alternative modalities such as CT or MRI [83, 84]. This distinction has significant ramifications when considering a patient for treatment such as surgical resection, neoadjuvant treatment, or palliation. This universal requirement for dispositive TNM staging may not be unequivocally valuable, especially if the results cannot always be trusted to act upon them. Before additional stringency can be applied to QIs tied to image acquisition and interpretation, EUS-based diagnostic criteria with high accuracy and high interobserver reliability must be established for many indications and circumstances.

EUS-Directed Tissue Sampling

EUS-based tissue acquisition is a domain where QI targets have the advantage of associated outcome-based benchmarks, and the ASGE suggests that endosonographers should obtain an adequate sample from solid lesions in greater than or equal to 85% of cases. As expected, the diagnostic accuracy of EUS-FNA does vary depending upon the organ of interest, and this variance should be considered when assessing quality targets [14]. In the setting of pancreatic tumors, EUS-FNA can be expected to demonstrate an overall diagnostic rate of approximately 71–85% based on multiple prospective and retrospective analyses [85, 86]. For sampling of malignant-appearing lymph nodes, such as in the case of esophageal adenocarcinoma, the sensitivity of FNA may be even higher (85%) [87, 88]. The recent proliferation of EUS-compatible biopsy (FNB) needles is of significant interest and may affect this paradigm going forward. FNB needles are multiple in format and include reverse bevel, forked-tip, and Franseen-type (serrated) devices. These needles offer conceptual advantages over traditional FNA, and there is a basis for the expectation that they will perform better. A recent randomized, crossover study suggested statistically significant differences in sensitivity (82% vs. 71%) and accuracy (84% vs. 75%) favoring a forked-tip FNB needle over FNA in solid pancreatic masses [89]. Data suggests the pooled diagnostic yield for forked-tip and Franseen-type FNB needles is approximately 93% for these lesions, which is comparable or better than traditional FNA yields [90]. Functionally, the latter two types of needle provide excellent histologic specimens, including tissue architecture. This allows for less equivocal diagnosis, and the additional quantity provides substrate for genetic sequencing or phenotyping—a potentially important factor in the milieu of future personalized cancer treatment [91].

Numerous factors may be expected to alter the performance of EUS tissue sampling, regardless of the needle chosen. These include variations in specimen processing, interpretation (i.e., assessment of atypical or suspicious cytopathology), the prevalence of comorbid chronic pancreatitis, and the technical aspects of the sampling itself [15]. The final category includes variables such as the number of passes performed, use of a stylet, suction format, and sampling technique [36, 92]. Suppose one simply examines suction as a variable. In that case, there are many options: high negative pressure, "wet suction," "stylet slow pull," and the concept of eliminating residual negative pressure (which can be accomplished by multiple means) [36]. It is easy to understand, then, how determining the precise "optimal approach" for any particular lesion is elusive—though we can reasonably expect that a given endosonographer should perform comparably to published benchmarks.

Of particular interest is the role of rapid, on-site evaluation (ROSE) at EUS. ROSE involves immediate assessment of cytological specimens (or touch preps) by a trained cytopathologist or cytotechnician. The purpose of ROSE is to provide real-time feedback regarding the sufficiency of the specimens obtained and establish a provisional diagnosis. ROSE was rapidly adopted following the development of EUS-FNA and has been continued based on observational and randomized data in support of its use [36, 93–95]. The principal advantage seen with the inclusion of ROSE is a reduction in the number of needle passes required to establish a diagnosis but not improvement in overall accuracy or a reduction in post-procedure complications [93, 94]. Recent randomized controlled trials comparing FNB with and without ROSE [96], as well as FNA with ROSE to FNB [97], suggest that FNB on its own is likely to produce similar diagnostic results, agnostic to the presence or absence of an on-site cytopathologist. The reality that ROSE is not readily available outside of high-volume, academic referral centers [98] may partially explain historically observed differences in FNA results by locality. Specifically, data suggest that in the era prior to FNB (through 2014), patients who underwent EUS tissue sampling at a free-standing suburban or rural center, with low procedure volume, were at greatest risk of needing a repeat biopsy [99]. Procedures performed in higher volume, hospital-based units were less likely to require repetition [99]. Given that FNB does not appear to require the use of ROSE for comparable success, it is conceivable that a wider transition toward FNB may be of greatest benefit to endoscopists at free-standing or lower-resourced centers.

There is an additional less tangible benefit to ROSE, however, apart from its connection with overall diagnostic accuracy. The concept of diagnosis in real time is implicit within the process of rapid evaluation. As long as the risk of false positive(s) is accounted for and only certainty is acted upon, immediate diagnosis can provide tangible advantages to the patient undergoing endoscopy. From the perspective of the endoscopist, having a certain diagnosis of malignancy in the setting of biliary obstruction may allow for the selection and insertion of an uncovered metal biliary stent via ERCP during the same anesthetic session as EUS. Without this information, the patient may be subject to a decompressive plastic stent, requiring revision at a prespecified interval. From the patient's perspective, immediate diagnosis can be incredibly important psychologically. Leaving the endoscopy center "with an answer" is important to patients, and there is measurably improved satisfaction linked to timely communication of a diagnosis—even if it is a bad one [100].

Quality in EUS: After the Endoscopy

The interval following endoscopy is no less important regarding quality assessment. This period includes drafting a procedure report, communication with the patient regarding the findings, instructions for follow-up, review of pathology or laboratory tests, and the recognition and management of adverse events [14, 101]. Appropriate attention to detail during this phase of an encounter for endosonography may be the most important when judging physician compliance with proposed QI benchmarks [22].

Writing the EUS Report

It has been previously noted that assessment of most of the ASGE/ACG proposed QIs for EUS relies almost entirely on the completeness of documentation [14, 22]. As such, drafting a qualifying report is critical when assessing a physician for compliance with recommended benchmarks under the present paradigm. It has been argued that a high-quality endoscopic report should be legible and systematic, includes *minimum standard terminology*, possesses *structured trees*, and contains *image documentation* of findings [102]. Despite these principles, and the aforementioned coupling of proposed QIs to documentation, there are only limited data regarding the quality of reporting in EUS [101].

In fact, the methods used by endosonographers to generate a report are often quite variable. A recent survey by Fusaroli et al., which included an international sample of 171 experienced endosonographers, revealed significant differences in practice regarding report generation [101]. Although 85% of physicians wrote their own EUS reports, 10% dictated them and 5% completed a report by "other means." Dictation was noted to be significantly more common in private practice (25%) than other settings, and only 75% of physicians used an electronic health record software to document EUS. Significant differences were noted in the use of digital images (72.5%), routine video capture (30%), and review before drafting a report (12%). In fact, 6.5% of physicians reported drafting the EUS report on a different day than the endoscopy, and 12% reported changing the structure of their report individually. These findings are especially dissonant when considering that respondents overwhelmingly felt that EUS reports should be more structured in the future and include both compulsory items and standardized terminology [101].

The widespread adoption of mandatory report items and standardized terminology can be facilitated by using endoscopy report documentation software. In ERCP, a procedure with comparable complexity and heterogeneity, the inclusion of mandatory structured data fields into standard workflow has been shown to allow the accurate extraction of priority QIs and avoid the need for intensive manual review [103]. This process can be successfully automated, which allows the generation of standardized, interim QI assessments (e.g., a "report card") that can be applied to an individual, a unit, or a health system. Although this type of approach remains in the pilot phase for ERCP, a similar process could be easily adapted to EUS and have several benefits. Such a system would not only promote individual compliance with proposed QIs to satisfy stakeholders but could provide a vehicle for larger-scale data collection regarding benchmarks. If the long-term goal of quality assessment in EUS is refinement and validation of provisional QIs, a national registry of information that can be tied to tangible patient outcomes is a necessary path forward. If broadly implemented, structured data derived from this type of report generation would allow assessment of the true population-level performance of EUS – knowledge which is presently lacking [15].

Adverse Events

As previously stated, adverse events associated with the performance of EUS should be rare. This is especially true in diagnostic cases without EUS-directed tissue sampling or other therapeutic maneuvers [47, 48]. Unlike many of the *process* QIs associated with EUS, the incidence of AEs following endosonography represents an important *outcome*-based QI with good supporting evidence [14]. Beyond ensuring that they occur only rarely, the timely recognition of adverse events is of critical concern. Perhaps the best example is luminal perforation, which should occur no more frequently than 1 in 1000 cases [49]. When perforation is recognized without a significant delay, action may be taken, which provides the patient with the best opportunity for a good outcome [104–106]. Although typically milder than visceral perforation, other AEs associated with EUS, such as bleeding and acute pancreatitis, may also benefit from prompt identification and management.

Misdiagnosis is another AE that is sometimes associated with EUS-directed tissue sampling. This can take the form of a false negative in the face of inadequate tissue or sampling error but can also be reflected by a false positive. False-negative results at the time of EUS can often result in either undertreatment or opportunity cost. This cost can be relatively innocuous (such as the need for repeat biopsy), or it can be gravely serious: growth of a small pancreatic tumor in the setting of chronic pancreatitis, such as to become unresectable. Depending upon circumstances, false positives have been demonstrated in between 1.1% and 5.3% of cases [107, 108]. Such errors are usually the result of pathologist misinterpretation and can be due to a confounding state such as chronic pancreatitis or IgG-4-related pancreaticobiliary disease. False positives, when they occur, can have devastating costs for an individual patient and may result in direct harm: for example, pursuing unnecessary chemotherapy or a pancreatoduodenectomy in a patient with mass-forming chronic pancreatitis. Although the interpretation of cytopathology is not the direct responsibility of the endosonographer, they have a critical role in the process. Clear communication of the clinical context, additional findings, and potential known confounders may assist the cytopathologist with interpretation. Further, in cases where equivocation occurs or misdiagnosis seems likely, EUS-directed FNB may be chosen in lieu of traditional FNA [109], and details of the clinical case should be reviewed in a multidisciplinary tumor board.

Communication with the Patient

The patient-physician relationship is a fundamental responsibility of any clinician. Although not specific to EUS, the frequency with which communication occurs post-procedure is considered a QI for endoscopy in general [14]. In specific, it is the responsibility of the endoscopist to determine criteria for discharge, provide instructions to the patient, and arrange a system of follow-up for relevant preceding findings. Communication with the patient's referring physician is also implied by way of the procedure documentation, as noted previously. Although this seems implicit, direct communication with the patient regarding the EUS findings is not universal, and many patients (up to 16%) may never receive a procedure report [101].

The value of this communication is perhaps best highlighted by the previous report by Siddiqui et al. [100] In this series, 131 patients were referred to two tertiary referral centers for EUS-directed assessment of a solid pancreatic mass. Given the open-access nature of EUS in this study, only 28% of patients were aware of their potential malignancy at the time of referral, and the overwhelming majority of patients (92%) had never previously met their endoscopist. Despite this, the majority of patients wanted to discuss the results with the endoscopist following EUS (76%) rather than wait to discuss it with their referring physician [100]. This discussion is a critically important responsibility for endosonographers and allows patients to shift focus from the uncertainty of diagnosis to a future plan of action. There is a tangible benefit to clear and informed communication in this setting that allows the patient and their family to better initiate the process of psychological adjustment following a new cancer diagnosis [110].

Conclusion

The concept of quality assessment and assurance in the delivery of medical care remains a focused national and international priority. Although significant progress has been made through establishing proposed quality indicators for EUS [14], endosonography remains significantly behind other areas of gastrointestinal endoscopy [13] when it comes to the refinement of validated, outcome-based quality metrics. Quality assessment in EUS is challenged explicitly by the heterogeneous nature of its indications, the complexity of its performance (including interobserver variability), and significant nonuniformity in the way results are documented and communicated. The present focus on priority quality indicators by GI professional societies (ASGE/ACG) is welcome, but significant challenges remain. Future efforts should be directed toward establishing EUS-based diagnostic criteria with high accuracy and interobserver reliability for multiple disease states, as well as promoting the development and adoption of minimum standard terminology and structured reporting for EUS. Only with these tools available will it be feasible to pursue validation of EUS-based QIs to the level of rigor applied to colorectal cancer screening.

References

1. Strohm WD, Phillip J, Hagenmueller F, et al. Ultrasonic tomography by means of an ultrasonic fiberendoscope. Endoscopy. 1980;12:241–4. Available at: https://pubmed.ncbi.nlm.nih.gov/7428729/. Accessed 11 May 2022.
2. Dimagno EP, Regan PT, Wilson DA, et al. Ultrasonic endoscope. Lancet. 1980;1:629–31. Available at: https://pubmed.ncbi.nlm.nih.gov/6102631/. Accessed 11 May 2022.
3. Peery AF, Crockett SD, Murphy CC, et al. Burden and cost of gastrointestinal, liver, and pancreatic diseases in the United States: update 2021. Gastroenterology. 2022;162:621–44. Available at: https://pubmed.ncbi.nlm.nih.gov/34678215/. Accessed 11 May 2022.
4. Dimaio CJ, Mishra G, McHenry L, et al. EUS core curriculum. Gastrointest Endosc. 2012;76:476–81. Available at: https://pubmed.ncbi.nlm.nih.gov/22898403/. Accessed 11 May 2022.
5. Yang D, Wagh MS, Draganov P, v. The status of training in new technologies in advanced endoscopy: from defining competence to credentialing and privileging. Gastrointest Endosc. 2020;92:1016.
6. Anon. ASGE|Diagnostic EUS training. Available at: https://www.asge.org/home/education/advanced-education-training/diagnostic-eus-training. Accessed 11 May 2022.
7. Wani S, Hall M, Keswani RN, et al. Variation in aptitude of trainees in endoscopic ultrasonography, based on cumulative sum analysis. Clin Gastroenterol Hepatol. 2015;13:1318–25.
8. Wachter RM. The end of the beginning: patient safety five years after "To err is human". Health Aff. 2004;23:534–45.
9. Anon. Crossing the quality chasm: a new health system for the 21st century. 2001. Available at: https://pubmed.ncbi.nlm.nih.gov/25057539/. Accessed 11 May 2022.
10. Barclay RL, Vicari JJ, Doughty AS, et al. Colonoscopic withdrawal times and adenoma detection during screening colonoscopy. N Engl J Med. 2006;355:2533–41. Available at: https://pubmed.ncbi.nlm.nih.gov/17167136/. Accessed 11 May 2022.
11. Lieberman D. A call to action — measuring the quality of colonoscopy. N Engl J Med. 2006;355:2588–9.

12. Kaminski MF, Wieszczy P, Rupinski M, et al. Increased rate of adenoma detection associates with reduced risk of colorectal cancer and death. Gastroenterology. 2017;153:98–105.
13. Shaukat A, Holub J, Pike IM, et al. Benchmarking adenoma detection rates for colonoscopy: results from a US-Based Registry. Am J Gastroenterol. 2021;116:1946–9. Available at: https://pubmed.ncbi.nlm.nih.gov/34158463/. Accessed 11 May 2022.
14. Wani S, Wallace MB, Cohen J, et al. Quality indicators for EUS. Gastrointest Endosc. 2015;81:67–80.
15. Pokala SK, Jones B, Wani S. Improving quality in EUS: a call for a national benchmarking registry. Gastrointest Endosc. 2021;94:75–7.
16. Chassin MR, Galvin RW, Donaldson MS. The urgent need to improve health care quality. Institute of Medicine National Roundtable on Health Care Quality. JAMA. 1998;280:1000–5. Available at: https://pubmed.ncbi.nlm.nih.gov/9749483/. Accessed 11 May 2022.
17. Eijkenaar F. Pay for performance in health care: an international overview of initiatives. Med Care Res Rev. 2012;69:251–76.
18. Gross WL, Cooper L, Boggs S, et al. Value-based care and strategic priorities. Anesthesiol Clin. 2017;35:725–31.
19. Jacobson BC, Chak A, Hoffman B, et al. Quality indicators for endoscopic ultrasonography. Am J Gastroenterol. 2006;101:898–901. Available at: https://pubmed.ncbi.nlm.nih.gov/16635234/. Accessed 11 May 2022.
20. Broazek JL, Akl EA, Compalati E, et al. Grading quality of evidence and strength of recommendations in clinical practice guidelines Part 3 of 3. The GRADE approach to developing recommendations. Allergy. 2011;66:588–95.
21. Schünemann HJ, Oxman AD, Brozek J, et al. GRADE: assessing the quality of evidence for diagnostic recommendations. Evid Based Med. 2008;13:162–3.
22. Coe SG, Raimondo M, Woodward TA, et al. Quality in EUS: an assessment of baseline compliance and performance improvement by using the American Society for Gastrointestinal Endoscopy-American College of Gastroenterology quality indicators. Gastrointest Endosc. 2009;69:195–201. Available at: https://pubmed.ncbi.nlm.nih.gov/19185684/. Accessed 11 May 2022.
23. Cassani L, Aihara H, Anand GS, et al. Core curriculum for EUS. Gastrointest Endosc. 2020;92:469–73. Available at: https://pubmed.ncbi.nlm.nih.gov/32713612/. Accessed 16 July 2022.
24. van Dam J, Brady PG, Freeman M, et al. Guidelines for training in electronic ultrasound: guidelines for clinical application. From the ASGE. American Society for Gastrointestinal Endoscopy. Gastrointest Endosc. 1999;49:829–33. Available at: https://pubmed.ncbi.nlm.nih.gov/10343245/. Accessed 16 July 2022.
25. Polkowski M, Larghi A, Weynand B, et al. Learning, techniques, and complications of endoscopic ultrasound (EUS)-guided sampling in gastroenterology: European Society of Gastrointestinal Endoscopy (ESGE) Technical Guideline. Endoscopy. 2012;44:190–205. Available at: https://pubmed.ncbi.nlm.nih.gov/22180307/. Accessed 16 July 2022.
26. Karstensen JG, Nayahangan LJ, Konge L, et al. A core curriculum for basic EUS skills: an international consensus using the Delphi methodology. Endosc Ultrasound. 2022;11:122–32. Available at: https://pubmed.ncbi.nlm.nih.gov/35488624/. Accessed 16 July 2022.
27. Wani S, Keswani RN, Petersen B, et al. Training in EUS and ERCP: standardizing methods to assess competence. Gastrointest Endosc. 2018;87:1371–82. Available at: http://www.giejournal.org/article/S0016510718301238/fulltext. Accessed 16 July 2022.
28. Johnson G, Webster G, Boškoski I, et al. Curriculum for ERCP and endoscopic ultrasound training in Europe: European Society of Gastrointestinal Endoscopy (ESGE) Position Statement. Endoscopy. 2021;53:1071–87. Available at: https://pubmed.ncbi.nlm.nih.gov/34311472/. Accessed 16 July 2022.
29. Wani S, Han S, Simon V, et al. Setting minimum standards for training in EUS and ERCP: results from a prospective multicenter study evaluating learning curves and competence among advanced endoscopy trainees. Gastrointest Endosc. 2019;89:1160–8.

30. Wani S, Keswani R, Hall M, et al. A prospective multicenter study evaluating learning curves and competence in endoscopic ultrasound and endoscopic retrograde cholangiopancreatography among advanced endoscopy trainees: the rapid assessment of trainee endoscopy skills study. Clin Gastroenterol Hepatol. 2017;15:1758–67. Available at: https://pubmed.ncbi.nlm.nih.gov/28625816/. Accessed 16 July 2022.
31. Wani S, Hall M, Wang AY, et al. Variation in learning curves and competence for ERCP among advanced endoscopy trainees by using cumulative sum analysis. Gastrointest Endosc. 2016;83:711–9.
32. Wani S, Keswani RN, Han S, et al. Competence in endoscopic ultrasound and endoscopic retrograde cholangiopancreatography, from training through independent practice. Gastroenterology. 2018;155:1483–94.
33. Broe M, Barry M, Patchett S, et al. Evaluating the clinical efficacy and cost effectiveness of direct access endoscopy. Surgeon. 2013;11:304–8. Available at: https://pubmed.ncbi.nlm.nih.gov/23510705/. Accessed 14 May 2022.
34. Smith CF, Tompson AC, Jones N, et al. Direct access cancer testing in primary care: a systematic review of use and clinical outcomes. Br J Gen Pract. 2018;68:e594–603. Available at: https://pubmed.ncbi.nlm.nih.gov/30104328/. Accessed 14 May 2022.
35. Dumonceau JM, Deprez PH, Jenssen C, et al. Indications, results, and clinical impact of endoscopic ultrasound (EUS)-guided sampling in gastroenterology: European Society of Gastrointestinal Endoscopy (ESGE) Clinical Guideline - Updated January 2017. Endoscopy. 2017;49:695–714.
36. Polkowski M, Jenssen C, Kaye P, et al. Technical aspects of endoscopic ultrasound (EUS)-guided sampling in gastroenterology: European Society of Gastrointestinal Endoscopy (ESGE) Technical Guideline - March 2017. Endoscopy. 2017;49:989–1006. Available at: https://pubmed.ncbi.nlm.nih.gov/28898917/. Accessed 29 April 2022.
37. Hallensleben ND, Umans DS, Bouwense SAW, et al. The diagnostic work-up and outcomes of 'presumed' idiopathic acute pancreatitis: a post-hoc analysis of a multicentre observational cohort. United European Gastroenterol J. 2020;8:340–50.
38. Wan J, Ouyang Y, Yu C, et al. Comparison of EUS with MRCP in idiopathic acute pancreatitis: a systematic review and meta-analysis. Gastrointest Endosc. 2018;87:1180–8.
39. Ortega AR, Gómez-Rodríguez R, Romero M, Fernández-Zapardiel S, del Mar Céspedes M, Carrobles J-M. Prospective comparison of endoscopic ultrasonography and magnetic resonance cholangiopancreatography in the etiological diagnosis of "idiopathic" acute pancreatitis. Pancreas. 2011;40:289–94. Available at: https://pubmed.ncbi.nlm.nih.gov/21206330/. Accessed 29 October 2021.
40. Meining A, Dittler HJ, Wolf A, et al. You get what you expect? A critical appraisal of imaging methodology in endosonographic cancer staging. Gut. 2002;50:599–603. Available at: https://pubmed.ncbi.nlm.nih.gov/11950802/. Accessed 14 May 2022.
41. Malik S, Kaushik N, Khalid A, et al. EUS yield in evaluating biliary dilatation in patients with normal serum liver enzymes. Dig Dis Sci. 2007;52:508–12. Available at: https://pubmed.ncbi.nlm.nih.gov/17211694/. Accessed 14 May 2022.
42. Dietrich CF, Arcidiacono PG, Braden B, et al. What should be known prior to performing EUS? Endosc Ultrasound. 2019;8:3–16. Available at: https://pubmed.ncbi.nlm.nih.gov/30777940/. Accessed 18 May 2022.
43. Dietrich C, Arcidiacono P, Braden B, et al. What should be known prior to performing EUS exams? (Part II). Endosc Ultrasound. 2019;8:360–9. Available at: https://pubmed.ncbi.nlm.nih.gov/31571619/. Accessed 29 April 2022.
44. Wallace MB, Hawes RH, Sahai AV, et al. Dilation of malignant esophageal stenosis to allow EUS guided fine-needle aspiration: safety and effect on patient management. Gastrointest Endosc. 2000;51:309–13. Available at: https://pubmed.ncbi.nlm.nih.gov/10699776/. Accessed 14 May 2022.
45. Mortensen MB, Fristrup C, Holm FS, et al. Prospective evaluation of patient tolerability, satisfaction with patient information, and complications in endoscopic ultrasonography.

Endoscopy. 2005;37:146–53. Available at: https://pubmed.ncbi.nlm.nih.gov/15692930/. Accessed 14 May 2022.
46. Lakhtakia S. Complications of diagnostic and therapeutic endoscopic ultrasound. Best Pract Res Clin Gastroenterol. 2016;30:807–23. Available at: https://pubmed.ncbi.nlm.nih.gov/27931638/. Accessed 14 May 2022.
47. Eloubeidi MA, Tamhane A, Varadarajulu S, et al. Frequency of major complications after EUS-guided FNA of solid pancreatic masses: a prospective evaluation. Gastrointest Endosc. 2006;63:622–9. Available at: https://pubmed.ncbi.nlm.nih.gov/16564863/. Accessed 14 May 2022.
48. Jacobson BC, Adler DG, Davila RE, et al. ASGE guideline: complications of EUS. Gastrointest Endosc. 2005;61:8–12. Available at: https://pubmed.ncbi.nlm.nih.gov/15672049/. Accessed 14 May 2022.
49. Jenssen C, Alvarez-Sánchez MV, Napoléon B, et al. Diagnostic endoscopic ultrasonography: assessment of safety and prevention of complications. World J Gastroenterol. 2012;18:4659–76. Available at: https://pubmed.ncbi.nlm.nih.gov/23002335/. Accessed 14 May 2022.
50. Wang KX, Ben QW, Jin ZD, et al. Assessment of morbidity and mortality associated with EUS-guided FNA: a systematic review. Gastrointest Endosc. 2011;73:283–90. Available at: https://pubmed.ncbi.nlm.nih.gov/21295642/. Accessed 14 May 2022.
51. Kojima H, Kitago M, Iwasaki E, et al. Peritoneal dissemination of pancreatic cancer caused by endoscopic ultrasound-guided fine needle aspiration: a case report and literature review. World J Gastroenterol. 2021;27:294–304.
52. Yane K, Kuwatani M, Yoshida M, et al. Non-negligible rate of needle tract seeding after endoscopic ultrasound-guided fine-needle aspiration for patients undergoing distal pancreatectomy for pancreatic cancer. Dig Endosc. 2020;32:801–11.
53. Matsui T, Nishikawa K, Yukimoto H, et al. Needle tract seeding following endoscopic ultrasound-guided fine-needle aspiration for pancreatic cancer: a report of two cases. World J Surg Oncol. 2019;17:134.
54. Sato N, Takano S, Yoshitomi H, et al. Needle tract seeding recurrence of pancreatic cancer in the gastric wall with paragastric lymph node metastasis after endoscopic ultrasound-guided fine needle aspiration followed by pancreatectomy: a case report and literature review. BMC Gastroenterol. 2020;20:13. Available at: https://pubmed.ncbi.nlm.nih.gov/31941458/. Accessed 14 May 2022.
55. Heimbach JK, Sanchez W, Rosen CB, et al. Trans-peritoneal fine needle aspiration biopsy of hilar cholangiocarcinoma is associated with disease dissemination. HPB. 2011;13:356–60. Available at: https://pubmed.ncbi.nlm.nih.gov/21492336/. Accessed 14 May 2022.
56. Malikowski T, Levy MJ, Gleeson FC, et al. Endoscopic ultrasound/fine needle aspiration is effective for lymph node staging in patients with cholangiocarcinoma. Hepatology. 2020;72:940–8.
57. Chafic AH, Dewitt J, LeBlanc JK, et al. Impact of preoperative endoscopic ultrasound-guided fine needle aspiration on postoperative recurrence and survival in cholangiocarcinoma patients. Endoscopy. 2013;45:883–9. Available at: https://pubmed.ncbi.nlm.nih.gov/24165813/. Accessed 14 May 2022.
58. van Wanrooij RLJ, Bronswijk M, Kunda R, et al. Therapeutic endoscopic ultrasound: European Society of Gastrointestinal Endoscopy (ESGE) technical review. Endoscopy. 2022;54:310–32. Available at: https://pubmed.ncbi.nlm.nih.gov/35114696/. Accessed 14 May 2022.
59. van der Merwe SW, van Wanrooij RLJ, Bronswijk M, et al. Therapeutic endoscopic ultrasound: European Society of Gastrointestinal Endoscopy (ESGE) Guideline. Endoscopy. 2022;54:185–205.
60. Lim H, Gong EJ, Min BH, et al. Clinical practice guideline for the management of antithrombotic agents in patients undergoing gastrointestinal endoscopy. Clin Endosc. 2020;53:663–77. Available at: https://pubmed.ncbi.nlm.nih.gov/33242928/. Accessed 18 May 2022.

61. Abraham NS, Barkun AN, Sauer BG, et al. American College of Gastroenterology-Canadian Association of Gastroenterology clinical practice guideline: management of anticoagulants and antiplatelets during acute gastrointestinal bleeding and the periendoscopic period. J Can Assoc Gastroenterol. 2022;5:100.
62. Acosta RD, Abraham NS, Chandrasekhara V, et al. The management of antithrombotic agents for patients undergoing GI endoscopy. Gastrointest Endosc. 2016;83:3–16. Available at: https://pubmed.ncbi.nlm.nih.gov/26621548/. Accessed 18 May 2022.
63. Kawakubo K, Yane K, Eto K, et al. A prospective multicenter study evaluating bleeding risk after endoscopic ultrasound-guided fine needle aspiration in patients prescribed antithrombotic agents. Gut Liver. 2018;12:353–9. Available at: https://pubmed.ncbi.nlm.nih.gov/29409308/. Accessed 18 May 2022.
64. Hamada T, Yasunaga H, Nakai Y, et al. Rarity of severe bleeding and perforation in endoscopic ultrasound-guided fine needle aspiration for submucosal tumors. Dig Dis Sci. 2013;58:2634–8. Available at: https://pubmed.ncbi.nlm.nih.gov/23695878/. Accessed 18 May 2022.
65. Varadarajulu S, Eloubeidi MA. Frequency and significance of acute intracystic hemorrhage during EUS-FNA of cystic lesions of the pancreas. Gastrointest Endosc. 2004;60:631–5. Available at: https://pubmed.ncbi.nlm.nih.gov/15472697/. Accessed 18 May 2022.
66. Kien-Fong VC, Chang F, Doig L, et al. A prospective control study of the safety and cellular yield of EUS-guided FNA or Trucut biopsy in patients taking aspirin, nonsteroidal anti-inflammatory drugs, or prophylactic low molecular weight heparin. Gastrointest Endosc. 2006;63:808–13. Available at: https://pubmed.ncbi.nlm.nih.gov/16650543/. Accessed 18 May 2022.
67. Nagata N, Yasunaga H, Matsui H, et al. Therapeutic endoscopy-related GI bleeding and thromboembolic events in patients using warfarin or direct oral anticoagulants: results from a large nationwide database analysis. Gut. 2018;67:1805–12. Available at: https://pubmed.ncbi.nlm.nih.gov/28874418/. Accessed 18 May 2022.
68. Khashab MA, Chithadi KV, Acosta RD, et al. Antibiotic prophylaxis for GI endoscopy. Gastrointest Endosc. 2015;81:81–9. Available at: https://pubmed.ncbi.nlm.nih.gov/25442089/. Accessed 18 May 2022.
69. Wiersema MJ, Vilmann P, Giovannini M, et al. Endosonography-guided fine-needle aspiration biopsy: diagnostic accuracy and complication assessment. Gastroenterology. 1997;112:1087–95. Available at: https://pubmed.ncbi.nlm.nih.gov/9097990/. Accessed 18 May 2022.
70. Facciorusso A, Buccino VR, Turco A, et al. Antibiotics do not decrease the rate of infection after endoscopic ultrasound fine-needle aspiration of pancreatic cysts. Dig Dis Sci. 2019;64:2308–15. Available at: https://pubmed.ncbi.nlm.nih.gov/31065897/. Accessed 18 May 2022.
71. Guarner-Argente C, Shah P, Buchner A, et al. Use of antimicrobials for EUS-guided FNA of pancreatic cysts: a retrospective, comparative analysis. Gastrointest Endosc. 2011;74:81–6. Available at: https://pubmed.ncbi.nlm.nih.gov/21704808/. Accessed 18 May 2022.
72. Facciorusso A, Buccino RV, Muscatiello N. How to measure quality in endoscopic ultrasound. Ann Transl Med. 2018;6:266. Available at: https://pubmed.ncbi.nlm.nih.gov/30094252/. Accessed 18 May 2022.
73. Kaneko M, Katanuma A, Maguchi H, et al. Prospective, randomized, comparative study of delineation capability of radial scanning and curved linear array endoscopic ultrasound for the pancreaticobiliary region. Endosc Int Open. 2014;2:E160–70. Available at: https://pubmed.ncbi.nlm.nih.gov/26134963/. Accessed 18 May 2022.
74. Sharma M, Hollerbach S, Fusaroli P, et al. General principles of image optimization in EUS. Endosc Ultrasound. 2021;10:168–84. Available at: https://pubmed.ncbi.nlm.nih.gov/33666178/. Accessed 18 May 2022.
75. Vila JJ, Jimnez FJ, Irisarri R, et al. Prospective observational study of the incidental findings on endoscopic ultrasonography: should a complete exploration always be performed? Scand J

Gastroenterol. 2009;44:1139–45. Available at: https://pubmed.ncbi.nlm.nih.gov/19585376/. Accessed 18 May 2022.
76. Yamamiya A, Irisawa A, Kashima K, et al. Interobserver reliability of endoscopic ultrasonography: literature review. Diagnostics. 2020;10:953.
77. Gress F, Schmitt C, Savides T, et al. Interobserver agreement for EUS in the evaluation and diagnosis of submucosal masses. Gastrointest Endosc. 2001;53:71–6. Available at: https://pubmed.ncbi.nlm.nih.gov/11154492/. Accessed 18 May 2022.
78. Fusaroli P, Buscarini E, Peyre S, et al. Interobserver agreement in staging gastric malt lymphoma by EUS. Gastrointest Endosc. 2002;55:662–8. Available at: https://pubmed.ncbi.nlm.nih.gov/11979247/. Accessed 18 May 2022.
79. Quispel R, Schutz HM, Hallensleben ND, et al. Do endosonographers agree on the presence of bile duct sludge and the subsequent need for intervention? Endosc Int Open. 2021;9:E911–7. Available at: https://pubmed.ncbi.nlm.nih.gov/34079877/. Accessed 18 May 2022.
80. Gonçalves B, Soares JB, Bastos P. Endoscopic ultrasound in the diagnosis and staging of pancreatic cancer. GE Port J Gastroenterol. 2015;22:161–71. Available at: https://pubmed.ncbi.nlm.nih.gov/28868399/. Accessed 18 May 2022.
81. Uberoi AS, Bhutani MS. Has the role of EUS in rectal cancer staging changed in the last decade? Endosc Ultrasound. 2018;7:366–70. Available at: https://pubmed.ncbi.nlm.nih.gov/30531023/. Accessed 18 May 2022.
82. Hajj II, Dewitt J, Sherman S, et al. Prospective evaluation of the performance and interobserver variation in endoscopic ultrasound staging of rectal cancer. Eur J Gastroenterol Hepatol. 2018;30:1013–8. Available at: https://pubmed.ncbi.nlm.nih.gov/29846267/. Accessed 18 May 2022.
83. Soriano A, Castells A, Ayuso C, et al. Preoperative staging and tumor resectability assessment of pancreatic cancer: prospective study comparing endoscopic ultrasonography, helical computed tomography, magnetic resonance imaging, and angiography. Am J Gastroenterol. 2004;99:492–501. Available at: https://pubmed.ncbi.nlm.nih.gov/15056091/. Accessed 18 May 2022.
84. Legmann P, Vignaux O, Dousset B, et al. Pancreatic tumors: comparison of dual-phase helical CT and endoscopic sonography. AJR Am J Roentgenol. 1998;170:1315–22. Available at: https://pubmed.ncbi.nlm.nih.gov/9574609/. Accessed 18 May 2022.
85. Hewitt MJ, McPhail MJW, Possamai L, et al. EUS-guided FNA for diagnosis of solid pancreatic neoplasms: a meta-analysis. Gastrointest Endosc. 2012;75:319–31. Available at: https://pubmed.ncbi.nlm.nih.gov/22248600/. Accessed 18 May 2022.
86. Savides TJ, Donohue M, Hunt G, et al. EUS-guided FNA diagnostic yield of malignancy in solid pancreatic masses: a benchmark for quality performance measurement. Gastrointest Endosc. 2007;66:277–82. Available at: https://pubmed.ncbi.nlm.nih.gov/17643700/. Accessed 18 May 2022.
87. Eloubeidi MA, Wallace MB, Reed CE, et al. The utility of EUS and EUS-guided fine needle aspiration in detecting celiac lymph node metastasis in patients with esophageal cancer: a single-center experience. Gastrointest Endosc. 2001;54:714–9. Available at: https://pubmed.ncbi.nlm.nih.gov/11726846/. Accessed 18 May 2022.
88. Vazquez-Sequeiros E, Norton LD, Clain JE, et al. Impact of EUS-guided fine-needle aspiration on lymph node staging in patients with esophageal carcinoma. Gastrointest Endosc. 2001;53:751–7. Available at: https://pubmed.ncbi.nlm.nih.gov/11375583/. Accessed 18 May 2022.
89. Oppong KW, Bekkali NLH, Leeds JS, et al. Fork-tip needle biopsy versus fine-needle aspiration in endoscopic ultrasound-guided sampling of solid pancreatic masses: a randomized crossover study. Endoscopy. 2020;52:454–61. Available at: https://pubmed.ncbi.nlm.nih.gov/32162287/. Accessed 18 May 2022.
90. Crinò SF, Grazie M, Manfrin E, et al. Randomized trial comparing fork-tip and side-fenestrated needles for EUS-guided fine-needle biopsy of solid pancreatic lesions. Gastrointest Endosc. 2020;92:648–58. Available at: https://pubmed.ncbi.nlm.nih.gov/32433914/. Accessed 18 May 2022.

91. Fujita A, Ryozawa S, Tanisaka Y, et al. Current status of needles in the optimization of endoscopic ultrasound-guided procedures. Diagnostics. 2020;10:463. Available at: https://pubmed.ncbi.nlm.nih.gov/32650628/. Accessed 18 May 2022.
92. Jani BS, Rzouq F, Saligram S, et al. Endoscopic ultrasound-guided fine-needle aspiration of pancreatic lesions: a systematic review of technical and procedural variables. N Am J Med Sci. 2016;8:1–11. Available at: https://pubmed.ncbi.nlm.nih.gov/27011940/. Accessed 29 April 2022.
93. Wani S, Mullady D, Early DS, et al. The clinical impact of immediate on-site cytopathology evaluation during endoscopic ultrasound-guided fine needle aspiration of pancreatic masses: a prospective multicenter randomized controlled trial. Am J Gastroenterol. 2015;110:1429–39. Available at: https://pubmed.ncbi.nlm.nih.gov/26346868/. Accessed 18 May 2022.
94. Lee LS, Nieto J, Watson RR, et al. Randomized noninferiority trial comparing diagnostic yield of cytopathologist-guided versus 7 passes for EUS-FNA of pancreatic masses. Dig Endosc. 2016;28:469–75. Available at: https://pubmed.ncbi.nlm.nih.gov/26694852/. Accessed 18 May 2022.
95. Kappelle WFW, van Leerdam ME, Schwartz MP, et al. Rapid on-site evaluation during endoscopic ultrasound-guided fine-needle aspiration of lymph nodes does not increase diagnostic yield: a randomized, multicenter trial. Am J Gastroenterol. 2018;113:677–85. Available at: https://pubmed.ncbi.nlm.nih.gov/29681624/. Accessed 18 May 2022.
96. Crinò SF, di Mitri R, Nguyen NQ, et al. Endoscopic ultrasound-guided fine-needle biopsy with or without rapid on-site evaluation for diagnosis of solid pancreatic lesions: a randomized controlled non-inferiority trial. Gastroenterology. 2021;161:899–909. Available at: https://pubmed.ncbi.nlm.nih.gov/34116031/. Accessed 18 May 2022.
97. Wang J, Wu X, Yin P, et al. Comparing endoscopic ultrasound (EUS)-guided fine needle aspiration (FNA) versus fine needle biopsy (FNB) in the diagnosis of solid lesions: study protocol for a randomized controlled trial. Trials. 2016;17:198.
98. Guo J, Sahai A, Teoh A, et al. An international, multi-institution survey on performing EUS-FNA and fine needle biopsy. Endosc Ultrasound. 2020;9:319–28. Available at: https://pubmed.ncbi.nlm.nih.gov/32883921/. Accessed 18 May 2022.
99. Huang RJ, Barakat MT, Park W, et al. Quality metrics in the performance of EUS: a population-based observational cohort of the United States. Gastrointest Endosc. 2021;94:68–74. Available at: https://pubmed.ncbi.nlm.nih.gov/33476611/. Accessed 29 April 2022.
100. Siddiqui UD, Rossi F, Padda MS, et al. Patient preferences after endoscopic ultrasound with fine needle aspiration (EUS-FNA) diagnosis of pancreas cancer: rapid communication valued over long-term relationships. Pancreas. 2011;40:680–1. Available at: https://pubmed.ncbi.nlm.nih.gov/21602735/. Accessed 29 April 2022.
101. Fusaroli P, Eloubeidi M, Calvanese C, et al. Quality of reporting in endoscopic ultrasound: results of an international multicenter survey (the QUOREUS study). Endosc Int Open. 2021;9:E1171. https://doi.org/10.1055/a-1482-7769.
102. Aabakken L, Barkun AN, Cotton PB, et al. Standardized endoscopic reporting. J Gastroenterol Hepatol. 2014;29:234–40. Available at: https://pubmed.ncbi.nlm.nih.gov/24329727/. Accessed 28 May 2022.
103. Coté GA, Elmunzer BJ, Forster E, et al. Development of an automated ERCP quality report card using structured data fields. Tech Innov Gastrointest Endosc. 2021;23:129–38. Available at: https://pubmed.ncbi.nlm.nih.gov/33928265/. Accessed 28 May 2022.
104. Dişibeyaz S, Öztaş E, Kuzu UB, et al. Closure of echoendoscope-related duodenal free wall perforation by placement of a covered metallic stent. Endosc Ultrasound. 2016;5:399.
105. Matsuoka M, Kobayashi K, Okura Y, et al. Endoscopic closure of an acute duodenal perforation occurring during endoscopic ultrasound using endoclips and polyglycolic acid sheets with fibrin glue. Case Rep Gastroenterol. 2021;15:253–61. Available at http://www.ncbi.nlm.nih.gov/pubmed/33790712. Accessed 28 May 2022.
106. Liu Y, Wang D, Li Z. Endoscopic closure for EUS and ERCP related duodenal perforation by endoclips. Gastroenterol Res Pract. 2016;2016:1051597. Available at: https://pubmed.ncbi.nlm.nih.gov/27703474/. Accessed 28 May 2022.

107. Gleeson FC, Kipp BR, Caudill JL, et al. False positive endoscopic ultrasound fine needle aspiration cytology: incidence and risk factors. Gut. 2010;59:586–93. Available at: https://pubmed.ncbi.nlm.nih.gov/20427392/. Accessed 28 May 2022.
108. Siddiqui AA, Kowalski TE, Shahid H, et al. False-positive EUS-guided FNA cytology for solid pancreatic lesions. Gastrointest Endosc. 2011;74:535–40.
109. Chen YI, Chatterjee A, Berger R, et al. Endoscopic ultrasound (EUS)-guided fine needle biopsy alone vs. EUS-guided fine needle aspiration with rapid onsite evaluation in pancreatic lesions: a multicenter randomized trial. Endoscopy. 2022;54:4–12. Available at: https://pubmed.ncbi.nlm.nih.gov/33506455/. Accessed 18 May 2022.
110. Butow PN, Kazemi JN, Beeney LJ, et al. When the diagnosis is cancer patient communication experiences and preferences. Cancer. 1996;77(12):2630–7.

Chapter 6
Quality in the Gastrointestinal Motility Laboratory

Brian Surjanhata and Kyle Staller

Table of Quality Measures/Metrics

Key Points

- Gastrointestinal motility testing can provide physiologic assessment of discrete contractile function and global motility to guide management options for a variety of burdensome diseases.
- Running a high-quality gastrointestinal motility laboratory has several components that include scheduling, staffing, physical space and equipment, and optimizing the patient experience.
- High demand for motility assessment highlights the importance of ensuring quality evaluations as these studies play a critical role in advancing patient care and our understanding of gastrointestinal dysmotility and disorders of gut-brain interaction.

B. Surjanhata · K. Staller (✉)
Center for Neurointestinal Health, GI Unit, Massachusetts General Hospital, Boston, MA, USA
e-mail: bsurjanhata@partners.org; kstaller@mgh.harvard.edu

J. D. Feuerstein, D. J. Stein (eds.), *Quality in Gastroenterology*, https://doi.org/10.1007/978-3-031-58492-3_6

Introduction

Gastrointestinal (GI) dysmotility and disorders of gut-brain interaction account for a significant number of consultations within clinical practice and have a considerable impact on healthcare costs as a result of testing, treatment, and ambulatory and hospital visits [1, 2]. Symptoms range from upper GI complaints such as dysphagia, gastroesophageal reflux, and symptoms suggestive of gastroparesis or dyspepsia to lower GI complaints including constipation, diarrhea, and fecal incontinence. When structural or inflammatory etiologies have been ruled out as clinically appropriate, the next step in evaluation may be GI motility testing which can guide management toward further medical or surgical management.

GI motility testing as a whole has two categories: transit evaluations that provide a global sense of motility and manometric evaluations that provide detailed assessment of contractile function. A typical GI motility laboratory offers manometric capabilities and, depending on the needs of the center or patient insurance base, ambulatory capsule-based or breath-test transit evaluations. A summary of testing that can be provided by an ambulatory GI motility lab is in Table 6.1. The goal of this chapter is not to discuss the indications or intricacies of interpretation but to highlight the components needed to establish an optimized GI motility lab as well as strategies to ensure the lab is providing high-quality evaluations to inform clinical decisions.

Table 6.1 Gastrointestinal motility diagnostic procedures offered within ambulatory motility labs settings

	Procedure	Indications
Basic	High-resolution esophageal manometry	• Dysphagia • Gastroesophageal reflux disease • Noncardiac chest pain • Evaluation prior to anti-reflux surgery • Lung transplant (pre-/post-) evaluation
	pH impedance	• Gastroesophageal reflux disease • Evaluation prior to anti-reflux surgery • Lung transplant (pre-/post-) evaluation
	Wireless pH capsule	• Gastroesophageal reflux disease
	High-resolution anorectal manometry	• Constipation • Fecal incontinence
	Wireless motility capsule	• Gastroparesis suspected • Constipation • Small bowel motility evaluation
	Hydrogen/methane breath testing	• Small intestinal bacterial overgrowth
	Gastric emptying breath testing	• Gastroparesis
Academic[a]	Antroduodenal manometry	• Gastroparesis • Small bowel dysmotility • Intestinal pseudo-obstruction
	Colonic manometry	• Constipation • Consideration of colectomy for very severe constipation subtype

[a] These procedures are typically performed at some tertiary care centers with special research interests and are becoming less utilized overall

Scheduling

A comprehensive and efficient lab starts with scheduling, striking the balance of having enough capacity to schedule referrals in a timely manner to inform clinical decisions, especially when surgery is anticipated, while having enough wait time to ensure all openings are filled in order to maximize clinical operations. The optimal time frame for this may be 2–3 weeks from referral.

Esophageal manometries should be scheduled in the morning to minimize the length of a patient's fasting status. The studies that are accompanied by pH impedance testing should be scheduled early in the week to account for the return of the probe and recorder within the 24-h time period. Other examinations that require fasting after midnight such as wireless motility capsule or breath testing should also be considered for morning sessions. This leaves anorectal manometries to be performed during the afternoon. Procedure slots should factor in time needed for check-in, evaluation of the patient (physical assessment of the patient, medical history review, brief interview of present symptoms), patient education, the procedure itself, any potential troubleshooting needed, and room turnover time. Generally, our center reserves 1 h per examination for esophageal manometry with or without pH impedance testing, anorectal manometry, or wireless motility capsule testing. In a typical week that has two rooms running, this results in about 70 cases per week.

Personnel

Running a quality motility lab is a team effort comprised of the director, a scheduling coordinator to guide patients prior to the studies, motility trained nurses and technicians to perform the studies, and physicians who are adept at interpretation and synthesize clinical recommendations. While assembling a team, recognize that these are uncomfortable procedures and patients have varied tolerance for discomfort and may have history of anxiety, trauma, or distrust of the medical system [1]. Therefore, staffing is not just about being able to perform duties but also finding the correct people capable of guiding patients through the procedure with a comforting bedside manner.

The director of the lab is typically a physician that is trained and clinically focused on GI motility. Assessment of qualifications should be based on review of the prospective director's curriculum vitae and prior experiences as there is no formal board certification for GI motility [3, 4]. In some centers, the director instead holds a PhD related in medical sciences but has an academic focus on GI motility, and there is available medical supervision of the lab by a physician [3]. The director serves multiple roles including purchasing equipment and lab supplies, overseeing maintenance of equipment, helping troubleshoot general operational and case issues, and updating procedure protocols to evaluate motility within present guidelines and functions as a liaison with administration and other disciplines. This helps ensure the lab runs efficiently and is able to meet the needs of the referring providers and the patients seeking care.

Motility trained registered nurses and technicians are typically the frontline providers administering the test. Training nurses and technicians is typically through direct teaching by physicians, peers, device company representatives, and seminars [5]. First, they should have enough of a foundation to be able to review referrals and understand the specific questions addressed to ensure that, in patients that are experiencing challenges during the procedure, a maneuver necessary to guide management is completed as best as possible. For example, in those that are being considered for anti-reflux surgery, ensuring that a high-quality multiple rapid swallow maneuver is performed can inform whether postoperative dysphagia may be a concern. They should also be able to recognize who may be clinically unfit to undergo the procedure at the time of presentation in order to be able to preserve patient safety. An example may be a patient with high suspicion for achalasia and who may not have been fasting for long enough—increasing risk for aspiration. Having a physician accessible can be helpful in triaging these decisions, though direct physician presence is unnecessary in all but the most unusual circumstances. Furthermore, the training and experience of the nurses and technicians should be at a level where they are able to troubleshoot or identify issues in real time. This includes ability to determine that the manometry catheters are placed correctly by identifying necessary anatomic landmarks. Recognizing whether repeating a maneuver is needed is also a mark of a well-experienced motility nurse or technician as this allows for more accurate information needed to guide clinical care. For example, excessive coughing during swallow maneuvers on esophageal manometry can make final interpretation technically challenging, and taking time to obtain extra swallows results in a more complete examination. Ensuring a smooth procedure may begin before the patient even arrives: staff may perform a pre-procedure phone call to review any preparations prior to the test, ensure the patient's arrival, and establish a therapeutic relationship to lessen periprocedural anxiety. During the procedure, careful documentation of any challenges arising during the case can help the interpreting provider understand the context of the findings reflected in the motility data.

All providers involved in interpretation must be able to not only provide correct manometric diagnosis through technical use of the motility software but also integrate a final clinical impression and recommendations based on the overall patient profile. While there is published guidance on interpreting various motility studies, making recommendations solely based on the study result may lead to further diagnostics or ineffective treatments, exposing patients to unnecessary risks. We argue that interpreting motility studies should not be in a vacuum but rather with the full understanding of symptoms prompting referral, medications taken during the study, and knowledge of the prior workup and results. For example, is an esophageal manometry revealing esophagogastric junction outlet obstruction a relevant finding in the context of dysphagia or chest pain or might this be a clinically irrelevant finding and is a result of body habitus or opiate use? If the situation is the latter, then complementary testing with timed barium swallow or functional lumen imaging probe may not be necessary, obviating further testing needs. In the case of anorectal manometry, an example may be recommending pelvic floor physical therapy mainly due to recent use of digital manipulation despite a normal balloon expulsion test and mildly abnormal dyssynergic pattern, therefore altering management recommendations despite the test suggesting otherwise. Presently, learning the art of interpreting motility studies is through direct mentorship, similar to how endoscopy is taught for trainees, but without formal competency milestones. There are ongoing efforts toward standardizing training and developing a formal credentialling process for motility interpretation [6, 7].

Physical Space

Creating an accessible and comfortable space for patients may increase the likelihood of completing studies successfully and improve patient satisfaction. The location of the motility laboratory can either be within office space or the endoscopy suite. This allows motility nurses and technicians easy access to providers in case there are issues to troubleshoot or concern for patient safety. Location of the motility laboratory in certain designated hospital or clinic spaces may be necessary due to local rules about where procedures may be performed. Recognizing the invasive nature of these procedures as well as the overlap of trauma history and psychosocial comorbidities in this patient population, designing the lab that provides a level of comfort while maintaining privacy is important. Rooms running invasive manometric studies should be private spaces separated by walls to allow for privacy. Noninvasive testing such as breath testing or capsule-based motility tests can be done in semiprivate areas separated by curtains if necessary. The room needs to be large enough to be able to accommodate the staff involved and the equipment to allow for maneuverability. A private bathroom, ideally adjoining the procedure room, should be available for patients (Fig. 6.1a).

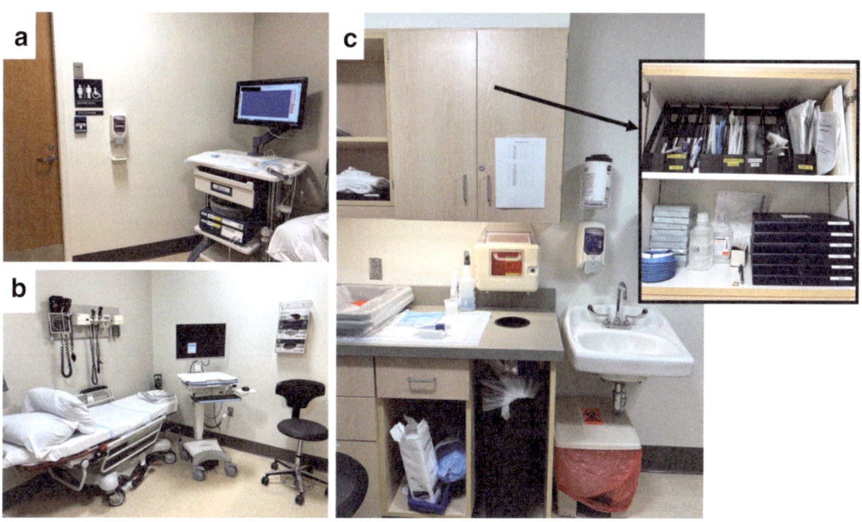

Fig. 6.1 A typical motility room includes (**a**) an adjoining bathroom, a motility procedure tower, (**b**) a stretcher able to assess a patient in supine and upright position, a mobile computer for the motility nurse or technician, personal protective equipment, (**c**) table space to arrange supplies, a sink with running water, receptacles for waste, and stocked cabinets with manometry supplies. (Figure sourced from original photos of the Massachusetts General Hospital GI Motility Lab taken by author Surjanhata)

The Equipment

The essential equipment for any motility lab room includes a mobile computer used by staff for periprocedural documentation, the manometry procedure tower, stocked cabinets with manometry supplies, a stretcher with ability to position the patient upright or supine, a sink with running water, emesis basins, and supplies to handle waste and soiled linens (Fig. 6.1b, c). The manometry procedure tower is purchased from the manometry supply vendor and houses the computer with the required software and the processing equipment that connects to the manometry catheters. High-resolution manometry catheters should be used for both esophageal and anorectal evaluation based on present guideline standards. Lidocaine jelly and spray to facilitate catheter insertion should be adequately stocked and stored in locked cabinets. The use of these medications should be documented in the electronic medical record during the procedure. A large volume referral center should ideally have the computer connected to the hospital network to be able to securely transfer and store raw manometry files on a shared drive that is accessible within the network and remain HIPAA compliant. This allows for decentralized access and remote reading, thereby facilitating interpretation in a timely manner. Additionally, as in any procedure room, access to oxygen and an emergency call button in case of medical emergency are essential. For staff, adequate access to personal protective equipment, including gloves, gowns, face shields, and a mask, is a must.

An important consideration also includes infection control between procedures. Generally, items that are permanent fixtures within the physical space, such as the mobile computer, manometry tower, or stretcher, should be cleaned within the standards of the hospital system's policies. Esophageal manometry, pH impedance, and anorectal manometry catheters are reusable and require a higher-level disinfection process, the details of which are beyond the scope of this chapter, to reduce cross-contamination and protect the fragile sensors [5]. There is a trend for most GI motility labs to prefer on-site sterilization rather than sending the fragile manometry catheters to an off-site facility. While this requires coordination between the director and the hospital system's infection control team and for frontline staff to pre-clean and wrap used catheters in biohazard bins prior to transporting to central processing, this allows for close oversight of infection control standards and helps guarantee consistent turnaround time for equipment. This centralized model requires advanced planning and effort but minimizes potential delays in lab operations related to disinfection.

Patient-Centered Approach

Manometry studies are invasive, uncomfortable, and sensitive examinations for patients and are not performed under sedation. Discomfort and intolerance are frequent causes of incomplete procedures. Therefore, approaching the manometry experience from a patient's viewpoint offers the best opportunity for success and completed studies. There are several strategies that can be employed to enhance the patient experience. First is establishing an open atmosphere for two-way communication. This starts with discussing the procedure steps at the beginning of the visit, even if education has been given during the initial clinic visit or via handout material prior to the visit. Continuous reassurance and coaching during the study are essential, especially during uncomfortable parts such as trans-nasal insertion of the esophageal manometry catheter. Further, it is important provide autonomy and remind patients that they are in the driver's seat and are allowed to give feedback including needing a break, the pace of the test, and whether they would like stop the study. Consideration of chaperones or gender-preferred providers for anorectal manometry may help ease some patients' concerns. Administering lidocaine spray for esophageal manometry may facilitate passage of the catheter. In certain situations, some clinicians ordering the study may elect to provide a small dose of a benzodiazepine in advance to help with procedure-related anxiety for esophageal manometry, akin to use during magnetic resonance imaging studies, although this would require the patient to have an escort home. Offering the opportunity to select background music may enhance a comforting environment for patients. If the patient is completing the study at home, such as pH impedance or wireless motility capsule testing, the patient should be discharged with verbal and written information on the study protocol, a contact number in case there are procedure-related symptoms or equipment issues, and when to return the equipment.

Documentation and Interpretation

Standard templates customized for the needs of the referral base and the practice should be used for reporting results and impressions, with the ability to free-text further input. All interpretation should be based on any present and available clinical standards that are integrated into templates. As of the time of this writing, esophageal manometry interpretation is presently based on Chicago Classification version 4.0 (2020), reflux evaluation based on Lyon Consensus (2018), and anorectal manometry based on London Classification (2019) [8–10]. The intricacies of these guidelines can be reviewed separately via the references. Templating documentation allows for consistent reporting and helps ensure guidelines are followed among a variety of clinicians interpreting the studies. Finalized documentation should be sent to referring providers within a week of completion to facilitate expeditious care.

Quality Metrics and Measures

There are no present set recommendations or guidelines to define how well a motility lab is being run. However, here we propose a few metrics to track and self-evaluate for continued improvement (Table 6.2):

Table 6.2 Proposed gastrointestinal laboratory quality metrics and measures

Metric	Benchmark	Some potential improvement areas
Number of weekly cases	• 90% of procedure slots have scheduled patients • >90% show rate	• Workflow of referrals and scheduling • Patient outreach
Completion rates	• 98% of patients scheduled fully complete protocol	• Pre-procedure patient education • Patient-centered experience
Accurate placement of manometry catheters	• 100% of esophageal manometry studies should have landmarks identified	• Education and training of staff • Open availability of providers to help troubleshoot
Template usage	• 100% of studies reported using a defined template	• Workflow optimization among motility providers
Timely report completion	• Studies interpreted within 1–2 weeks of procedure date	• Decentralized access to motility studies and software • Workflow optimization among motility providers

1. **Number of weekly cases**: is each slot being filled based on the referral numbers with a high show rate? A deficiency here may suggest that there is a workflow issue between referral receipt and ability to schedule or that there are insufficient reminders to patients prior to appointments.
2. **Completion rates**: are the majority of patients arriving for their study have had adequate pre-procedure preparation and able to finish the entire study protocol? Poor completion rates may suggest need to enhance pre-procedure education and outreach or improve the patient-centered experience.
3. **Accurate catheter placement**: are pertinent esophageal landmarks such as the upper and lower esophageal sphincters and the diaphragmatic crura appropriately used to place the catheter correctly during esophageal manometry and appropriate stabilization of the catheter in the anal canal during anorectal manometry? Incorrectly placed catheters may reflect gaps in foundational and technical knowledge among frontline staff.
4. **Templates**: are standardized templates for studies being used by all interpreting physicians within the practice?
5. **Timely completed reports:** are finalized interpretations with recommendations available within 1–2 weeks of the procedure?

Concluding Remarks

GI motility testing has become an important part of evaluation for many patients presenting for GI consultation including dysphagia, gastroesophageal reflux, dyspepsia- or gastroparesis-like symptoms, abdominal pain, bloating, constipation, and fecal incontinence. Running an efficient GI motility laboratory has several components including a coordinated schedule scheme, assembling a well-informed team, having updated and streamlined equipment, and optimizing the patient experience in efforts to achieve a higher study completion rate. Increasing demand for motility testing highlights the importance of ensuring quality output from a motility laboratory, as these studies play a critical role in advancing our understanding of a variety of burdensome diseases.

Disclosures Brian Surjanhata has no disclosures to report.
Kyle Staller has served as a consultant to Anji, Arena, Boston Pharmaceuticals, Gelesis, GI Supply, Sanofi, and Shire/Takeda and has received research support from Ironwood and Urovant.

References

1. Chang L. Review article: epidemiology and quality of life in functional gastrointestinal disorders. Aliment Pharmacol Ther. 2004;20(Suppl 7):31–9.
2. Sperber AD, Bangdiwala SI, Drossman DA, Ghoshal UC, Simren M, Tack J, et al. Worldwide prevalence and burden of functional gastrointestinal disorders, results of Rome Foundation Global Study. Gastroenterology. 2021;160(1):99–114.e3.
3. Parkman HP, Orr WC. The gastrointestinal motility laboratory. Gastrointest Endosc Clin N Am. 2009;19(1):171–84, viii.
4. Yadlapati R, Chen JW, Khan A. How to set up a successful motility lab. Gastroenterology. 2020;158(5):1202–10.
5. Baker JR, Curtin BF, Moshiree B, Rao SSC. Organizing and developing a GI motility lab in community practice: challenges and rewards. Curr Gastroenterol Rep. 2022;24(6):73–87.
6. Yadlapati R, Keswani RN, Pandolfino JE. Competency based medical education in gastrointestinal motility. Neurogastroenterol Motil. 2016;28(10):1460–4.
7. Gyawali CP, Savarino E, Lazarescu A, Bor S, Patel A, Dickman R, et al. Curriculum for neurogastroenterology and motility training: a report from the joint ANMS-ESNM task force. Neurogastroenterol Motil. 2018;30(9):e13341.
8. Yadlapati R, Kahrilas PJ, Fox MR, Bredenoord AJ, Prakash Gyawali C, Roman S, et al. Esophageal motility disorders on high-resolution manometry: Chicago classification version 4.0©. Neurogastroenterol Motil. 2021;33(1):e14058.
9. Gyawali CP, Kahrilas PJ, Savarino E, Zerbib F, Mion F, Smout AJPM, et al. Modern diagnosis of GERD: the Lyon Consensus. Gut. 2018;67(7):1351–62.
10. Carrington EV, Heinrich H, Knowles CH, Fox M, Rao S, Altomare DF, et al. The International Anorectal Physiology Working Group (IAPWG) recommendations: standardized testing protocol and the London classification for disorders of anorectal function. Neurogastroenterol Motil. 2020;32(1):e13679.

Chapter 7
Quality in Capsule Endoscopy

Samuel J. Miller and Daniel S. Mishkin

Table of Quality Measures/Metrics

Key Points

- Physician education and experience are important to help readers identify normal and abnormal findings.
- Appropriate reporting of the capsule findings to better direct referring providers with the management of their patients.
- Recognize the importance of the indication to help interpret the capsule findings as well as the clinical scenario to provide recommendations.
- Understand the appropriateness and availability of complementary testing.
- Be aware of strategies to optimize diagnostic yield for individual clinical scenarios.

S. J. Miller
Gastro Health, Framingham, MA, USA
e-mail: sjmille1@bidmc.harvard.edu

D. S. Mishkin (✉)
Division of Gastroenterology, Atrius Health, Boston, MA, USA
e-mail: Daniel_Mishkin@AtriusHealth.org

J. D. Feuerstein, D. J. Stein (eds.), *Quality in Gastroenterology*,
https://doi.org/10.1007/978-3-031-58492-3_7

Small bowel video capsule endoscopy (SB-VCE) is an attractive testing modality for many physicians and patients given that it is relatively noninvasive and low risk and allows for direct visualization of the small bowel mucosa that is typically unreachable by standard esophagogastroduodenoscopy or colonoscopy. This technology is one of the newer diagnostic modalities in the field of gastroenterology, as the first capsule was approved by the FDA in 2000 [1]. At this time, SB-VCE is a necessary testing modality in the field of gastroenterology and is not universally performed by all gastroenterologists.

Overview of Capsule Systems

Over the years, there have been multiple capsule endoscopy companies and cameras designed to evaluate dedicated areas of the gastrointestinal tract. This chapter will review the quality issues related to such small intestinal evaluations. Healthcare teams should become familiar with the pros and cons of the various systems that are available in your area of practice, specifically the various different hardware and software combinations. We are fortunate that, over the years, this technology continues to improve with wider field of view, increased and even variable camera frame rates, prolonged battery life, additional cameras, and even capsules that have forward, backward, and 360-degree panoramic views around the belly of the device [2]. Some have incorporated a two-way data transmission for real-time adjustments of light intensity and capsule rates, while others can be controlled with an external magnet which may help target the identification of a lesion and also facilitate gastric emptying [3]. The data is generally stored via the use of wireless transmissions to an external storage device.

While there are differences in the hardware, there are also differences between the software systems that download the videos and the ways in which the images are viewed. In addition, some software systems have aids that can help detect abnormalities for a more expedient review [2]. We encourage capsule readers to be aware of the differences between various capsule hardware and software, in order to optimize the use of technologies that provide more efficient and accurate reads, in an effort to perform high-quality SB-VCE.

Physician Training

The quality of an SB-VCE study is variably influenced by the competency of the capsule reader, which appears to be associated with prior experience reading SB-VCE and with other endoscopic procedures. Several studies have formally demonstrated that interobserver agreement on small bowel findings, small bowel polyp detection rate, small bowel polyp sizing, and detection of subtle lesions were all improved in operators with prior experience reading SB-VCE and performance of other endoscopic procedures [4–7]. In light of these findings, it is generally accepted that formal training is required to perform high-quality SB-VCE though the exact recommendations for training vary between organizations and have evolved over the past two decades.

In 2005, the American Society for Gastrointestinal Endoscopy (ASGE) released a guideline statement suggesting that standard training in SB-VCE should be considered separately from training in other endoscopic techniques. A practitioner considered competent in SB-VCE should have completed 24 months of gastroenterology fellowship, should have completed training in upper endoscopy and colonoscopy, and concluded formal SB-VCE training including didactic teaching of 8 h or more and a hands-on course [8, 9]. There was also a recommendation that a trainee complete a certain number of directly supervised SB-VCEs though the exact number of recommended studies has evolved over time; the most recent ASGE guidelines from 2017 suggest that trainees should perform 20 directly observed SB-VCEs, with a goal of 90% correlation in their findings with a credentialed SB-VCE reader [10]. The American College of Gastroenterology (ACG) released a consensus statement in the same year that reiterated the recommendations of the ASGE and again acknowledged that SB-VCE should be performed only by readers who had completed adequate training and demonstrated competency in SB-VCE through performance of supervised SB-VCE [5]. However, these statements are recommendations and based primarily on expert opinion and not robust data. In 2019, the European Society of Gastrointestinal Endoscopy (ESGE) guidelines suggested that 30–50 studies are required to be considered competent [11]. The ESGE subsequently published a curriculum that includes a number of capsule cases and combined didactic and hands-on training that are required to perform high-quality SB-VCE [12]. This robust program, which includes direct observation, proctoring, and test videos, demonstrated competency in trainees, when compared to attending physicians, after 20 cases. Another study suggested 25 cases was where the learning curve flattened and competency was achieved [13].

As we continue to address the optimal number of cases needed to achieve true competency, and read independently, it still remains unknown how many yearly cases must be performed to maintain one's skillset, and whether there is a role for refresher courses in the future, in order to do so.

Pre-procedural Evaluations

In many practices, SB-VCE is performed by a small subset of gastroenterologists. Therefore, SB-VCE may be ordered by gastroenterologists who do not perform SB-VCE or physicians from another specialty, such as primary care or surgery. As a result, a high-quality SB-VCE requires an appropriate indication and careful patient selection, preparation, execution, and interpretation of results to inform clinical care.

Common Indications for the procedure include the evaluation of overt and obscure sources of gastrointestinal bleeding in the small bowel, iron deficiency anemia, diagnosis and staging of small bowel Crohn's disease, identification of small bowel malignancies, screening for polyps in patients with known polyposis syndromes, diagnosis and staging of other small bowel enteropathies such as suspected or refractory celiac disease, and to further evaluate abnormal small intestinal imaging [14–18]. At times, additional indications may be clinically appropriate, even though it may be of lower yield, such as diarrhea or abdominal pain. It is strongly recommended that the reader be aware of the indication for the capsule referral as it may affect the interpretation.

SB-VCE is contraindicated in patients under 2 years of age and in patients with known or suspected gastrointestinal obstruction, stricture, or fistula, due to concerns regarding capsule retention, as discussed below. Historically, SB-VCE has also been contraindicated in patients with implanted electromedical devices, such as cardiac pacemakers, though more recent literature suggests that SB-VCE may be performed in this patient population without additional precautions [19, 20]. However, the ESGE no longer considers it a contraindication, and the American Gastroenterological Association (AGA) generally endorses use in patients with pacemakers [20].

Pregnancy is a relative contraindication for SB-VCE. There is a theoretical risk of capsule retention from reduced gastrointestinal motility and pressure on the gastrointestinal tract from the gravid uterus, though this has not been formally studied, and there have been case reports of successful SB-VCE use to identify gastrointestinal bleeding in pregnancy [21, 22]. Swallowing disorders are also recognized as a relative contraindication to SB-VCE, though this can be mitigated with the use of a capsule delivery device, if needed. Finally, SB-VCE is contraindicated in patients who are planned to undergo magnetic resonance imaging (MRI), and patients should proceed with the MRI first, and then SB-VCE, once it has been documented that the capsule has passed out of the body, clinically or radiographically. The theoretical risk of retained video capsule at the time of an MRI can result in bowel injury related to MRI forces exerted on the capsule, as well as potential interference in the MRI study. However, several case reports of patients undergoing MRI with retained capsules discussed no adverse events related to capsule retention [23].

A high-quality SB-VCE is generally preceded by an overnight fast, usually beginning the night prior to the procedure, though some centers advocate for a clear liquid diet for the 24 h prior to the procedure, while others recommend a bowel preparation. Significant controversy remains over the use of a full or partial bowel preparation with or without purgative medications the day before the procedure, as the present body of literature has demonstrated conflicting evidence [24, 25]. In theory, a bowel preparation would serve to optimize visualization of the mucosa and thus improve diagnostic yield. It is also potentially conferring benefit by encouraging a faster small intestinal transit time resulting in a more complete evaluation of the small intestine. With the conflicting data, many weigh the patient preference of not wanting to take a bowel prep with these theoretical benefits.

Patients are recommended to avoid iron supplementation for at least 3 days prior to the procedure, as it may create the appearance of melena in the small bowel lumen [26]. Patients should also be instructed to wear loose fitting clothes in order to be able to accommodate the data recording device worn for the duration of the study.

Prior to swallowing the capsule, providers should confirm that the capsule is paired appropriately with the recording device. The capsule should then be swallowed by the patient in a seated position with a sip of water; some literature suggests that adding simethicone to the water improves visualization of the mucosa by reducing bubbles in the small bowel [25, 27]. Some authors advise that the administration of a prokinetic agent, such as metoclopramide or erythromycin, improves the quality of capsule studies, especially in populations of patients with slowed gut motility such as diabetics or patients on psychoactive medications; one large meta-analysis suggests that prokinetic agents do improve completion rate of SB-VCE (i.e., the percentage of capsules that reach the cecum) but have little impact on diagnostic yield [28, 29].

Patients that have difficulty swallowing, delayed gastric emptying, or altered anatomy in the upper gastrointestinal tract are not necessarily unable to have SB-VCE, though these issues should make one question if endoscopic capsule placement may be needed. The use of a capsule deployment device can mitigate these potential barriers and is generally employed after an initial failed attempt to ingest the capsule in typical fashion [30]. The AdvanCE device is one such device which includes a disposable catheter that is preloaded through the gastroscope instrument channel and therefore requires an upper endoscopy to be completed. A specialized capsule cup is screwed onto the distal end of the catheter as it exits the scope instrument channel, and the activated video capsule is loaded into the cup. Providers should ensure that the capsule is appropriately paired to the recording device before placement. After a complete upper endoscopy, the endoscope is withdrawn and loaded with the accessory deployment device before reinserting the gastroscope with the leading capsule delivery device into the mouth and then to the desired anatomical location where it will be deployed, typically in the duodenum. The capsule is released by a spring-loaded mechanism which is activated using a thumb ring in the handle at the proximal end of the catheter, similar to a snare handle.

Perhaps the most feared complication of SB-VCE is capsule retention, which is defined by the video capsule remaining in the gastrointestinal tract for greater than 2 weeks, or requiring a procedural intervention to remove it [31]. Retained capsules have been linked with bowel obstruction and perforation, though the absolute risk of either of these complications is low [32–35]. A high-quality SB-VCE requires that patients are appropriately evaluated for their risk of retention before their procedure; if the risk is deemed to be high, additional testing may be needed such as cross-sectional imaging or a patency capsule endoscopy to be performed prior to a formal SB-VCE. Such risk factors include a history of gastrointestinal obstruction, abdominal surgeries, Crohn's disease, chronic nonsteroidal anti-inflammatory drug use, abdominal or pelvic radiation, or symptoms that could potentially be a harbinger of a partial or complete small bowel obstruction. The indication for SB-VCE is also important to review, as the risk of retention is somewhat dependent on the procedural indication. For instance, in one meta-analysis, the incidence of capsule retention during SB-VCE was found to be 1.2% when performed to evaluate gastrointestinal bleeding, while the incidence was 2.6% and 2.1% when evaluating Crohn's disease and for neoplasms, respectively [31]. It has been suggested that the target should be for 2% or lower overall retention rate, irrespective of the indication, and this should be audited yearly [11]. This information can be used to appropriately counsel the patient on the relative risks and benefits of the SB-VCE and also should inform a clinician's decision on whether to pursue additional testing.

If there is significant concern for a possible stricture or potential for capsule retention, a patency capsule endoscopy should be performed prior to formal SB-VCE. The patency capsule, which is similar in size to the video capsule, consists of a metal radiofrequency identification tag surrounded by an absorbable material and a small amount of barium [2]. The patency capsule is swallowed by the patient, and after 30 h, the capsule begins to dissolve, leaving only the miniscule metal radiofrequency identification tag and the outer casing. To assess for passage of the patency capsule, an abdominal X-ray or a spot CT scan can be used to assess the location of the patency capsule and verify if it has passed through the small intestine or not. Studies have suggested that successful passage of the patency capsule into the colon or out of the body, without symptoms of obstruction, after 30 h indicates that the video capsule will pass through the small bowel successfully and that SB-VCE can be safely performed with a very low risk of capsule retention [36, 37]. Though exceedingly rare, there have been case reports of small bowel obstruction with the patency capsule [38].

While a possible capsule retention can be suspected should the device have limited to no movement in the same area of the small intestine with or without associated luminal contents, or if the capsule remains in the small intestine at the end of the recording, this does not necessarily mean the capsule is retained. The capsule may have a delay in passage but still pass naturally. For example, failure of the video capsule to reach the colon can be seen in up to 16–30% of SB-VCE in different studies, simply due to delayed transit [31, 39, 40]. Therefore, in an asymptomatic patient, it is recommended that an abdominal X-ray be obtained at 2 weeks to verify passage. However, in a patient who is at higher-than-average risk for capsule retention, or if they have any concerning symptoms, imaging should be obtained even earlier. It should be noted that, if the capsule does reach the cecum during the SB-VCE, there is no need to confirm passage into the rectum as there have been no reported cases of capsule retention in the colon.

If capsule retention does occur, timely assessment and treatment are essential quality metrics. The ideal approach is dependent on locally available expertise, the location of the capsule, and the likely pathology leading to capsule retention. Options typically include surgical removal, endoscopic removal, or medical therapy in the setting of enteropathies [41]. For example, in patients with active Crohn's disease, this can be best managed medically and/or endoscopically. For suspected

NSAID enteropathy, if the patient remains asymptomatic, stopping the offending medication may help the capsule pass naturally. However, if a neoplasm is suspected, the potential treatment plan may need to include a surgical intervention, performed in an expedited fashion if there is a retained video capsule, as the definitive treatment is generally surgical. Irrespective of the management strategy, each case of capsule retention should be addressed promptly, as part of a high-quality SB-VCE program.

Reporting the Procedure Results

Most providers will only be reviewing the finalized SB-VCE report, though, if possible, a gastroenterologist will most likely want to see images of significant clinical findings. Therefore, it is important to know how to complete a report that communicates the necessary information including the indication, identification of the appropriate landmarks, descriptions of the findings and their possible locations if needed, and a treatment plan. In addition, having an appropriate expectation for the timing of a capsule read is important, as one should try to read capsules as soon as the videos have been processed and not delay it for an extended period of time. For example, it would be inappropriate to leave a capsule unread for a patient who may be actively bleeding.

The first important step for a provider reading an SB-VCE is to identify the landmarks, recognizing that there are limited definitive ones in the small intestine. The first of such landmarks is the identification of the stomach as the capsule passes the gastroesophageal junction and the appearance of the gastric rugae. The first duodenal image should also be marked and should be the last time the capsule passes through the pylorus, as the capsule can sometimes pass into the duodenum and regurgitate back into the stomach before eventually advancing distally. As the capsule passes through the duodenum, the ampulla of Vater may be appreciated but may also be difficult to visualize. In the normal small intestine, there are no specific landmarks until the cecum is reached, which should be annotated. Documentation of these landmarks assists with communication of results as they can help indirectly estimate a potential finding's location, when time between findings and landmarks is calculated.

The ability to provide additional comments about the adequacy of mucosal visualization is another important feature to document. Similar to the need to document the bowel preparation on a colonoscopy, additional information should be provided to ensure that the bowel is sufficiently clean to visualize the mucosa adequately; if not, this may affect diagnostic yield. In addition, there is some concern that too rapid a passage can also lead to an incomplete evaluation as it has been suspected that a small bowel transit time of less than 2 h can increase the risk of a missed lesion [42].

A high-quality SB-VCE should also use consistent terms to describe normal and abnormal findings and take each unique patient presentation into consideration, thereby allowing for optimal interpretation by ordering physicians and determination of appropriate next steps in clinical care. A standard lexicon of terms for describing small bowel findings, known as the "capsule endoscopy structured terminology" (CEST), was compiled by experts in SB-VCE after review of 766 cases with both normal and abnormal findings [43]. Using this lexicon, small bowel lesions are ideally categorized as flat (angioectasia, spot, and plaque), protruding (mass/tumor, polyp, nodule, and venous structure), and excavated lesions (ulcer, erosion, aphtha, scar, and diverticulum). More diffuse findings are classified as villous abnormalities (atrophic and abnormal villi) or mucosal abnormalities (erythematous, pale, edematous, granular, and nodular). Discrete luminal findings are described accordingly as well (stenosis, dilation, and surgical anastomosis). The use of precise language and consideration of a specific patient's clinical scenario is especially relevant to the performance of high-quality SB-VCE, as the clinical implications and follow-up recommendations after the study may be heavily influenced by how findings are described. For instance, the differentiation of an "angioectasia" from a "red spot" is critical in an SB-VCE performed for evaluation of gastrointestinal bleeding, as an angioectasia has a higher risk of bleeding than a red spot, and thus may warrant performance of additional endoscopic procedures for therapeutic purposes, rather than watchful waiting. Similarly, a protruding venous structure noted in a patient with cirrhosis and portal hypertension could be suggestive of a small bowel varix, whereas in a patient without these conditions, an analogous lesion would be classified as a benign entity, such as a venous bleb. The precise differentiation between excavated lesions also remains clinically relevant. For instance, ulcerations may be suggestive of early inflammatory bowel disease in the appropriate patient population, whereas the clinical relevance of single erosions or a few aphthae is less clear, especially if patients are using enterotoxic medications, such as nonsteroidal anti-inflammatories [44]. Clearly, while each SB-VCE may present a unique array of small bowel findings, attempts at standard reporting of normal and abnormal results are essential to perform a high-quality SB-VCE that will produce meaningful information to direct patient care.

Providing Recommendations

When an abnormality is found, or even in the absence of clinically significant findings, referring providers may be seeking guidance from the provider performing SB-VCE on appropriate next steps in the patient's clinical care. Therefore, it is important to communicate well with the referring provider and be aware of what additional services are available at their center, as well as the diagnostic yield of additional modalities, relative to SB-VCE.

Complementary testing with endoscopic techniques is typically considered in the context of obscure gastrointestinal bleeding, though it is also considered in the evaluation of small bowel enteropathies and neoplasms. The diagnostic yield was found to be 56% for SB-VCE compared to 26% for push enteroscopy in one pooled analysis containing 396 patients, while a subsequent, smaller study showed more modest findings, though also in favor of SB-VCE with regard to diagnostic yield (50% vs. 24%) [45, 46]. Double-balloon enteroscopy (DBE), which allows more complete visualization of the small bowel when compared to push enteroscopy, has also been evaluated against SB-VCE for detection of obscure gastrointestinal bleeding. Retrospective studies have generally suggested that the diagnostic yield of these modalities is similar (64% for DBE and 54% for SB-VCE, respectively), and a prospective study evaluating agreement between SB-VCE and DBE findings suggested that, overall, the concordance between SB-VCE and DBE is moderate, as measured by kappa coefficient. However, this study stratified concordance for each type of lesion identified and noted that concordance was higher for vascular and inflammatory lesions than for neoplasias [47, 48]. Several small studies support the notion that DBE is superior to SB-VCE with regard to diagnostic yield when evaluating for small bowel neoplasias. One small study of 183 patients demonstrated 18 patients had small bowel mass lesions identified on DBE; 15 of these patients had SB-VCE, of which only 5 identified the mass [49]. An even smaller study showed similar findings, with DBE identifying more patients with small bowel masses and more masses per patient than SB-VCE [50]. Though less well studied, the use of DBE compared to SB-VCE in evaluation of small bowel enteropathies has been evaluated, with one study reporting a superior diagnostic yield when evaluating Crohn's disease in DBE over SB-VCE, though in different patient cohorts (52% vs. 29%, respectively) [51]. Regardless of the indication, it is prudent to recognize that no test is perfect, and while the deep enteroscopies can also perform biopsies, tattoos, and other therapeutic maneuvers, it is more invasive and may require both anterograde and retrograde procedures to be complete, if necessary.

Imaging tests also can serve as complementary modalities to SB-VCE, when evaluating small bowel pathology. With regard to diagnostic yield of obscure gastrointestinal bleeding, SB-VCE has outperformed small bowel barium radiography for clinically significant findings greater than or equal to 30%, due to the ability to visualize additional vascular and inflammatory lesions [45]. For evaluation of small bowel neoplasia, SB-VCE has been compared to both small bowel follow-through and magnetic resonance enterography (MRE). SB-VCE outperformed small bowel follow-through in a small study of patients with gastrointestinal polyposis syndromes, with a superior diagnostic yield (27% vs. 12.5%) and a greater number of polyps detected overall. When evaluated against MRE for screening of small bowel neoplasms in patients with familial adenomatous polyposis and Peutz-Jeghers syndrome, SB-VCE was found to have a similar diagnostic yield for polyps >15 mm in size but a superior sensitivity for detecting smaller lesions [52]. Of note, MRE does provide additional information regarding anatomic location and extraintestinal pathology, which confers another advantage to this modality. The use of SB-VCE as compared to various radiologic modalities has also been evaluated with regard to diagnosis and monitoring of Crohn's disease, with variable results [53]. One small study of 41 patients comparing CT enterography, small bowel follow-through, SB-VCE, and ileocolonoscopy showed no significant difference in sensitivity for active disease detection, yet it did suggest that SB-VCE was less specific in this regard. However, a similarly sized study showed that SB-VCE was more sensitive than small bowel follow-through and CT scan in diagnosis of Crohn's disease [54]. Essentially, high-quality SB-VCE remains a superior diagnostic modality in certain clinical contexts; it is important to consider the use of available radiologic methods and other endoscopic procedures as alternative and complementary tests, as deemed appropriate.

Additional Ways to Improve Quality

Physicians should always try and stay up to date and improve their skills to stay ahead of the curve. Below are a few suggestions that are based on clinical experience that may help improve quality and efficiency performing SB-VCE:

- Ensure the reader is allocating enough time for the capsule read and is not rushing or distracted.
- Recognize one's abilities and try to test oneself, with regard to the speed at which a reader can view a recorded capsule video, and still identify abnormalities. It is not advised to read at very high frame rates as there is even data to suggest that reading at a frame rate of >20 frames per second is associated with an increased chance of missing a lesion [55]. This will evolve over time with experience and also depends somewhat on the individual video and differing segments of the gastrointestinal tract.
- Do not hesitate to order a repeat SB-VCE as this may allow providers and patients to benefit from both recordings. This may be relevant if the prep was suboptimal or the capsule passed through the small intestine too quickly. However, it may also be relevant if a patient has a persistent problem that requires additional investigation. For example, the diagnostic yield of SB-VCE after suspected bleed may be higher when administered closer to the clinical bleed [56, 57]. Therefore a prior negative study should not negate the need for a repeat SB-VCE test in the correct clinical context.
- Capsule readers should follow up on patients with abnormalities that may require additional testing or interventions to confirm the findings. This will help capsule readers continue to learn from the cases they have read.
- Review all complications, such as capsule retentions, and assess if it may have been avoided or even predicted, given the clinical scenario.
- Identify another provider that one can discuss cases as well as review images or videos with, should there be uncertainty about the findings. With more experience, this will become less frequent, but even seasoned providers may benefit from a second opinion in difficult cases.

Conclusion

For any center performing high-quality SB-VCE procedures, it is obvious that appropriate equipment and careful patient selection is required to ensure that SB-VCE studies have superior diagnostic yield and minimal risk of complication for patients. Furthermore, physicians performing SB-VCE should have standard training and use precise language to describe findings to avoid ambiguity. Additional endoscopic and radiographic modalities should always be considered for complementary or alternative testing, if appropriate and available. Ideally, a high-quality center should ideally be able to share images in order to solicit additional clinical opinions in cases with uncertain pathology, or when complementary testing fails to clarify a diagnosis. Ultimately, these elements should optimize clinicians' ability to make a clear diagnosis and not simply describe findings, with the goal of advancing a patient's clinical care. Referring physicians should be promptly informed of findings, diagnostic impressions, and clinical recommendations, such that next steps in diagnosis and management can be optimally determined.

Quality Metrics

- Awareness of the hardware and software of the SB-VCE system being used.
- Ensuring physician credentialing—adequate experience +/− training.
- Appropriate indication selection.
- Awareness of known contraindications and risks of capsule retention.
- Appropriate preparation and troubleshooting for individual patient needs.
- Reporting the capsule findings appropriately, consistently, and promptly.
- Awareness of appropriate and available complementary testing.

References

1. Mishkin DS, Chuttani R, Croffie J, Disario J, Liu J, Shah R, Somogyi L, Tierney W, Wong Kee Song LM, Petersen BT. ASGE technology status evaluation report: wireless capsule endoscopy. Gastrointest Endosc. 2006;63:539–45. https://doi.org/10.1016/j.gie.2006.01.014.
2. Melson J, Trikudanathan G, Abu Dayyeh BK, Bhutani MS, Chandrasekhara V, Jirapinyo P, Krishnan K, Kumta NA, Pannala R, Parsi MA, Sethi A, Trindade AJ, Watson RR, Maple JT, Lichtenstein DR. Video capsule endoscopy. Gastrointest Endosc. 2021;93(4):784–96. https://doi.org/10.1016/j.gie.2020.12.001.
3. Luo YY, Pan J, Chen YZ, Jiang X, Zou WB, Qian YY, Zhou W, Liu X, Li ZS, Liao Z. Magnetic steering of capsule endoscopy improves small bowel capsule endoscopy completion rate. Dig Dis Sci. 2019;64:1908–15. https://doi.org/10.1007/s10620-019-5479-z.
4. Petroniene R, Dubcenco E, Baker JP, Ottaway CA, Tang SJ, Zanati SA, Streutker CJ, Gardiner GW, Warren RE, Jeejeebhoy KN. Given capsule endoscopy in celiac disease: evaluation of diagnostic accuracy and interobserver agreement. Am J Gastroenterol. 2005;100:685–94. https://doi.org/10.1111/j.1572-0241.2005.41069.x.

5. Postgate A, Tekkis P, Fitzpatrick A, Bassett P, Fraser C. The impact of experience on polyp detection and sizing accuracy at capsule endoscopy: implications for training from an animal model study. Endoscopy. 2008;40:496–501. https://doi.org/10.1055/s-2007-995590.
6. Jang BI, Lee SH, Moon JS, Cheung DY, Lee IS, Kim JO, Cheon JH, Park CH, Byeon JS, Park YS, Shim KN, Kim YS, Kim KJ, Lee KJ, Ryu JK, Chang DK, Chun HJ, Choi MG. Interobserver agreement on the interpretation of capsule endoscopy findings based on capsule endoscopy structured terminology: a multicenter study by the Korean Gut Image Study Group. Scand J Gastroenterol. 2010;45:370–4. https://doi.org/10.3109/00365520903521574.
7. Pezzoli A, Cannizzaro R, Pennazio M, Rondonotti E, Zancanella L, Fusetti N, Simoni M, Cantoni F, Melina R, Alberani A, Caravelli G, Villa F, Chilovi F, Casetti T, Iaquinto G, D'imperio N, Gullini S. Interobserver agreement in describing video capsule endoscopy findings: a multicentre prospective study. Dig Liver Dis. 2011;43:126–31. https://doi.org/10.1016/j.dld.2010.07.007.
8. Koffas A, Laskaratos FM, Epstein O. Training in video capsule endoscopy: current status and unmet needs. World J Gastrointest Endosc. 2019;11(6):395–402. https://doi.org/10.4253/wjge.v11.i6.395.
9. Faigel DO, Baron TH, Adler DG, Davila RE, Egan J, Hirota WK, Jacobson BC, Leighton JA, Qureshi W, Rajan E, Zuckerman MJ, Fanelli R, Wheeler-Harbaugh J, ASGE. ASGE guideline: guidelines for credentialing and granting privileges for capsule endoscopy. Gastrointest Endosc. 2005;61:503–5. https://doi.org/10.1016/S0016-5107(04)02781-6.
10. Faulx AL, Lightdale JR, Acosta RD, Agrawal D, Bruining DH, Chandrasekhara V, Eloubeidi MA, Gurudu SR, Kelsey L, Khashab MA, Kothari S, Muthusamy VR, Qumseya BJ, Shaukat A, Wang A, Wani SB, Yang J, DeWitt JM. Guidelines for privileging, credentialing, and proctoring to perform GI endoscopy. Gastrointest Endosc. 2017;2017(85):273–81. https://doi.org/10.1016/j.gie.2016.10.036.
11. Spada C, McNamara D, Despott EJ, Adler S, Cash BD, Fernández-Urién I, Ivekovic H, Keuchel M, McAlindon N, Saurin JC, Panter S, Bellisario C, Minozzi S, Senore C, Bennett C, Bretthauer M, Dinis-Ribeiro M, Domagk D, Hassan C, Kaminski MF, Rees CJ, Valori R, Bisschops R, Rutter MD. Performance measures for small-bowel endoscopy: a European Society of Gastrointestinal Endoscopy (ESGE) quality improvement initiative. Endoscopy. 2019;51:574–98. https://doi.org/10.1055/a-0889-9586.
12. Sidhu R, Zammit SC, Baltes P, Carretero C, Despott EJ, Murino A, Dray X, Sanders DS, Keuchel M, Dekker E, East JE, Johnson G, Pimentel-Nunes P, Arvanitakis M, Ponchon T, Dinis-Ribeiro M, Bisschops R. Curriculum for small-bowel capsule endoscopy and device-assisted enteroscopy training in Europe: European Society of Gastrointestinal Endoscopy (ESGE) position statement. Endoscopy. 2020;52:669–86. https://doi.org/10.1055/a-1185-1289.
13. Rajan E, Martinez M, Gorospe E, Al Bawardy B, Dobashi A, Mara KC, Hansel SL, Bruining DH, Murray JA, Leggett CL, Nehra V, Iyer PG, Pasha SF, Leighton JA, Shiff AD, Gurudu SR, Raffals LE, Lavey C, Katzka DA, Chen CH. Prospective multicenter study to evaluate capsule endoscopy competency using a validated assessment tool. Gastrointest Endosc. 2020;91:1140–5. https://doi.org/10.1016/j.gie.2019.12.024.
14. ASGE Standards of Practice Committee, Early DS, Ben-Menachem T, Decker GA, Evans JA, Fanelli RD, Fisher DA, Fukami N, Hwang JH, Jain R, Jue TL, Khan KM, Malpas PM, Maple JT, Sharaf RS, Dominitz JA, Cash BD. Appropriate use of GI endoscopy. Gastrointest Endosc. 2012;75:1127–31. https://doi.org/10.1016/j.gie.2012.01.011.
15. Pennazio M, Spada C, Eliakim R, Keuchel M, May A, Mulder CJ, Rondonotti E, Adler SN, Albert J, Baltes P, Barbaro F, Cellier C, Charton JP, Delvaux M, Despott EJ, Domagk D, Klein A, McAlindon M, Rosa B, Rowse G, Sanders DS, Saurin JC, Sidhu R, Dumonceau JM, Hassan C, Gralnek IM. Small-bowel capsule endoscopy and device-assisted enteroscopy for diagnosis and treatment of small-bowel disorders: European Society of Gastrointestinal Endoscopy (ESGE) clinical guideline. Endoscopy. 2015;47:352–76. https://doi.org/10.1055/s-0034-1391855.
16. Yung DE, Koulaouzidis A, Avni T, Kopylov U, Giannakou A, Rondonotti E, Pennazio M, Eliakim R, Toth E, Plevris JN. Clinical outcomes of negative small-bowel capsule endos-

copy for small-bowel bleeding: a systematic review and meta-analysis. Gastrointest Endosc. 2017;85:305–317.e2. https://doi.org/10.1016/j.gie.2016.08.027.

17. Dionisio PM, Gurudu SR, Leighton JA, Leontiadis GI, Fleischer DE, Hara AK, Heigh RI, Shiff AD, Sharma VK. Capsule endoscopy has a significantly higher diagnostic yield in patients with suspected and established small-bowel Crohn's disease: a meta-analysis. Am J Gastroenterol. 2010;105:1240–8. https://doi.org/10.1038/ajg.2009.713.
18. Hall BJ, Holleran GE, Smith SM, Mahmud N, McNamara DA. A prospective 12-week mucosal healing assessment of small bowel Crohn's disease as detected by capsule endoscopy. Eur J Gastroenterol Hepatol. 2014;26:1253–9. https://doi.org/10.1097/MEG.0000000000000194.
19. Stanich PP, Kleinman B, Betkerur K, Mehta Oza N, Porter K, Meyer MM. Video capsule endoscopy is successful and effective in outpatients with implantable cardiac devices. Dig Endosc. 2014;26:726–30. https://doi.org/10.1111/den.12288.
20. Enns RA, Hookey L, Armstrong D, Bernstein CN, Heitman SJ, Teshima C, Leontiadis GI, Tse F, Sadowski D. Clinical practice guidelines for the use of video capsule endoscopy. Gastroenterology. 2017;152:497–514. https://doi.org/10.1053/j.gastro.2016.12.032.
21. Savas N. Gastrointestinal endoscopy in pregnancy. World J Gastroenterol. 2014;20:15241–52. https://doi.org/10.3748/wjg.v20.i41.15241.
22. Hogan RB, Ahmad N, Hogan RB III, Hensley SD, Phillips P, Doolittle P, Reimund E. Video capsule endoscopy detection of jejunal carcinoid in life-threatening hemorrhage, first trimester pregnancy. Gastrointest Endosc. 2007;66:205–7. https://doi.org/10.1016/j.gie.2006.11.021.
23. Bandorski D, Kurniawan N, Baltes P, Hoeltgen R, Hecker M, Stunder D, Keuchel M. Contraindications for video capsule endoscopy. World J Gastroenterol. 2016;22(45):9898–908. https://doi.org/10.3748/wjg.v22.i45.9898.
24. Gkolfakis P, Tziatzios G, Dimitriadis GD, Triantafyllou K. Meta-analysis of randomized controlled trials challenging the usefulness of purgative preparation before small-bowel video capsule endoscopy. Endoscopy. 2018;50:671–83. https://doi.org/10.1055/s-0043-125207.
25. Wei W, Ge ZZ, Lu H, Gao YJ, Hu YB, Xiao SD. Purgative bowel cleansing combined with simethicone improves capsule endoscopy imaging. Am J Gastroenterol. 2008;103:77–82. https://doi.org/10.1111/j.1572-0241.2007.01633.x.
26. Hanscom M, Stead C, Feldman H, Marya NB, Cave D. Video capsule endoscopy and device-assisted enteroscopy. Dig Dis Sci. 2022;67:1539–52. https://doi.org/10.1007/s10620-021-07085-0.
27. Fang YH, Chen CX, Zhang BL. Effect of small bowel preparation with simethicone on capsule endoscopy. J Zhejiang Univ Sci B. 2009;10:46–51. https://doi.org/10.1631/jzus.B0820148.
28. Costache RS, Lulache AI, Jinga M, Vlăduț C, Costache DO, Radu FI. Use of prokinetics and other quality factors in capsule endoscopy—old and new insights (review). Exp Ther Med. 2020;20:2484–8. https://doi.org/10.3892/etm.2020.8960.
29. Koulaouzidis A, Giannakou A, Yung DE, Dabos KJ, Plevris JN. Do prokinetics influence the completion rate in small-bowel capsule endoscopy? A systematic review and meta-analysis. Curr Med Res Opin. 2013;29:1171–85. https://doi.org/10.1185/03007995.2013.818532.
30. Holden JP, Dureja P, Pfau PR, Schwartz DC, Reichelderfer M, Judd RH, Danko I, Iyer LV, Gopal DV. Endoscopic placement of the small-bowel video capsule by using a capsule endoscope delivery device. Gastrointest Endosc. 2007;65:842–7. https://doi.org/10.1016/j.gie.2007.01.033.
31. Liao Z, Gao R, Xu C, Li ZS. Indications and detection, completion, and retention rates of small-bowel capsule endoscopy: a systematic review. Gastrointest Endosc. 2010;71:280–6. https://doi.org/10.1016/j.gie.2009.09.031.
32. Repici A, Barbon V, De Angelis C, Luigiano C, De Caro G, Hervoso C, Danese S, Preatoni P, Pagano N, Comunale S, Pennazio M, Rizzetto M. Acute small-bowel perforation secondary to capsule endoscopy. Gastrointest Endosc. 2008;67:180–3. https://doi.org/10.1016/j.gie.2007.05.044.
33. Um S, Poblete H, Zavotsky J. Small bowel perforation caused by an impacted endocapsule. Endoscopy. 2008;40(Suppl 2):E122–3. https://doi.org/10.1055/s-2007-995694.

34. Lin OS, Brandabur JJ, Schembre DB, Soon MS, Kozarek RA. Acute symptomatic small bowel obstruction due to capsule impaction. Gastrointest Endosc. 2007;65:725–8. https://doi.org/10.1016/j.gie.2006.11.033.
35. Pham T, Miller A, La Paglia D, Cham A. Small bowel obstruction with perforation secondary to PillCam. Case Rep Gastrointest Med. 2018;2018:9081742. https://doi.org/10.1155/2018/9081742.
36. Herrerias JM, Leighton JA, Costamagna G, Infantolino A, Eliakim R, Fischer D, Rubin DT, Manten HD, Scapa E, Morgan DR, Bergwerk AJ, Koslowsky B, Adler SN. Agile patency system eliminates risk of capsule retention in patients with known intestinal strictures who undergo capsule endoscopy. Gastrointest Endosc. 2008;67:902–9. https://doi.org/10.1016/j.gie.2007.10.063.
37. Spada C, Shah SK, Riccioni ME, Spera G, Marchese M, Iacopini F, Familiari P, Costamagna G. Video capsule endoscopy in patients with known or suspected small bowel stricture previously tested with the dissolving patency capsule. J Clin Gastroenterol. 2007;41:576–82. https://doi.org/10.1097/01.mcg.0000225633.14663.64.
38. Rasmussen B, Nathan T, Jensen MD. Symptomatic patency capsule retention in suspected Crohn's disease. J Crohns Colitis. 2016;10:1445–7. https://doi.org/10.1093/ecco-jcc/jjw105.
39. Höög CM, Bark LÅ, Arkani J, Gorsetman J, Broström O, Sjöqvist U. Capsule retentions and incomplete capsule endoscopy examinations: an analysis of 2300 examinations. Gastroenterol Res Pract. 2012;2012:518718. https://doi.org/10.1155/2012/518718.
40. Westerhof J, Weersma RK, Hoedemaker RA, Koornstra JJ. Completion rate of small bowel capsule endoscopy is higher after erythromycin compared to domperidone. BMC Gastroenterol. 2014;14:162. https://doi.org/10.1186/1471-230X-14-162.
41. Tanaka S, Mitsui K, Shirakawa K, Tatsuguchi A, Nakamura T, Hayashi Y, Sakamoto C, Terano A. Successful retrieval of video capsule endoscopy retained at ileal stenosis of Crohn's disease using double-balloon endoscopy. J Gastroenterol Hepatol. 2006;21:922–3. https://doi.org/10.1111/j.1440-1746.2006.04120.x.
42. Buscaglia JM, Kapoor S, Clarke JO, Bucobo JC, Giday SA, Magno P, Yong E, Mullin GE. Enhanced diagnostic yield with prolonged small bowel transit time during capsule endoscopy. Int J Med Sci. 2008;5:303–8. https://doi.org/10.7150/ijms.5.303.
43. Korman LY, Delvaux M, Gay G, Hagenmuller F, Keuchel M, Friedman S, Weinstein M, Shetzline M, Cave D, de Franchis R. Capsule endoscopy structured terminology (CEST): proposal of a standardized and structured terminology for reporting capsule endoscopy procedures. Endoscopy. 2005;37:951–9. https://doi.org/10.1055/s-2005-870329.
44. Mow WS, Lo SK, Targan SR, Dubinsky MC, Treyzon L, Abreu-Martin MT, Papadakis KA, Vasiliauskas EA. Initial experience with wireless capsule enteroscopy in the diagnosis and management of inflammatory bowel disease. Clin Gastroenterol Hepatol. 2004;2:31–40. https://doi.org/10.1016/s1542-3565(03)00289-1.
45. Triester SL, Leighton JA, Leontiadis GI, Fleischer DE, Hara AK, Heigh RI, Shiff AD, Sharma VK. A meta-analysis of the yield of capsule endoscopy compared to other diagnostic modalities in patients with obscure gastrointestinal bleeding. Am J Gastroenterol. 2005;100:2407–18. https://doi.org/10.1111/j.1572-0241.2005.00274.x.
46. Arakawa D, Ohmiya N, Nakamura M, Honda W, Shirai O, Itoh A, Hirooka Y, Niwa Y, Maeda O, Ando T, Goto H. Outcome after enteroscopy for patients with obscure GI bleeding: diagnostic comparison between double-balloon endoscopy and videocapsule endoscopy. Gastrointest Endosc. 2009;69:866–74. https://doi.org/10.1016/j.gie.2008.06.008.
47. Marmo R, Rotondano G, Casetti T, Manes G, Chilovi F, Sprujevnik T, Bianco MA, Brancaccio ML, Imbesi V, Benvenuti S, Pennazio M. Degree of concordance between double-balloon enteroscopy and capsule endoscopy in obscure gastrointestinal bleeding: a multicenter study. Endoscopy. 2009;41:587–92. https://doi.org/10.1055/s-0029-1214896.
48. Ross A, Mehdizadeh S, Tokar J, Leighton JA, Kamal A, Chen A, Schembre D, Chen G, Binmoeller K, Kozarek R, Waxman I, Dye C, Gerson L, Harrison ME, Haluszka O, Lo S,

Semrad C. Double balloon enteroscopy detects small bowel mass lesions missed by capsule endoscopy. Dig Dis Sci. 2008;53:2140–3. https://doi.org/10.1007/s10620-007-0110-0.
49. Matsumoto T, Esaki M, Moriyama T, Nakamura S, Iida M. Comparison of capsule endoscopy and enteroscopy with the double-balloon method in patients with obscure bleeding and polyposis. Endoscopy. 2005;37:827–32. https://doi.org/10.1055/s-2005-870207.
50. Sidhu R, McAlindon ME, Drew K, Hardcastle S, Cameron IC, Sanders DS. Evaluating the role of small-bowel endoscopy in clinical practice: the largest single-centre experience. Eur J Gastroenterol Hepatol. 2012;24:513–9. https://doi.org/10.1097/MEG.0b013e328350fb05.
51. Saperas E, Dot J, Videla S, Alvarez-Castells A, Perez-Lafuente M, Armengol JR, Malagelada JR. Capsule endoscopy versus computed tomographic or standard angiography for the diagnosis of obscure gastrointestinal bleeding. Am J Gastroenterol. 2007;102:731–7. https://doi.org/10.1111/j.1572-0241.2007.01058.x.
52. Caspari R, von Falkenhausen M, Krautmacher C, Schild H, Heller J, Sauerbruch T. Comparison of capsule endoscopy and magnetic resonance imaging for the detection of polyps of the small intestine in patients with familial adenomatous polyposis or with Peutz-Jeghers' syndrome. Endoscopy. 2004;36:1054–9. https://doi.org/10.1055/s-2004-826041.
53. Solem CA, Loftus EV Jr, Fletcher JG, Baron TH, Gostout CJ, Petersen BT, Tremaine WJ, Egan LJ, Faubion WA, Schroeder KW, Pardi DS, Hanson KA, Jewell DA, Barlow JM, Fidler JL, Huprich JE, Johnson CD, Harmsen WS, Zinsmeister AR, Sandborn WJ. Small-bowel imaging in Crohn's disease: a prospective, blinded, 4-way comparison trial. Gastrointest Endosc. 2008;68:255–66. https://doi.org/10.1016/j.gie.2008.02.017.
54. Jensen MD, Nathan T, Rafaelsen SR, Kjeldsen J. Diagnostic accuracy of capsule endoscopy for small bowel Crohn's disease is superior to that of MR enterography or CT enterography. Clin Gastroenterol Hepatol. 2011;9:124–9. https://doi.org/10.1016/j.cgh.2010.10.019.
55. Zheng Y, Hawkins L, Wolff J, Goloubeva O, Goldberg E. Detection of lesions during capsule endoscopy: physician performance is disappointing. Am J Gastroenterol. 2012;107:554–60. https://doi.org/10.1038/ajg.2011.461.
56. Singh A, Marshall C, Chaudhuri B, Okoli C, Foley A, Person SD, Bhattacharya K, Cave DR. Timing of video capsule endoscopy relative to overt obscure GI bleeding: implications from a retrospective study. Gastrointest Endosc. 2013;77:761–6. https://doi.org/10.1016/j.gie.2012.11.041.
57. Gomes C, Pinho R, Rodrigues A, Ponte A, Silva J, Rodrigues JP, Sousa M, Silva JC, Carvalho J. Impact of the timing of capsule endoscopy in overt obscure gastrointestinal bleeding on yield and rebleeding rate—is sooner than 14 d advisable? World J Gastrointest Endosc. 2018;10:74–82. https://doi.org/10.4253/wjge.v10.i4.74.

Chapter 8
Quality Care in Celiac Disease

Claire Jansson-Knodell and Alberto Rubio-Tapia

Table of Quality Measures/Metrics

C. Jansson-Knodell · A. Rubio-Tapia (✉)
Celiac Disease Program, Division of Gastroenterology, Hepatology, and Nutrition, Digestive Disease Institute, Cleveland Clinic, Cleveland, OH, USA
e-mail: janssoc@ccf.org; rubiota@ccf.org

J. D. Feuerstein, D. J. Stein (eds.), *Quality in Gastroenterology*, https://doi.org/10.1007/978-3-031-58492-3_8

Key Points

- Quality care starts by making a proper diagnosis of celiac disease as gluten ingestion can cause symptoms in patients with a number of other conditions that do not have the same morbidity and mortality risk as celiac disease.
- Diagnosis represents the beginning, not the end, of gastroenterologist involvement in the management of celiac disease.
- The role of the dietitian is vital when it comes to partnering with patients and providing education on the gluten-free diet.
- Regular follow-up and monitoring is the key to providing high-quality care for celiac disease patients.

Introduction to Celiac Disease

Celiac disease is an immune-mediated enteropathy that develops in genetically susceptible individuals after exposure to dietary gluten. It is a common disorder with a prevalence of around 1% in population-based studies [1, 2]. The flattening of the small intestine villi decreases the surface area available for absorption resulting in a malabsorptive state. The accompanying inflammation exacerbates the situation by causing net fluid secretion which leads to diarrhea. Symptoms other than diarrhea can include abdominal pain, bloating, weight loss, vitamin and micronutrient deficiencies, and a host of other ailments [3]. The multitude of possible presentations and overlap with other gastrointestinal and autoimmune conditions make it a challenging illness to diagnose. Treatment of celiac disease is a strict lifelong gluten-free diet. Alternative treatments are under investigation, but the lack of therapeutics beyond diet makes it a challenging illness to treat. Dietitians with their knowledge and expertise in the gluten-free diet are a key resource in celiac disease care. This chapter will describe quality care for the diagnosis and management of celiac disease.

Diagnosis

It is imperative to provide patients with an accurate diagnosis of celiac disease. There are many conditions where patients feel unwell after ingesting gluten beyond celiac disease (see Table 8.1). In non-celiac gluten sensitivity, irritable bowel syndrome (IBS) with fructan intolerance, and other food intolerances, the gluten-free diet is helpful but not as essential as in celiac disease. Strict dietary adherence may lead to symptom resolution, but it does not have the same clinical outcome and mortality benefits in these conditions. Namely, non-celiac gluten sensitivity, IBS, and food intolerance do not have the same malabsorptive nature, association with nutritional deficiencies, risk for concomitant autoimmune diseases, and increased chance of developing complications. Confirmation of the diagnosis with appropriate distinction between other conditions and celiac disease is the first step in providing high-quality care to these patients.

Table 8.1 Description of selected clinical conditions responsive to gluten-free diet

Condition	Characteristics
Celiac disease	Small intestine damage with villous atrophy and subsequent malabsorption of nutrients
Non-celiac gluten sensitivity	Reaction to gluten that is not immunologic or allergic but results in intestinal and extraintestinal symptoms [4, 5]
Irritable bowel syndrome	Response to gluten and other wheat components such as fructans; amylase trypsin inhibitors and fermentable oligo-, di-, monosaccharide, and polyols have been implicated in IBS pathogenesis [6]
Wheat allergy	IgE-mediated response that can include respiratory, dermal, circulatory, and other symptoms after ingestion, skin contact, or inhalation of the allergen [7]
Dermatitis herpetiformis	Vesiculobullous, pruritic, and localized skin lesions on extensor surfaces as the result of IgA antibodies deposited in the superficial papillary dermis; gastrointestinal symptoms less common [8, 9]
Gluten ataxia	Autoimmune disease characterized by cerebellar injury affecting Purkinje cells from cross-reactivity between gluten-related antibodies and antigenic epitopes at Purkinje cell level [10, 11]

Serology Testing

Achieving a high-quality diagnosis begins with the testing strategy (see Fig. 8.1). The tissue transglutaminase immunoglobulin A (TTG-IgA) is the screening test of choice in celiac disease [13]. TTG-IgA has been extensively studied and performs well in both primary care and referral settings [14]. Its sensitivity approaches 95%, and its specificity ranges from 96% to 100% [15]. While performance differences exist in the various test kits that are commercially available, the TTG-IgA exhibits consistency in its sensitivity and specificity performance [15, 16]. For this reason, it should be the preferred initial test for celiac disease. It must be accompanied by a total IgA level. If an IgA deficiency is uncovered, the TTG-IgA is no longer a valid screening test, and IgG-based testing should be performed; this can be in the form of TTG-IgG or deamidated gliadin peptide (DGP-IgG) testing [17, 18]. All diagnostic laboratory testing for celiac serology should be done on patients eating a gluten-containing diet. Ingestion of gluten is necessary for TTG antibody detection. Reducing or eliminating gluten from the diet leads to decreasing or normalized levels of all celiac-associated antibody tests. Precise timing for this reduction is unknown; therefore, it is essential that testing is conducted while an individual is eating gluten.

Test panels featuring multiple antibodies are available, but we advocate for the use of TTG-IgA over this approach to simplify the initial assessment for celiac disease. This strategy avoids the problem of ambiguous or mixed results which can result in misdiagnosis of celiac disease. Underdiagnosis can occur if the panel is interpreted as positive for celiac disease only when all antibody results are positive; sensitivity is lost in this manner [14]. Overdiagnosis can occur if any positive antibody result is viewed as positive for celiac disease; specificity is at stake with this interpretation leading to additional unnecessary and costly testing such as

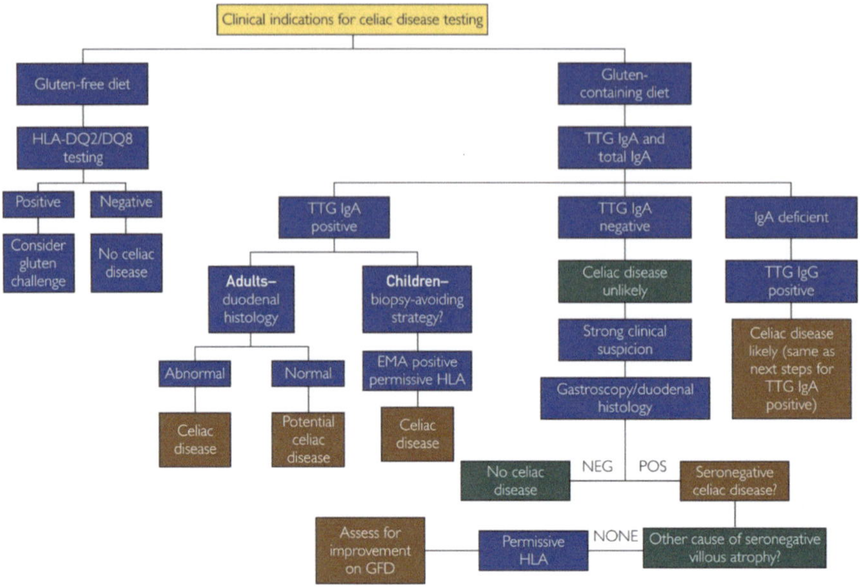

Fig. 8.1 A proposed diagnostic algorithm for celiac disease [12]. (This figure was published in Mayo Clinic Proceedings, volume 94, issue 12, Amy S Oxentenko and Alberto Rubio-Tapia, "Celiac Disease," 2556–2571, Copyright Elsevier (2019). Permission received for reproduction)

endoscopy [19]. Diagnostic accuracy is paramount given the only available treatment is a lifelong gluten-free diet.

Certain antibody tests used in the past are no longer recommended for the screening or diagnosis of celiac disease. These include anti-gliadin antibodies (AGA) and anti-reticulin antibodies (ARA) [13, 16]. Their sensitivity, specificity, positive predictive value, and negative predictive value are inferior to the TTG-IgA. If a patient's diagnosis or the clinical suspicion is based on one of these tests, the initial step should be to repeat celiac serology with a recommended blood test such as the TTG-IgA.

Biopsy

Once the screening test is suggestive of celiac disease, it must be followed by a confirmatory biopsy of the small intestine during esophagogastroduodenoscopy (EGD). Proper biopsy technique and sampling are essential for diagnosis as the histologic changes of celiac disease are patchy [13, 20, 21]. Multiple biopsy specimens are required. Multiple locations should be sampled including the duodenal bulb [20, 22, 23]. Studies indicate that endoscopists are imperfect when it comes to obtaining these biopsies from a number and location standpoint which can create downstream diagnostic and patient care implications [24–27]. Since a higher number of biopsies increases the confidence we have in arriving at a celiac disease diagnosis, a specific biopsy technique is recommended [24, 28]. In one study, diagnostic yield more than doubled (0.7–1.8%) with a greater number of biopsies taken; unfortunately, this occurred less than 40% of the time [26]. Guidelines advise at least four biopsies from the post-bulbar or distal duodenum and one to two biopsies from the duodenal bulb at either the 9 o'clock or 12 o'clock location [13, 29]. The idea behind this positioning of the bulb biopsies is to minimize the Brunner gland sampling and any confounding effects of peptic duodenitis by avoiding locations where fluid pools. The bulb biopsy is not to be missed as research indicates around 10% of patients with suspected celiac disease had villous atrophy only in the bulb [20, 22, 23]. Biopsies should be taken even when the endoscopic appearance of the mucosa is normal. Endoscopic evidence of villous atrophy may be present in the form of reduction in folds, scalloping, fissuring, and nodularity but does not have sufficient sensitivity to preclude biopsy [30]. A standard biopsy forceps can be used [31]. Ideally only one biopsy should be taken per pass [32]. Specimens can be placed to float freely in formalin or mounted on fiber-free paper to assist with orientation [21, 33].

Increased intraepithelial lymphocytes, crypt hyperplasia, and villous flattening, blunting, or atrophy comprise the features of celiac disease on biopsy. Characteristic histologic findings should be reported by pathology using the Marsh or Corazza classification (see Table 8.2) [34, 35]. Lymphocytic infiltration is presently defined as >25 intraepithelial lymphocytes per 100 epithelial cells. Crypt hyperplasia can be noted by an increase in the crypt-to-villi ratio. Villous changes range from partial, subtotal, to total villous atrophy although interobserver agreement is poor between pathologists [36]. A positive serology coupled with villous atrophy on biopsy secures the diagnosis of celiac disease, but the diagnosis is also a consideration with lesser degrees of intestinal injury (e.g., positive TTG-IgA and Marsh 1–2) [13].

As TTG-IgA testing may be subject to verification bias, it is important when the clinical suspicion is high to biopsy and not to rely on the negative TTG-IgA alone [37]. Seronegative celiac disease needs to be a diagnostic consideration in those with suggestive symptoms and villous atrophy on biopsy. This seronegative (normal TTG-IgA) subgroup accounts for about 5–16% of patients with celiac disease [19, 38, 39]. Human leukocyte antigen (HLA) typing revealing DQ2 or DQ8 genetics and histologic response to the gluten-free diet can help establish the diagnosis of seronegative celiac disease. A gluten challenge to demonstrate gluten-induced damage may be necessary in selected cases with seronegative celiac disease.

Table 8.2 Criteria for Marsh and Corazza pathology classifications [34, 35]

Marsh	IELs Marsh/Corazza	Crypts	Villi	Corazza
Type 0	<40	Normal	Normal	
Type 1	>40/>25	Normal	Normal	Grade A
Type 2	>40/>25	Hypertrophic	Normal	
Type 3	>40/>25	Hypertrophic	Partial to subtotal	Grade B1
	>40/>25	Hypertrophic	Total	Grade B2
Type 4	>40	Normal	Total	

IELs, intraepithelial lymphocytes (per 100 enterocytes)

Non-biopsy Diagnosis

A biopsy-sparing approach can be considered in the pediatric population [29]. If the TTG-IgA is greater than or equal to ten times the upper limit of normal and the family is agreeable, diagnosis can be confirmed if a second blood test is positive for endomysial antibodies (EMA-IgA) [29]. In previous iterations of pediatric guidelines, HLA typing showing genetic predisposition and symptoms was obligatory, but this is no longer the case. Further research is needed to determine if this strategy could be applicable to adults.

Response to Gluten Withdrawal

Response to a gluten-free diet without testing is not an appropriate approach to the evaluation of celiac disease. A growing number of individuals follow a gluten-free diet for various reasons. In the United States, it is estimated that 0.5–2% of the population eats gluten-free [40, 41]. In the United Kingdom, 1–2% of individuals avoid gluten [42]. In Australia, a population-based survey, after excluding patients diagnosed with celiac disease, found that 7% report adverse gastrointestinal symptoms following wheat consumption [43]. Very few patients in this group claimed to have a formally diagnosed condition requiring food avoidance [43]. Wheat is frequently noted to be a troublesome food in those who report a food intolerance [44]. Symptoms alone cannot distinguish those with celiac disease from those with other disorders. Irritable bowel syndrome coexists with celiac disease in 38% of celiac patients [45]. The positive predictive value for celiac disease of symptom improvement after removal of gluten from the diet is only 36% [46]. Additionally, the positive predictive value for celiac disease of symptom recurrence and exacerbation after reintroduction of gluten is even less useful at 28% [46]. A double-blind, randomized controlled trial showed that gluten ingestion causes bloating and abdominal pain even in the absence of celiac disease [47]. It is unreliable and not in the patient's best interest to use response to gluten as a screening or confirmatory test for celiac disease.

Previously Gluten-Free

For patients already following a gluten-free diet without a prior celiac disease diagnosis, ensuring an accurate diagnosis is key. Patients can either undergo genetic testing while continuing the gluten-free diet or do a gluten challenge before standard celiac disease testing as described in the above section (see Fig. 8.1). These genotypes are not influenced by a patient's diet and can be checked on a normal or a gluten-free diet. HLA-DQ2 and DQ8 are the most important genetic risk factors for celiac disease and are found in 95% and 5% of celiac patients, respectively [48, 49]. The absence of these HLA haplotypes makes celiac disease highly unlikely with a negative predictive value approaching 100% [50]. The positive predictive value is quite low at 12% because HLA-DQ2 is commonly encountered in the general Caucasian population; as such, genetic testing is not helpful to make a positive diagnosis but to exclude a celiac diagnosis when absent [50].

If genetic testing reveals DQ2 or DQ8, the next step is a gluten challenge. Ingestion of at least 3 g of gluten per day (equivalent to the amount in about one slice of gluten-containing bread) for as short a time as 2 weeks is likely sufficient to trigger serologic and histologic changes that are diagnostic of celiac disease [51]. This method of gluten challenge led to either serologic or histologic changes in 90% of patients, meaning the false negative rate is around 10% using this dose and duration of gluten [51]. Therefore, if the patient's tolerance to the challenge is acceptable, the duration can be extended to 6–8 weeks to improve diagnostic precision. A gluten challenge is strongly indicated to obtain an accurate diagnosis in those patients who have already embarked on a gluten-free diet without a prior formal assessment for celiac disease.

Management

Diagnosis marks the beginning, not the end, of physician involvement in the care of celiac disease patients. This section will summarize how we treat a patient with high quality for their gastroenterology care (see Table 8.3).

Clinic Visit

The goal of the initial clinic visit after uncovering celiac disease is to review the new diagnosis with the patient. Education is provided on the pathophysiology of celiac disease, its multitude of potential symptoms and presentations, and the presently

Table 8.3 Quality care metrics for celiac disease

Celiac disease quality measures
Dietitian referral
Gastroenterologist physician follow-up
Follow-up serology
Nutritional markers
DXA bone density scan
Advise first-degree family member screening
Discuss vaccines
Follow-up EGD after 2 years of GFD to check for mucosal healing

available dietary treatment. Baseline laboratories should be obtained. We recommend checking a complete blood count, ferritin, vitamin D, vitamin B12, folate, zinc, albumin, TSH, liver chemistries (AST and ALT), and hepatitis B surface antibody. Any abnormal levels should be followed over time to monitor for improvement after treatment of celiac disease. For any deficiencies uncovered, these should be replaced appropriately; we expect some of these to improve as the intestine heals and absorptive capacity increases. A dual-energy absorptiometry scan (DXA) is advised to assess bone health given celiac disease is a malabsorptive condition associated with lower bone mineral density and higher risk of fractures [52, 53]. Preventive health is also emphasized with recommendations for vaccination against the following diseases: herpes zoster (strongly recommended for age >50 years old and/or any age with refractory celiac disease, may be considered for younger patients too after shared decision-making), influenza (any age, yearly), pneumococcal (any age, PCV20 one booster dose), COVID-19 (any age, complete immunization with booster), and hepatitis B if not immune (any age). Physicians may consider vaccine administration during the office visit to improve compliance based on availability in the clinic. This initial visit is also a good time to discuss the importance of family member screening. Most importantly, it is an opportunity to provide a referral to our partners the registered dietitians and emphasize the need to collaborate with them for treatment.

Dietitian Consult

The dietitian plays a key role in the management of celiac disease. We advise a consult at diagnosis to provide education on the gluten-free diet. Eliminating dietary gluten is presently the only available treatment for celiac disease—this makes the dietitian a vital member of the team. There are medications being developed that will hopefully prevent the intestinal damage caused by gluten in the future in a safe and reliable fashion. For now, a strict lifelong gluten-free diet is the recommended treatment for celiac disease.

The registered dietitian will perform a nutritional assessment and review the main sources of gluten which include wheat, barley, and rye [54]. They will evaluate the patient's ability to implement this dietary change. When considering the patient's capacity to achieve this, the dietitian considers socioeconomic barriers, access to gluten-free foods, label reading, food preparation, and avoidance of cross-contamination skills [54]. They should address restaurant safety and review medications, cosmetic, and household products that contain gluten. The registered dietitian individualizes their comprehensive nutrition assessment, education, and treatment plans for each patient. Dietitians possess a wealth of knowledge and provide patients with excellent educational materials and resources [54]. They will review that gluten-free is defined as <20 ppm of gluten because complete elimination is aspirational given the possibility of contamination with trace amounts of gluten.

Collaborating with a dietitian has been shown to improve our care of celiac disease patients with better adherence to a gluten-free diet. When patients and families have better knowledge of celiac disease and dietary management, compliance with a gluten-free diet improves [55–58]. This dietary knowledge and these management skills can take time to acquire. Research shows that it can take 6 months to master distinguishing between gluten-free and gluten-containing foods [59]. It can take 1–2 years to articulate and explain a gluten-free diet and celiac disease to others [59]. It can take between 3 and 5 years to identify medications and supplements that contain gluten [59]. It takes >5 years to learn to manage international travel and remain adherent to the gluten-free diet [59]. This research suggests that learning and adhering to a gluten-free diet is a time-intensive process and occurs in a sequential fashion. Skills are first acquired that are used in the home, then socially, then at work, and then in novel settings [59]. Awareness of this timeline for skill acquisition emphasizes the complexity of celiac disease management and the opportunities for dietitian support along the way. This information is valuable to support patients in a proactive fashion and express empathy with the difficulties of following a gluten-free diet.

Benefits of a Gluten-Free Diet

There are numerous benefits of a gluten-free diet. These include symptom resolution, serology normalization, healing of villi, improvement of nutritional parameters, and decreased morbidity and mortality. For most patients with celiac disease, eliminating gluten in the diet leads to symptomatic improvement. In a majority of cases, this improvement is rapid and substantial. Diarrhea responds to gluten elimination typically within days with resolution occurring at a mean of 4 weeks [60]. Bloating, abdominal pain, nausea, and vomiting also resolve with exclusion of gluten [60]. In a survey of biopsy-proven celiac disease patients, rate of bloating improved from 73% to 4%, abdominal pain 79% to 3%, and nausea or vomiting 44% to 9% with the introduction of a gluten-free diet [60]. Dietary noncompliance is the leading cause of nonresponse for patients with celiac disease [61]. Reintroduction or inadvertent exposure tends to result in less severe symptoms in those adherent to a gluten-free diet compared to non-adherent patients [62]. The impact of a gluten-free diet on symptoms is profound in a vast majority of cases.

Serology testing also exhibits improvement on a gluten-free diet. Decrease from baseline numbers is expected over a period of months. We recommended monitoring of serology after starting a gluten-free diet at 3, 6, and 12 months during the first year and every 6–12 months thereafter. TTG and DGP antibodies decreased significantly in a cohort of patients followed after their diagnosis and implementation of dietary treatment [63]. Antibody concentration dropped by 1 year and continued to decline years later in strictly compliant patients indicating celiac-specific antibody monitoring is a reliable way to measure long-term compliance [63]. In another study of adult patients, endomysial antibody positivity was found less frequently in those strictly compliant with a gluten-free diet [64]. Higher titers of tissue transglutaminase antibodies were observed in noncompliant adults compared to compliant adults with celiac disease [65]. In a study of 2245 celiac patients, only 1% had persistently positive tissue transglutaminase antibodies at 5-year follow-up [66]. Serology normalization is another benefit of the gluten-free diet.

Poor compliance with the gluten-free diet is strongly associated with ongoing mucosal injury [67]. Mucosal recovery is often achieved (95%) in children diagnosed with celiac disease but can be more difficult to achieve in adults [68]. Those who follow a strict gluten-free diet have a greater chance of healing their small intestine. In fact, celiac patients on a strict long-term gluten-free diet have been observed to have similar villous height-to-crypt depth as control subjects [69]. Mucosal morphology can take time to normalize and dietary compliance facilitates that greatly [69]. A good histopathologic response is a benefit of the gluten-free diet and strongly associated with a decreased risk of bone disease and lymphoma [70, 71]. We suggest a follow-up duodenal biopsy after 2 years of following a gluten-free diet in adults to check for mucosal healing as a goal of treatment with the gluten-free diet.

Treating celiac disease improves various nutritional parameters. These include body mass index and weight [72]. Previously abnormal laboratory markers including hemoglobin, albumin, iron, calcium, and zinc all improve while following a gluten-free diet [73, 74]. Bone mineral density has also been shown to respond in a positive fashion to elimination of gluten in both adults and children [52, 75–77].

Adherence to a gluten-free diet reduces the risk of developing adverse health outcomes associated with celiac disease. Malignancy rates including for enteropathy-associated T-cell lymphoma, small bowel adenocarcinoma, esophageal cancer, colon cancer, hepatobiliary cancer, pancreatic cancer, and lymphoma are higher in celiac disease compared to the general population [78, 79]. Mortality was also modestly higher in celiac patients with a hazard ratio of 1.17 [79]. When compared to first-degree relative controls, excess mortality was seen in celiac patients [80]. This risk can be mitigated by adherence to the gluten-free diet as the standardized mortality ratio decreased with good dietary compliance [80].

Adherence to a gluten-free diet has also been shown to improve quality of life among celiac disease patients. Higher quality of life scores across multiple dimensions were seen in compliant celiac disease patients compared to noncompliant patients [81, 82]. Studies have also demonstrated higher well-being scores in children who are adherent to the gluten-free diet [83].

Following a gluten-free diet improves symptoms, normalizes serology, heals intestinal mucosa, improves nutritional status, protects from adverse outcomes, and enhances quality of life. Achieving mucosal healing can prevent complications or ameliorate downstream effects of celiac disease indicating that a careful long-term follow-up strategy is scientifically supported [84].

Physician Follow-Up

Celiac disease patients require follow-up with a gastroenterologist and a dietitian. Research shows that a minority of patients with celiac disease get the follow-up they need; at 1 year only 41% of patients had a follow-up visit, 3% met with a

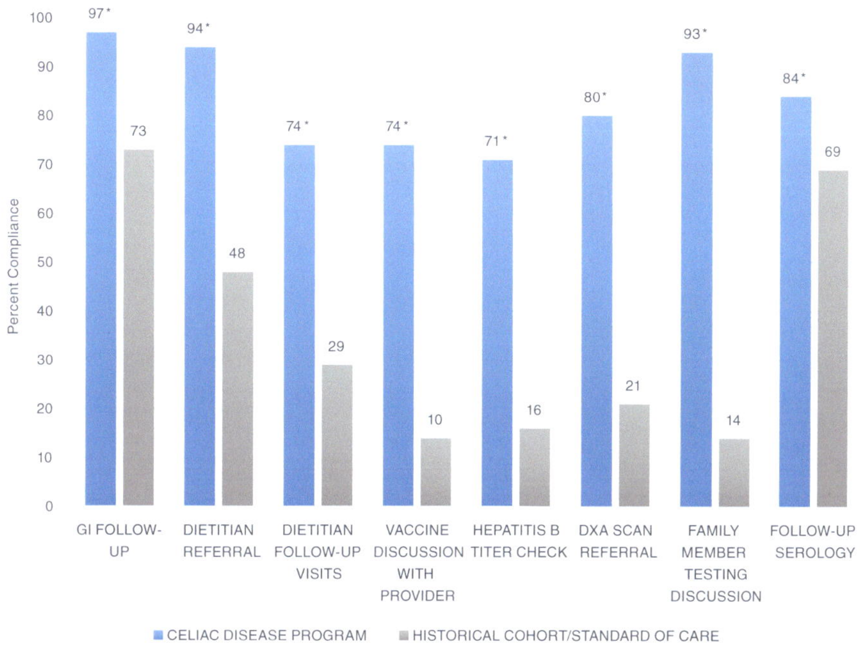

Fig. 8.2 Quality celiac care metrics for patients receiving care in the Celiac Disease Program at Cleveland Clinic compared to a historical cohort seen in general gastroenterology. *Indicates statistical significance. (Published in abstract form: Ford, A., Jansson-Knodell, C., Cavagnaro, S., Rubio-Tapia, A. Ready for Primetime! A Dedicated Celiac Disease Program Improves Celiac Care Quality Metrics in Real Life. *Gastroenterology*. 162(7): S354–S355. May, 2022)

registered dietitian, and 22% had a repeat serologic test [85]. There is definite room for improvement. The National Institutes of Health and the American Gastroenterological Association recommend patient care by a "physician and a dietitian" [86, 87]. Following in a specialty celiac disease program improves patient outcomes (see Fig. 8.2). Care in a celiac disease program outperformed even general gastroenterology care in terms of dietitian referral, serial serology, getting family members screened, and clinical follow-up visits.

We share here the strategy we use in our celiac disease program for high-quality care of newly diagnosed patients (see Fig. 8.3). We recommend a visit at diagnosis, at 3–6 months, at 12 months, and annually thereafter. Earlier visits are encouraged for difficult-to-manage symptoms, continued weight loss, or other pressing concerns. At each visit, symptoms should be reviewed, response to gluten-free diet, and bowel patterns with information on frequency and consistency with the use of the Bristol stool form scale for objectivity. Serology markers should be obtained at each visit. A repeat esophagogastroduodenoscopy is due after 2 years on the gluten-free diet to assess for return to normal of villi. Abnormal labs should be repeated in a serial fashion. Dietitian involvement is essential at diagnosis and as frequent as needed during follow-up to ensure the patient is appropriately adapting to the dietary change. Review with a skilled dietitian is the gold standard for gluten-free diet monitoring [88]. Further consultation with the dietitian can be offered at each visit and should be encouraged if the patient is experiencing any particular dietary

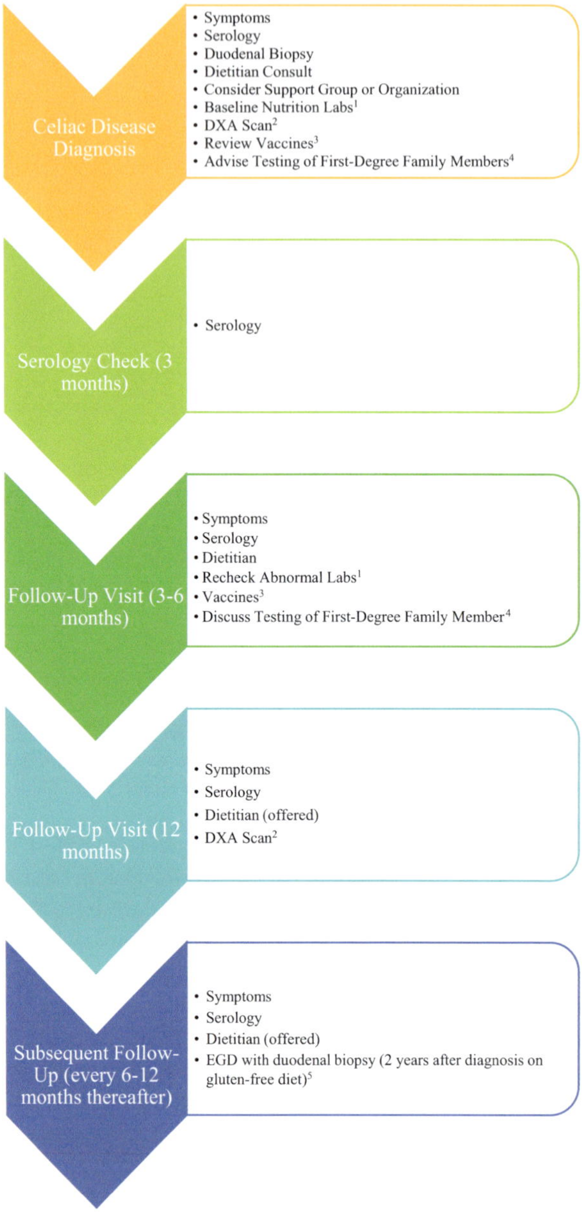

Fig. 8.3 A proposed follow-up algorithm for adults with newly diagnosed celiac disease. (1) No consensus. At our celiac disease program, we check CBC, ferritin, vitamin D, vitamin B12, folate, zinc, albumin, TSH, AST, ALT, and hepatitis B S Ab; (2) DXA, dual-energy absorptiometry, at diagnosis or within 1 year; (3) herpes zoster, influenza, pneumococcal, COVID-19, and hepatitis B, consider vaccine administration during office visit to improve compliance; (4) we recommend testing all first-degree family members given higher prevalence and revisit this recommendation during follow-up; (5) after confirmation of mucosal healing, clinical follow-up every year may be reasonable

challenges. Examples may include insufficient fiber intake, excess weight gain, cross-contamination concerns, and approach to social and travel settings. Testing of first-degree family members must be discussed at diagnosis and reviewed during follow-up. Vaccines and bone health form the crux of health maintenance discussions. DXA scan is advised within 1 year of diagnosis. Specialty care within gastroenterology practice is essential. Patients find celiac disease specific groups or organizations and gastroenterologists to be excellent sources of information outperforming family physicians [89]. A comprehensive approach with ongoing follow-up delivers high-quality care to celiac disease patients.

Family Member Screening

Celiac disease has a clear genetic predisposition. The frequency of disease is higher in those with first-degree family member who carries the diagnosis [90]. Siblings were at high risk, and this risk is highest in monozygous twins. Families that have multiple relatives affected are at higher risk [91]. Prevalence estimates range from 10% to 20% for those with a first-degree family member with celiac disease [90, 91]. This epidemiological data has clear clinical implications. Celiac disease patients should inform family members of the potentially increased risk of disease and the recommendation for testing. We encourage first-degree family member testing for all of our celiac disease patients.

Conclusion

High-quality care is what every celiac patient deserves. This chapter reviews the diagnosis and management of celiac disease patients. It gives an overview of diagnosis with the use of serology and biopsy. It provides the rationale for ensuring an accurate diagnosis. Management is addressed highlighting the role of the gastroenterologist and dietitian in patient care. We share our proposed follow-up of celiac patients. This chapter provides a framework for a high-quality diagnosis and long-term clinical care of patients with celiac disease.

References

1. Jansson-Knodell CL, Hujoel IA, West CP, Taneja V, Prokop LJ, Rubio-Tapia A, et al. Sex difference in celiac disease in undiagnosed populations: a systematic review and meta-analysis. Clin Gastroenterol Hepatol. 2019;17(10):1954–68.e13.
2. Singh P, Arora A, Strand TA, Leffler DA, Catassi C, Green PH, et al. Global prevalence of celiac disease: systematic review and meta-analysis. Clin Gastroenterol Hepatol. 2018;16(6):823–36.e2.

3. Bledsoe AC, King KS, Larson JJ, Snyder M, Absah I, Choung RS, et al. Micronutrient deficiencies are common in contemporary celiac disease despite lack of overt malabsorption symptoms. Mayo Clin Proc. 2019;94(7):1253–60.
4. Casella G, Villanacci V, Di Bella C, Bassotti G, Bold J, Rostami K. Non celiac gluten sensitivity and diagnostic challenges. Gastroenterol Hepatol Bed Bench. 2018;11(3):197–202.
5. Mansueto P, Seidita A, D'Alcamo A, Carroccio A. Non-celiac gluten sensitivity: literature review. J Am Coll Nutr. 2014;33(1):39–54.
6. Koumbi L, Giouleme O, Vassilopoulou E. Non-celiac gluten sensitivity and irritable bowel disease: looking for the culprits. Curr Dev Nutr. 2020;4(12):nzaa176.
7. Cianferoni A. Wheat allergy: diagnosis and management. J Asthma Allergy. 2016;9:13–25.
8. Collin P, Salmi TT, Hervonen K, Kaukinen K, Reunala T. Dermatitis herpetiformis: a cutaneous manifestation of coeliac disease. Ann Med. 2017;49(1):23–31.
9. Reunala T, Hervonen K, Salmi T. Dermatitis herpetiformis: an update on diagnosis and management. Am J Clin Dermatol. 2021;22(3):329–38.
10. Ghezzi A, Filippi M, Falini A, Zaffaroni M. Cerebral involvement in celiac disease: a serial MRI study in a patient with brainstem and cerebellar symptoms. Neurology. 1997;49(5):1447–50.
11. Hadjivassiliou M, Sanders DD, Aeschlimann DP. Gluten-related disorders: gluten ataxia. Dig Dis. 2015;33(2):264–8.
12. Oxentenko AS, Rubio-Tapia A. Celiac disease. Mayo Clin Proc. 2019;94(12):2556–71.
13. Rubio-Tapia A, Hill ID, Kelly CP, Calderwood AH, Murray JA. ACG clinical guidelines: diagnosis and management of celiac disease. Am J Gastroenterol. 2013;108(5):656–76; quiz 77.
14. van der Windt DA, Jellema P, Mulder CJ, Kneepkens CM, van der Horst HE. Diagnostic testing for celiac disease among patients with abdominal symptoms: a systematic review. JAMA. 2010;303(17):1738–46.
15. Li M, Yu L, Tiberti C, Bonamico M, Taki I, Miao D, et al. A report on the international transglutaminase autoantibody workshop for celiac disease. Am J Gastroenterol. 2009;104(1):154–63.
16. Leffler DA, Schuppan D. Update on serologic testing in celiac disease. Am J Gastroenterol. 2010;105(12):2520–4.
17. Villalta D, Alessio MG, Tampoia M, Tonutti E, Brusca I, Bagnasco M, et al. Testing for IgG class antibodies in celiac disease patients with selective IgA deficiency. A comparison of the diagnostic accuracy of 9 IgG anti-tissue transglutaminase, 1 IgG anti-gliadin and 1 IgG anti-deaminated gliadin peptide antibody assays. Clin Chim Acta. 2007;382(1–2):95–9.
18. Villalta D, Tonutti E, Prause C, Koletzko S, Uhlig HH, Vermeersch P, et al. IgG antibodies against deamidated gliadin peptides for diagnosis of celiac disease in patients with IgA deficiency. Clin Chem. 2010;56(3):464–8.
19. Rashtak S, Ettore MW, Homburger HA, Murray JA. Combination testing for antibodies in the diagnosis of coeliac disease: comparison of multiplex immunoassay and ELISA methods. Aliment Pharmacol Ther. 2008;28(6):805–13.
20. Bonamico M, Mariani P, Thanasi E, Ferri M, Nenna R, Tiberti C, et al. Patchy villous atrophy of the duodenum in childhood celiac disease. J Pediatr Gastroenterol Nutr. 2004;38(2):204–7.
21. Ravelli A, Bolognini S, Gambarotti M, Villanacci V. Variability of histologic lesions in relation to biopsy site in gluten-sensitive enteropathy. Am J Gastroenterol. 2005;100(1):177–85.
22. Evans KE, Aziz I, Cross SS, Sahota GR, Hopper AD, Hadjivassiliou M, et al. A prospective study of duodenal bulb biopsy in newly diagnosed and established adult celiac disease. Am J Gastroenterol. 2011;106(10):1837–742.
23. Gonzalez S, Gupta A, Cheng J, Tennyson C, Lewis SK, Bhagat G, et al. Prospective study of the role of duodenal bulb biopsies in the diagnosis of celiac disease. Gastrointest Endosc. 2010;72(4):758–65.
24. Jansson-Knodell CL, Kessler WR. The role of female endoscopists: are women gastroenterologists better at obtaining biopsies for celiac disease than men? Scand J Gastroenterol. 2021;56(4):505–7.
25. Lebwohl B, Genta RM, Kapel RC, Sheehan D, Lerner NS, Green PH, et al. Procedure volume influences adherence to celiac disease guidelines. Eur J Gastroenterol Hepatol. 2013;25(11):1273–8.

26. Lebwohl B, Kapel RC, Neugut AI, Green PH, Genta RM. Adherence to biopsy guidelines increases celiac disease diagnosis. Gastrointest Endosc. 2011;74(1):103–9.
27. Ofei S, Boyle B, Ediger T, Hill I. Adherence to endoscopy biopsy guidelines for celiac disease. J Pediatr Gastroenterol Nutr. 2015;61(4):440–4.
28. Pais WP, Duerksen DR, Pettigrew NM, Bernstein CN. How many duodenal biopsy specimens are required to make a diagnosis of celiac disease? Gastrointest Endosc. 2008;67(7):1082–7.
29. Husby S, Koletzko S, Korponay-Szabo I, Kurppa K, Mearin ML, Ribes-Koninckx C, et al. European Society Paediatric Gastroenterology, Hepatology and Nutrition guidelines for diagnosing coeliac disease 2020. J Pediatr Gastroenterol Nutr. 2020;70(1):141–56.
30. Dickey W, Hughes D. Disappointing sensitivity of endoscopic markers for villous atrophy in a high-risk population: implications for celiac disease diagnosis during routine endoscopy. Am J Gastroenterol. 2001;96(7):2126–8.
31. Dandalides SM, Carey WD, Petras R, Achkar E. Endoscopic small bowel mucosal biopsy: a controlled trial evaluating forceps size and biopsy location in the diagnosis of normal and abnormal mucosal architecture. Gastrointest Endosc. 1989;35(3):197–200.
32. Latorre M, Lagana SM, Freedberg DE, Lewis SK, Lebwohl B, Bhagat G, et al. Endoscopic biopsy technique in the diagnosis of celiac disease: one bite or two? Gastrointest Endosc. 2015;81(5):1228–33.
33. Ludvigsson JF, Bai JC, Biagi F, Card TR, Ciacci C, Ciclitira PJ, et al. Diagnosis and management of adult coeliac disease: guidelines from the British Society of Gastroenterology. Gut. 2014;63(8):1210–28.
34. Marsh MN. Gluten, major histocompatibility complex, and the small intestine. A molecular and immunobiologic approach to the spectrum of gluten sensitivity ('celiac sprue'). Gastroenterology. 1992;102(1):330–54.
35. Corazza GR, Villanacci V. Coeliac disease. J Clin Pathol. 2005;58(6):573–4.
36. Corazza GR, Villanacci V, Zambelli C, Milione M, Luinetti O, Vindigni C, et al. Comparison of the interobserver reproducibility with different histologic criteria used in celiac disease. Clin Gastroenterol Hepatol. 2007;5(7):838–43.
37. Hujoel IA, Jansson-Knodell CL, Hujoel PP, Hujoel MLA, Choung RS, Murray JA, et al. Estimating the impact of verification bias on celiac disease testing. J Clin Gastroenterol. 2021;55(4):327–34.
38. Lewis NR, Scott BB. Meta-analysis: deamidated gliadin peptide antibody and tissue transglutaminase antibody compared as screening tests for coeliac disease. Aliment Pharmacol Ther. 2010;31(1):73–81.
39. Schiepatti A, Sanders DS, Baiardi P, Caio G, Ciacci C, Kaukinen K, et al. Nomenclature and diagnosis of seronegative coeliac disease and chronic non-coeliac enteropathies in adults: the Paris consensus. Gut. 2022;71:2218.
40. Choung RS, Unalp-Arida A, Ruhl CE, Brantner TL, Everhart JE, Murray JA. Less hidden celiac disease but increased gluten avoidance without a diagnosis in the United States: findings from the National Health and Nutrition Examination Surveys from 2009 to 2014. Mayo Clin proceedings; 2016.
41. DiGiacomo DV, Tennyson CA, Green PH, Demmer RT. Prevalence of gluten-free diet adherence among individuals without celiac disease in the USA: results from the Continuous National Health and Nutrition Examination Survey 2009-2010. Scand J Gastroenterol. 2013;48(8):921–5.
42. Littlejohns TJ, Chong AY, Allen NE, Arnold M, Bradbury KE, Mentzer AJ, et al. Genetic, lifestyle, and health-related characteristics of adults without celiac disease who follow a gluten-free diet: a population-based study of 124,447 participants. Am J Clin Nutr. 2021;113(3):622–9.
43. Golley S, Corsini N, Topping D, Morell M, Mohr P. Motivations for avoiding wheat consumption in Australia: results from a population survey. Public Health Nutr. 2015;18(3):490–9.
44. Jansson-Knodell CL, White M, Lockett C, Xu H, Shin A. High prevalence of food intolerances among US internet users. Public Health Nutr. 2021;24(3):531–5.
45. Sainsbury A, Sanders DS, Ford AC. Prevalence of irritable bowel syndrome-type symptoms in patients with celiac disease: a meta-analysis. Clin Gastroenterol Hepatol. 2013;11(4):359–65.e1.

46. Campanella J, Biagi F, Bianchi PI, Zanellati G, Marchese A, Corazza GR. Clinical response to gluten withdrawal is not an indicator of coeliac disease. Scand J Gastroenterol. 2008;43(11):1311–4.
47. Biesiekierski JR, Newnham ED, Irving PM, Barrett JS, Haines M, Doecke JD, et al. Gluten causes gastrointestinal symptoms in subjects without celiac disease: a double-blind randomized placebo-controlled trial. Am J Gastroenterol. 2011;106(3):508–14; quiz 15.
48. Lundin KE, Gjertsen HA, Scott H, Sollid LM, Thorsby E. Function of DQ2 and DQ8 as HLA susceptibility molecules in celiac disease. Hum Immunol. 1994;41(1):24–7.
49. Sollid LM, Markussen G, Ek J, Gjerde H, Vartdal F, Thorsby E. Evidence for a primary association of celiac disease to a particular HLA-DQ alpha/beta heterodimer. J Exp Med. 1989;169(1):345–50.
50. Hadithi M, von Blomberg BM, Crusius JB, Bloemena E, Kostense PJ, Meijer JW, et al. Accuracy of serologic tests and HLA-DQ typing for diagnosing celiac disease. Ann Intern Med. 2007;147(5):294–302.
51. Leffler D, Schuppan D, Pallav K, Najarian R, Goldsmith JD, Hansen J, et al. Kinetics of the histological, serological and symptomatic responses to gluten challenge in adults with coeliac disease. Gut. 2013;62(7):996–1004.
52. Bai JC, Gonzalez D, Mautalen C, Mazure R, Pedreira S, Vazquez H, et al. Long-term effect of gluten restriction on bone mineral density of patients with coeliac disease. Aliment Pharmacol Ther. 1997;11(1):157–64.
53. Vasquez H, Mazure R, Gonzalez D, Flores D, Pedreira S, Niveloni S, et al. Risk of fractures in celiac disease patients: a cross-sectional, case-control study. Am J Gastroenterol. 2000;95(1):183–9.
54. Celiac disease (CD) 2021 evidence-based nutrition practice guideline from Academy of Nutrition and Dietetics 2021. pp. 1–23. https://adaevidencelibrary.com/topic.cfm?menu=3677&cat=5988. Accessed 20 Jun 2022.
55. Charalampopoulos D, Panayiotou J, Chouliaras G, Zellos A, Kyritsi E, Roma E. Determinants of adherence to gluten-free diet in Greek children with coeliac disease: a cross-sectional study. Eur J Clin Nutr. 2013;67(6):615–9.
56. Jackson PT, Glasgow JF, Thom R. Parents' understanding of coeliac disease and diet. Arch Dis Child. 1985;60(7):672–4.
57. Leffler DA, Edwards-George J, Dennis M, Schuppan D, Cook F, Franko DL, et al. Factors that influence adherence to a gluten-free diet in adults with celiac disease. Dig Dis Sci. 2008;53(6):1573–81.
58. Sdepanian VL, de Morais MB, Fagundes-Neto U. Celiac disease: evaluation of compliance to gluten-free diet and knowledge of disease in patients registered at the Brazilian Celiac Association (ACA). Arq Gastroenterol. 2001;38(4):232–9.
59. Clerx EM, Silvester J, Leffler D, DeGroote M, Fishman LN. Sequence of acquisition of self-management skills to follow a gluten-free diet by adults with celiac disease. Dig Liver Dis. 2019;51(8):1096–100.
60. Murray JA, Watson T, Clearman B, Mitros F. Effect of a gluten-free diet on gastrointestinal symptoms in celiac disease. Am J Clin Nutr. 2004;79(4):669–73.
61. See J, Murray JA. Gluten-free diet: the medical and nutrition management of celiac disease. Nutr Clin Pract. 2006;21(1):1–15.
62. Barratt SM, Leeds JS, Sanders DS. Factors influencing the type, timing and severity of symptomatic responses to dietary gluten in patients with biopsy-proven coeliac disease. J Gastrointestin Liver Dis. 2013;22(4):391–6.
63. Nachman F, Sugai E, Vazquez H, Gonzalez A, Andrenacci P, Niveloni S, et al. Serological tests for celiac disease as indicators of long-term compliance with the gluten-free diet. Eur J Gastroenterol Hepatol. 2011;23(6):473–80.
64. Hopman EG, von Blomberg ME, Batstra MR, Morreau H, Dekker FW, Koning F, et al. Gluten tolerance in adult patients with celiac disease 20 years after diagnosis? Eur J Gastroenterol Hepatol. 2008;20(5):423–9.

65. Kahramanoglu Aksoy E, Akpinar MY, Pirincci Sapmaz F, Dogan O, Uzman M, Nazligul Y. Thymic stromal lymphopoietin levels are increased in patients with celiac disease. Bosn J Basic Med Sci. 2019;19(3):282–7.
66. Zanini B, Lanzarotto F, Mora A, Bertolazzi S, Turini D, Cesana B, et al. Five year time course of celiac disease serology during gluten free diet: results of a community based "CD-Watch" program. Dig Liver Dis. 2010;42(12):865–70.
67. Rubio-Tapia A, Rahim MW, See JA, Lahr BD, Wu TT, Murray JA. Mucosal recovery and mortality in adults with celiac disease after treatment with a gluten-free diet. Am J Gastroenterol. 2010;105(6):1412–20.
68. Wahab PJ, Meijer JW, Mulder CJ. Histologic follow-up of people with celiac disease on a gluten-free diet: slow and incomplete recovery. Am J Clin Pathol. 2002;118(3):459–63.
69. Collin P, Maki M, Kaukinen K. Complete small intestine mucosal recovery is obtainable in the treatment of celiac disease. Gastrointest Endosc. 2004;59(1):158–9; author reply 9–60.
70. Lebwohl B, Michaelsson K, Green PH, Ludvigsson JF. Persistent mucosal damage and risk of fracture in celiac disease. J Clin Endocrinol Metab. 2014;99(2):609–16.
71. Lebwohl B, Granath F, Ekbom A, Smedby KE, Murray JA, Neugut AI, et al. Mucosal healing and risk for lymphoproliferative malignancy in celiac disease: a population-based cohort study. Ann Intern Med. 2013;159(3):169–75.
72. Barera G, Mora S, Brambilla P, Ricotti A, Menni L, Beccio S, et al. Body composition in children with celiac disease and the effects of a gluten-free diet: a prospective case-control study. Am J Clin Nutr. 2000;72(1):71–5.
73. Rajpoot P, Sharma A, Harikrishnan S, Baruah BJ, Ahuja V, Makharia GK. Adherence to gluten-free diet and barriers to adherence in patients with celiac disease. Indian J Gastroenterol. 2015;34(5):380–6.
74. Rea F, Polito C, Marotta A, Di Toro A, Iovene A, Collini R, et al. Restoration of body composition in celiac children after one year of gluten-free diet. J Pediatr Gastroenterol Nutr. 1996;23(4):408–12.
75. Sategna-Guidetti C, Grosso SB, Grosso S, Mengozzi G, Aimo G, Zaccaria T, et al. The effects of 1-year gluten withdrawal on bone mass, bone metabolism and nutritional status in newly-diagnosed adult coeliac disease patients. Aliment Pharmacol Ther. 2000;14(1):35–43.
76. Blazina S, Bratanic N, Campa AS, Blagus R, Orel R. Bone mineral density and importance of strict gluten-free diet in children and adolescents with celiac disease. Bone. 2010;47(3):598–603.
77. Heyman R, Guggenbuhl P, Corbel A, Bridoux-Henno L, Tourtelier Y, Balencon-Morival M, et al. Effect of a gluten-free diet on bone mineral density in children with celiac disease. Gastroenterol Clin Biol. 2009;33(2):109–14.
78. Askling J, Linet M, Gridley G, Halstensen TS, Ekstrom K, Ekbom A. Cancer incidence in a population-based cohort of individuals hospitalized with celiac disease or dermatitis herpetiformis. Gastroenterology. 2002;123(5):1428–35.
79. West J, Logan RF, Smith CJ, Hubbard RB, Card TR. Malignancy and mortality in people with coeliac disease: population based cohort study. BMJ. 2004;329(7468):716–9.
80. Corrao G, Corazza GR, Bagnardi V, Brusco G, Ciacci C, Cottone M, et al. Mortality in patients with coeliac disease and their relatives: a cohort study. Lancet. 2001;358(9279):356–61.
81. Casellas F, Rodrigo L, Vivancos JL, Riestra S, Pantiga C, Baudet JS, et al. Factors that impact health-related quality of life in adults with celiac disease: a multicenter study. World J Gastroenterol. 2008;14(1):46–52.
82. Usai P, Manca R, Cuomo R, Lai MA, Boi MF. Effect of gluten-free diet and co-morbidity of irritable bowel syndrome-type symptoms on health-related quality of life in adult coeliac patients. Dig Liver Dis. 2007;39(9):824–8.
83. Wagner G, Berger G, Sinnreich U, Grylli V, Schober E, Huber WD, et al. Quality of life in adolescents with treated coeliac disease: influence of compliance and age at diagnosis. J Pediatr Gastroenterol Nutr. 2008;47(5):555–61.

84. Haines ML, Anderson RP, Gibson PR. Systematic review: the evidence base for long-term management of coeliac disease. Aliment Pharmacol Ther. 2008;28(9):1042–66.
85. Herman ML, Rubio-Tapia A, Lahr BD, Larson JJ, Van Dyke CT, Murray JA. Patients with celiac disease are not followed up adequately. Clin Gastroenterol Hepatol. 2012;10(8):893–9.e1.
86. National Institutes of Health Consensus development conference statement on celiac disease, June 28–30, 2004. Gastroenterology. 2005;128(4 Suppl 1):S1–9.
87. Rostom A, Murray JA, Kagnoff MF. American Gastroenterological Association (AGA) Institute technical review on the diagnosis and management of celiac disease. Gastroenterology. 2006;131(6):1981–2002.
88. Simpson S, Thompson T. Nutrition assessment in celiac disease. Gastrointest Endosc Clin N Am. 2012;22(4):797–809.
89. Rashid M, Cranney A, Zarkadas M, Graham ID, Switzer C, Case S, et al. Celiac disease: evaluation of the diagnosis and dietary compliance in Canadian children. Pediatrics. 2005;116(6):e754–9.
90. Rubio-Tapia A, Van Dyke CT, Lahr BD, Zinsmeister AR, El-Youssef M, Moore SB, et al. Predictors of family risk for celiac disease: a population-based study. Clin Gastroenterol Hepatol. 2008;6(9):983–7.
91. Book L, Zone JJ, Neuhausen SL. Prevalence of celiac disease among relatives of sib pairs with celiac disease in U.S. families. Am J Gastroenterol. 2003;98(2):377–81.

Chapter 9
Quality in Colorectal Cancer Screening

Afshin A. Khan, Carole Macaron, Carol A. Burke, and Aparajita Singh

Table of Quality Measures/Metrics

A. A. Khan · A. Singh (✉)
Division of Gastroenterology, University of California San Francisco,
San Francisco, CA, USA
e-mail: afshin.khan@ucsf.edu; khana13@ccf.org; aparajita.singh@ucsf.edu

C. Macaron · C. A. Burke
Department of Gastroenterology, Hepatology and Nutrition, Cleveland Clinic,
Cleveland, OH, USA
e-mail: macaroc@ccf.org; burkec1@ccf.org

J. D. Feuerstein, D. J. Stein (eds.), *Quality in Gastroenterology*,
https://doi.org/10.1007/978-3-031-58492-3_9

Key Points

- Multiple tests are approved for CRC screening but their effectiveness, acceptability, safety, and cost vary.
- Despite the availability of various screening modalities, about one-third of the eligible US population is unscreened.
- Organized CRC screening programs are more likely to succeed in improving the uptake, quality, and adherence to CRC screening than opportunistic programs.
- The quality of screening programs requires objective metrics, continuous monitoring of compliance with benchmarks, and investigation and remediation of the process to achieve the highest patient outcomes.
- Mail and phone reminders, patient navigation, and elimination of cost sharing along with provider-level interventions are associated with improved adherence.
- Practices should implement quality assurance program to monitor for underuse, misuse, and overuse of the CRC screening process.

Introduction

The cumulative lifetime risk of colorectal cancer (CRC) in the United States of America (USA) is 4% and lags only behind lung, breast, and prostate cancer as the third leading cause of cancer death [1]. Since the year 2000, CRC incidence and mortality have declined primarily due to an increased uptake in CRC screening in addition to improved treatment for CRC [2, 3]. Improving the process of CRC screening by establishing quality metrics for the continuum of care will enhance the benefit of screening programs.

CRC risk stratification is the first step in ensuring the quality of CRC screening and cancer prevention. In the USA, approximately 102–107 million people are considered average-risk for CRC, of whom 43–45 million people are eligible for CRC screening [4]. Individuals with a higher than average CRC risk warrant special consideration and alterations in approaches to CRC prevention and should not be managed according to average-risk CRC screening recommendations. Data demonstrates a 3–5× increase in CRC risk in individuals with a family history of ≥1 first-degree relative with CRC younger than 60 years of age or CRC in ≥2 first-degree relatives at any age, a personal history of inflammatory bowel disease or primary sclerosing cholangitis, or a personal history of advanced adenomatous or serrated polyps. The highest risk (>20%) for CRC includes individuals with a germline pathogenic variant or colorectal phenotype associated with a hereditary CRC syndrome or serrated polyposis syndrome. To facilitate the identification of higher than average-risk individuals, an accurate, three-generation family cancer history with special attention to ages at cancer diagnosis and death and advanced adenomatous and serrated polyps should be documented [5].

Once the eligible patient or population is identified, education must be provided to the screenee to ensure awareness of the benefit of screening including advantages and disadvantages of each modality available. An exploration of differences between one- and two-step screening tests, ascertainment of the screenee willingness to undergo timely diagnostic colonoscopy for the evaluation of positive results from a two-step test, and adherence to recommended follow-up of a negative test are mandatory. The quality of screening programs requires objective metrics, continuous monitoring of compliance with benchmarks, and investigation and remediation of the process to achieve the highest patient outcomes.

CRC screening is recommended for asymptomatic, average-risk individuals. Age is a major risk factor for CRC, whereby incidence rates increase dramatically with age, with rates doubling every 5 years until 50 years of age and increasing by 30% after 55 years with each 5-year interval thereafter [6]. In most recent years, however, CRC is impacting younger individuals, with a declining incidence rate in older population, owing partly to increased screening uptake in this age group [2]. The median age of CRC diagnosis has shifted from 72 years between 2001 and 2005 to 66 years between 2015 and 2016 [6]. CRC incidence and mortality have also begun to increase in individuals <50 years old, termed as early-age onset CRC (EAO-CRC) [7]. Unlike late-onset CRC (LO-CRC), EAO-CRC manifests differently in terms of its pathology, anatomical distribution, biology, and epidemiology [8]. Current increases in incidence rates of CRC in 45–49-year-olds reflect trends noted in 50-year-olds in the 1990s prior to the uptake of CRC screening. This has influenced the American College of Gastroenterology (ACG), American Cancer Society (ACS), the United States Multi-Society Task Force (USMSTF), and the United States Preventive Services Task Force (USPSTF) to recommend CRC screening starting at age 45, previously recommended at age 50 [7]. It is estimated that lowering the age of screening to 45 from 50 years has added 19 million adults to the screening population [4]. Therefore, it is of paramount importance to utilize the appropriate resource for the right screenee.

Underuse, Misuse, and Overuse of Screening

Underuse, misuse, and overuse of screening can negatively impact the efficacy and quality of the CRC screening programs, limit resource availability, and cause potential harm to the individuals. CRC screening is underused when individuals eligible for screening do not undergo screening or do not adhere to screening at appropriate intervals. Offering inappropriate screening options, for example, FIT (fecal immunochemical test) instead of colonoscopy, to individuals at high risk of CRC such as a personal or family history of CRC or advanced adenoma is an example of misuse. Repeating a stool test after it is positive instead of timely referral to colonoscopy is another example of misuse of screening.

Providing testing to individuals not due for CRC screening or to those with limited life expectancy is an example of overuse of screening. Studies have reported overuse of screening among recipients of Medicare and Veterans Affairs medical systems [9, 10]. Practice audit process should be established to monitor for underuse, misuse, and overuse of screening modalities. Organized screening programs have shown to have some protection against these forms of harms of screening [11].

Colorectal Cancer Screening Modalities

Multiple modalities are approved for CRC screening (Table 9.1). They can be considered as one-step or two-step tests. Colonoscopy is a one-step test that completes the screening process by being both diagnostic and therapeutic whereby polyps can also be removed. Two-step tests are the ones wherein a positive test requires a follow-up colonoscopy. They include fecal- and blood-based tests, CT colonography, and capsule colonoscopy.

Table 9.1 Recommended colorectal cancer screening options along with their screening intervals

Society	Age recommendations	Screening tools (interval recommendations)
USPSTF	45–75 (grade A)	HSgFOBT (annually) FIT (annually) Multi-target stool DNA (q1–3 years) Colonoscopy (q10 years) CT colonography (q5 years) FS (q5 years) FS with FIT (FS q10 years plus FIT annually)
ACS	45–75	HSgFOBT (annually) FIT (annually) Multi-target stool DNA (q3 years) Colonoscopy (q10 years) FS (q5 years)
USMSTF	45–75 (strong)	**Tier 1** Colonoscopy (q10 years) FIT (annually) **Tier 2** CT colonography (q5 years) FS (q10 years) **Tier 3** Capsule colonoscopy (q5 years)
ACP	45–75	HSgFOBT (q2 years) FIT (q2 years) Colonoscopy (q10 years) FS with FIT (FS q10 years plus FIT q2 years)
NCCN	45–75	HSgFOBT (annually) FIT (annually) Multi-target stool DNA (q3 years) Colonoscopy (q10 years) CT colonography (q5 years) FS (q5 years)

USPSTF, United States Preventive Services Task Force; ACS, American Cancer Society; USMSTF, United States Multi-Society Task Force; ACP, American College of Physicians; NCCN, National Comprehensive Cancer Network; HSgFOBT, high-sensitivity guaiac fecal occult blood testing; FIT, fecal immunochemical test; FS, flexible sigmoidoscopy

Note: adapted from *Screening and prevention of colorectal cancer* by Kanth and Inadomi, 2021, 374. Copyright 2021 BMJ [12]

The USPSTF does not recommend a preferred screening method, while the USMSTF recommends colonoscopy and stool FIT as their preferred options. The USMSTF suggests flexible sigmoidoscopy, multi-target stool DNA test, CT colonography, and capsule colonoscopy be offered to those unwilling or unable to undergo colonoscopy or FIT [13, 14].

Stool-Based FIT

In the USA, CRC screening is most often opportunistic, often offered by a primary care provider (PCP) at a routine office visit. Stool-based tests are typically offered sequentially to patients who decline colonoscopy. For those considering these non-invasive at-home stool tests, key requirements should be discussed and emphasized with patients including the need for regular (annually or biennial) exams if negative and a timely follow-up colonoscopy if the test is positive.

When organizing a FIT-based screening program, practices face several challenges to set up key elements at multiple levels of the program: (1) provider and participant, (2) choice and type of stool test and processing laboratory units, and (3) navigation system to follow up on positive screening stool tests to ensure completion of timely colonoscopy following a positive test (Fig. 9.1). These key processes provide several opportunities for quality measurement and improvement.

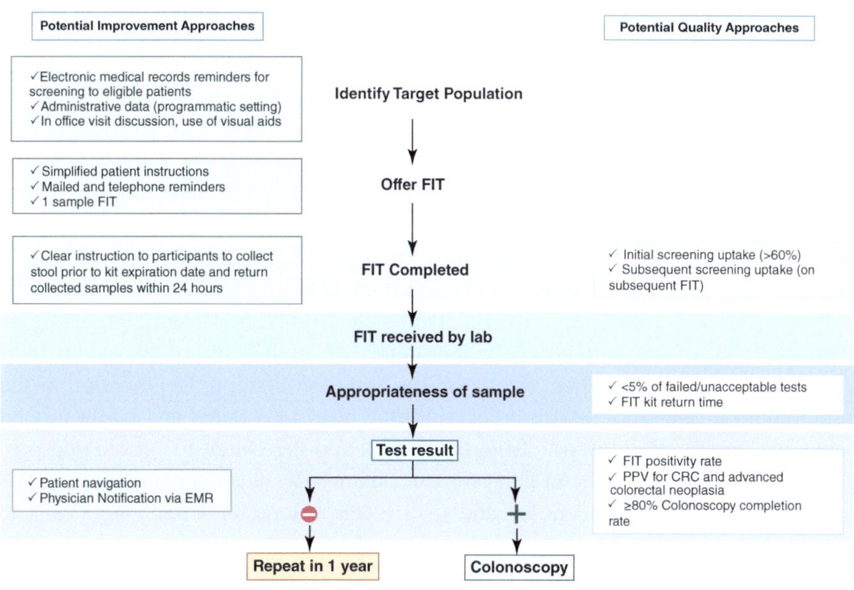

Fig. 9.1 Improvement and quality measures associated with FIT

FIT Quality Issues

Optimization of FIT Screening Uptake

In a programmatic screening program, eligible patients are identified using administrative data, and pre-invitation letters are usually sent to patients prior to mailing the stool test kit. Several approaches have been described in the literature to optimize outreach such as simplified instructions for stool test kit and mailed and telephone reminders. In a systematic review and meta-analysis of 73 US trials, repeated mailed fecal blood tests with patient navigation were associated with an increased annual test completion (relative risk, 2.09; 95% CI, 1.91–2.29) [13]. A large randomized controlled trial showed that electronic message sent via electronic health records (EHR) prior to mailing FIT increased uptake of CRC screening in 5.5% of the enlisted population [15].

In the opportunistic setting, use of electronic medical records reminders to offer screening to eligible patients, discussion of CRC screening options at routine clinic visits using decision aids, and conversation cards have been suggested by societies and experts to enhance shared decision-making around screening [16]. Compared to usual care, the combination of a video-based CRC screening decision aid immediately before their PCP encounter and patient navigation in a primary care safety net setting helped patients to more likely complete a CRC screening test within 6 months of the index visit (adjusted difference 40 percentage points; 95% CI, 29–51 percentage points). Patient-provider contact and engagement was shown to be one of the strongest predictors of screening uptake [17].

Optimization of Patient Preparation of the FIT and Instruction on Prompt Return of Completed Tests

The USMSTF recommends the use of a single-sample FIT over the traditional three-card gFOBT owing to its increased sensitivity for CRC and advanced colorectal neoplasia detection and its superior adherence. FIT is easier to complete and does not require dietary or medication adjustment. Thus, patient instructions can be greatly simplified. Instructions should also be clear on effective sampling using an unexpired FIT kit and emphasize the importance of rapid return of the specimen to the laboratory for processing, ideally on the day of collection. Degradation of the hemoglobin in the stool before processing may lead to a failed test and a missed screening opportunity. Reports from the French and the Dutch FIT screening programs showed that processing delays greater than 7–10 days increased false negative tests for advanced adenoma and to a lesser extent for CRC [18, 19]. The USMSTF suggests that participants should be informed about the importance of fast return of the kit, preferably within 24 h of collection [19]. Programs are advised to monitor their kit return time and should request a repeat test in case the return time was beyond the range of acceptability based on the kit manufacturer.

Optimization of Choice of FIT, Number of Samples, and Interval for Repeat Testing

Quantitative FITs are preferred over qualitative FITs. Large national screening programs in Europe often rely on quantitative FITs due to their consistent performance characteristic for CRC and advanced adenoma. In countries with limited colonoscopy resources, the fecal hemoglobin threshold can be adjusted to improve positive predictive value of colonoscopy and better meet endoscopic resources. Similarly, in countries with adequate colonoscopy access, FIT threshold can be lowered to 10 μg/g of stool, thus increasing its sensitivity to 91% and specificity to 90% [20].

Evidence supports the use of a single FIT compared to two- or three-sample FITs as the pooled performed characteristics of FIT for CRC were similar regardless of the number of FIT samples [21]. This helps increase patient participation as we know from FIT vs. three-card gFOBT trials; participation was more than 20% higher in the FIT group [22].

The ideal interval for FIT-based screening is unclear. Most population-based screening programs outside of the USA use biennial screening. In the Dutch screening program, the number of advanced neoplasia found at repeat screening was not affected when testing interval varied over 1–3 years [22]. Three ongoing RCTs (CONFIRM, COLOPREV, and SCREESCO trials) are comparing colonoscopy to annual or biennial FIT for the risk of CRC incidence and mortality.

Optimization of Positive FIT Results Follow-Up

Timely follow-up colonoscopy after a positive FIT is critical for the success of the FIT-based screening program. Although a completion colonoscopy target of 80% has been advised, this benchmark is not reached in many instances for several reasons: lack of physician referral, nonadherence to referrals of colonoscopy due to financial issues, transportation, and other structural barriers. A recent retrospective review at a large, integrated health system that uses FIT as the main screening method found that 8% of patients dying from CRC had an abnormal FIT screening result without appropriate follow-up (odds ratio, 7.26; 95% CI, 5.26–10.03) which highlights the need for interventions to improve timely follow-up colonoscopy after an abnormal result, thus optimizing the effectiveness of screening in preventing deaths from CRC [17]. Patient navigators who can provide one-on-one education and individually address structural barriers and provider notification of positive FIT results via EHR may improve follow-up after a positive stool test [23].

Longer time delays between a positive FIT and diagnostic colonoscopy are associated with worse outcomes. In a recently published systematic review, colonoscopy performed >9 months vs. within 1 month from positive FIT was associated with a higher incidence of CRC [adjusted odds ratios (AORs) of 1.75 and 1.48 in the largest 2 studies] and a higher incidence of advanced stage CRC at diagnosis, with AORs of 2.79 and 1.55, respectively [24].

Recommended Quality Metrics for FIT

The USMSTF has suggested specific quality-management standards for FIT-based programs:

- FIT completion rate of >60% of individuals offered screenings.
- Proportion of returned FIT that cannot be processed of less than 5%.
- Colonoscopy completion rate for those with positive FIT of 80% or greater.
- Adenoma detection rate greater than 45% in men and 35% in women on colonoscopies performed in patients with positive FIT using a threshold of 20 μg/g hemoglobin/g dry stool or less.

Experts have suggested additional key metrics for noninvasive CRC screening tests [5]:

- Ninety percent or greater of noninvasive test should be completed within 1 year of ordering the test.
- Patients who do not complete a noninvasive screening test within 1 month should undergo outreach to improve compliance.
- Outreach should be attempted in all participants within 2 weeks of the test result.
- Participants with negative test results should be informed of the appropriate recall interval and how the recall will happen.
- All participants with positive test results should be offered a colonoscopy date within 6 months.
- Percentage of colonoscopy performed after a positive noninvasive test/number of colonoscopies recommended should be 95% or greater.

Multi-target DNA Test Quality Issues

In the USA, multi-target stool DNA (mt-sDNA) test was approved by the Food and Drug Administration (FDA) in 2014 for average-risk screening. The performance characteristic study on mt-sDNA reported test accuracy by age [25]. The company (Exact Sciences) controls the distribution, receipt, processing, and result reporting of the test and quality control of its screening test. mt-sDNA is costly compared to FIT alone which limited thus far its applicability in a large-scale CRC screening outreach program.

Based on the DeeP-C study, about 14% of individuals with positive mt-sDNA will have a negative colonoscopy [25]. Other than possible missed lesions on colonoscopy, concerns over an increase in aerodigestive cancers outside of the colon have been raised. However, recent studies showed that relative to SEER, aerodigestive cancer incidence is reduced in patients with positive mt-sDNA and negative colonoscopy [26, 27].

Colonoscopy Quality Issues

Colonoscopy is recommended as a Tier 1 CRC screening test by USMSTF and a commonly performed procedure in the USA. Colonoscopy requires bowel preparation and dietary modification prior to the procedure. Most of the colonoscopies are done under sedation in the USA, which require the patient to be accompanied by an adult upon discharge. Being a one-step test, colonoscopy allows not just the detection but removal of the precancerous polyps in the same setting. Limitation of the colonoscopy includes the possibility of procedural complications of aspiration, perforation, bleeding, and infection, especially among those with underlying cardiovascular conditions. Over-detection of adenomas that would not have progressed to cancer is a potential harm of colonoscopy screening, but no research has directly assessed their health implications [28, 29]. Missed lesions and post-colonoscopy CRC (PCCRC) are some other major drawbacks of colonoscopy. In some studies, the prevalence of PCCRC has been reported to be up to 3.7–8.6% which can be prevented with improving procedural factors in colonoscopy [30]. A robust quality assurance program in improving colonoscopy is thus essential to reducing PCCRC.

Colonoscopy is the preferred diagnostic test for patients with positive tests from other screening methods. High-quality colonoscopy is crucial for the effectiveness of any screening method. The USMSTF on Colorectal Cancer has defined several colonoscopy quality metrics including adenoma detection rate, cecal intubation rate, and withdrawal time among others. These colonoscopy-specific quality metrics are discussed in detail in a different chapter.

Role of Artificial Intelligence in Colonoscopy

Artificial intelligence (AI) has been increasingly used in different facets of medicine including for detection of polyps during colonoscopy. AI is employed endoscopically to distinguish hyperplastic polyps from premalignant lesions, using real-time computer-aided detection (CADe) whereby red boxes appear on the screen to help identify potential polyps [31]. Randomized controlled trials have shown increased adenoma detection rate (ADR) with AI [32]. Additionally, AI can also alert endoscopists regarding blind spots and excess speeds during withdrawal. This can theoretically lead to increased detection of premalignant lesions, hence resulting in reduction in CRC incidence and CRC-related mortality. However, AI may result in overdiagnosis leading to frequent colonoscopies with potential for treatment complications. This can be circumvented by utilizing and improving AI tools including computer-aided diagnosis (CADx) which helps classify polyps into histology of diminutive lesions which may not need to be removed, hence avoiding complications and pathology-associated costs. AI can be used to train low-performing endoscopists to increase ADR in an effort to improve quality of colonoscopies [33]. However, not all endoscopists may benefit from using AI as studies have shown that those with high ADRs have near-zero post-colonoscopy CRC without utilizing AI [34]. Despite the potential pitfalls and need for further development and improvement, AI can be used to standardize procedure documentation, increase adenoma detection rates, and aid in automatically notifying patients and PCP regarding results and assign appropriate interval time [35].

Sigmoidoscopy Quality Issues

Data from randomized controlled trials and observational studies provide sufficient evidence demonstrating that a single screening sigmoidoscopy reduces CRC incidence and mortality [14, 36, 37]. While overall ADR was 12.1% in the UK Flexible Sigmoidoscopy Screening Trial, wide variation in ADRs was observed, ranging from 8.6% to 15.9% ($p < 0.0001$), mostly attributed to variation in the performance of the endoscopists [38, 39]. Similar to colonoscopy, low ADR by endoscopists performing flexible sigmoidoscopy increases the risk for interval distal cancer [40]. A recent study suggested that insertion of the scope to the splenic flexure and achieving a withdrawal time from the splenic flexure of at least 3.25 min improve ADR [41]. ADR increased from 8.2% for endoscopists with <2.5 min estimated splenic flexure withdrawal time to 9.9% for endoscopists with 3.25–3.99 min estimated withdrawal time, and 10.0% for ≥4 min estimated splenic flexure withdrawal time (p trend = 0.021).

Quality improvement targets have been published for screening flexible sigmoidoscopy. They include completion of adequate follow-up colonoscopy on more than 90% of patients in whom it is indicated and documentation of depth of insertion in cm and of the quality of bowel preparation [42].

CT Colonography Quality Issues

CT colonography (CTC) is recommended as a two-step screening test for CRC screening and has reasonable accuracy to detect CRC and adenoma. USMSTF suggests CT colonography as a screening test for individuals unable or unwilling to undergo colonoscopy or FIT and it should be repeated every 5 years (Table 9.1). This can be preferred approach for those with significant cardiovascular risk factors for sedation, for example, before cardiac or pulmonary transplant setting. Benefits include CTC being a less invasive test, not requiring sedation, and therefore having lower risk of complications than colonoscopy. However, some bowel preparation is still required and a positive result should be followed up with a colonoscopy. Extra-colonic findings can be detected in 1.3–11.4% of examinations [14]. With new techniques requiring less radiation (1–5 mSv), the risk of radiation exposure may no longer be a significant concern [14, 43].

Adequate colonic preparation, insufflation, and often fecal tagging are essential for accurate test results. Rate of inadequate exams due to limited preparation or insufflation should be monitored. CT Colonography Reporting and Data System, or "C-RADS," has been proposed for standardized reporting systems to minimize variability in reporting and comparisons.

Quality indicators comparable to colonoscopy are yet to be established for CTC. Similar to colonoscopy, adequate training and rigorous quality control of examination performance are essential for optimizing the efficacy of CTC. The radiologists should have expertise to detect subtle colonic lesions and have specialty interest in CRC screening. Accreditation training programs for radiologists have been proposed. The practice should also be monitored to avoid unnecessary referral of healthy asymptomatic individuals for further testing for extra-colonic findings which can potentially cause harm and increase cost of care [44].

Blood-Based Test Quality Issues

Blood-based tests can be a desirable option by many given their convenience and ease. It is minimally invasive with fewer risks of complications. It can be added to routine blood draw. Repeat interval is unknown and positive results require colonoscopy. Long-term reduction in CRC incidence and mortality remains unknown. It may potentially improve patient adherence.

The only FDA-approved blood-based screening option currently available is a Septin 9 PCR test known as Epi proColon® (Epigenomics) which detects methylation of the promoter region of Septin 9 DNA. The USPSTF recommendation for CRC screening does not include blood tests. Despite its convenience, Septin 9 is not considered a preferred CRC screening method by any society and ACG recommends against using it [13]. The USPSTF currently endorses Septin 9 for average-risk adults ≥50 years who have declined other USPSTF-endorsed CRC screening modalities. Sensitivity and specificity for CRC detection for Septin 9 have been reported to be 62% and 90% in a recent systematic review, but sensitivity for advanced adenoma detection was significantly lower to 11% [45].

Colon Capsule Endoscopy Quality Issues

Colon capsule endoscopy is a newer noninvasive modality that does require bowel preparation, but no medication adjustment or sedation is required. It is painless and has minimal risk of complications. The technology has improved sensitivity and specificity with second-generation cameras [46]. In a 2016 meta-analysis, second-generation capsule cameras detected polyps >10 mm with 87% sensitivity (95% CI,

81–91%) and 95.3% specificity (95% CI, 91.5–97.5%) and identified all 11 invasive cancers detected by colonoscopy [46]. In a recent study, the sensitivity of second-generation capsule for polyps ≥6 mm, polyps ≥10 mm, and adenomas ≥10 mm was 79% (95% CI: 62–91%), 88% (95% CI: 62–98%), and 100% (95% CI: 72–100%), respectively [47]. If a lesion is detected, an optical colonoscopy and repeat bowel preparation are required. Colon capsule endoscopy is not recommended for CRC screening by any of the societies. It is approved by the US FDA for use only in patients who had an incomplete colonoscopy for technical or other reasons. More research is needed to determine accuracy and efficacy of this emerging technology in order to potentially improve CRC screening acceptance and adherence [14]. Quality metrics regarding quality of bowel preparation, timely excretion rate of the capsule before the battery expires, standardization of image reading process, and adherence with a follow-up colonoscopy if a test is found positive would be some of the potential quality assurance steps.

Intervention to Maximize Adherence to CRC Screening

The effectiveness of CRC screening is not simply limited to the efficacy of screening options available but encompasses other elements including access to screening, awareness of its importance, adherence to the screening choice selected, and appropriate follow-up of both positive and negative tests. Quality metrics must be established, measured, and adhered to at an individual, provider, and systems level to increase the efficacy of CRC screening.

Individual-Level Interventions

In order to propose quality metrics for CRC screening on an individual level, one must understand the pattern in differences in adherence to CRC screening and preference for different CRC screening modalities among different population subgroups.

Optimizing adherence to CRC screening Non-adherence to CRC screening contributes to CRC related morbidity and mortality [48]. Despite strong recommendations from all major medical societies, only 66% of all eligible adults in the US are up to date on testing. Adherence varies among minority race/ethnicity groups, insurance status (uninsured at 30% or insured by Medicaid at 53%) [6], socioeconomic status (SES), education, and geographical location, to name a few. Only 52% of individuals with less than high school level education are up-to-date on screening. Within the USA, there is substantial variability in CRC screening by state ranging from 60% in Wyoming to 76% in Massachusetts in all adults aged ≥50, in 2018 [6]. Less than 55% of individuals living below the federal poverty line are up-to-date on screening. People with low SES who are Medicare beneficiaries are less likely to have supplemental insurance to cover their share of cost associated with colonoscopy which has led to reduced CRC screening uptake [49]. Co-pays and deductibles are major barrier to screening. Recently, several states including Kentucky (2016), Oregon (2017), and California (2021) have enacted policies to eliminate cost sharing. Furthermore, as of 2022, federal guidance was issued which eliminated cost sharing for follow-up colonoscopy after a positive CRC screening test [50].

Preference for CRC screening modality Different CRC screening tests carry different effectiveness, safety, and cost profile with varying degree of adherence. Steering patients to one preferred strategy, for example, colonoscopy, has been shown to lead to reduced uptake, especially in some racial-ethnic groups who prefer stool-based testing [51]. It is important to understand patient preferences to best tailor intervention efforts to different segments of the population. Furthermore, it must be emphasized that the best CRC screening is the one that increases adherence in the individual [52]. Research has shown that offering multiple CRC screening modalities increases individual participation and acknowledges their preferences [16, 51, 53]. According to one study, FOBT is more likely opted for by women, especially married women, and those whose partners have also undergone screening [17]. Another study also pointed for a preference for stool-based tests among women who showed higher uptake for FIT compared to men who chose colonoscopy [18]. A national survey assessing patients' preference for type of CRC screening found an overall preference for stool-based tests over colonoscopy [19]. Prior exposure or experience with stool-based tests also increased adherence to a similar test over colonoscopy, preferably mt-sDNA over FIT/gFOBT. Uninsured individuals also opted for stool-based tests over colonoscopy, highlighting financial barriers to colonoscopy. There is mixed data about preference for a certain CRC screening modality among different racial-ethnic groups. Some studies have shown a preference for colonoscopy among non-Hispanic White (NHW), while racial-ethnic minorities opt for stool-based tests [51]. There are other studies that highlight preference for colonoscopy among racial-ethnic minorities [20]. These differences in study findings may be partly explained by differences in preferences in different subpopulations included in these studies and partly explained by different dissemination of information about CRC screening modalities among racial-ethnic minorities compared to NHW and access to different modalities.

While adherence to CRC screening can be increased by tailoring population-specific strategies, there are other quality metrics that have been shown to increase adherence across different populations (Fig. 9.2). This includes educational materials tailored to overcome language/cultural barriers, EHR alerts and reminders, invitation letters (either by the hospital or insurance company at the recommended intervals), and public service announcements, all of which have been shown to increase awareness and uptake of CRC screening [21–23]. Other factors such as patient navigation tailored specifically to the target population, mailing FIT kits, easy access to bowel preparation material, and/or FOBT kits also increase uptake by up to 20% [24, 54].

INDIVIDUAL LEVEL	SYSTEM LEVEL	PROVIDER LEVEL
Positive Factors • Mailing Fit Kit • Culturally appropriate educational materials with attention to language barriers • Electronic health records reminders • Invitation letters by insurance or providers • Easy access to bowel preparation • Participating in other cancer screenings • Family history of cancer or personal history of cancer • Having regular access to care • Having private insurance • Being non-hispanic white • Having high level of education Negative Factors • Low education • Racial ethnic minorities • Low income • Reduced access to care • Being acultured in the US including English proficiency, being foreign born, years living in the US	• Organized and funded screening programs • Insurance coverage for CRC screening and subsequent treatment • Public Service announcements targeted to increase awareness • Improving access to CRC screening tests	• Primary care provider's recommendaion • Effective patient provider cmmunication • Counseling and educating about importance of CRC screening and options available • Availability of patient navigator in helping patients with understanding or finishing screening

Fig. 9.2 Factors that impact colorectal cancer screening uptake

Provider-Level Interventions

Patients with no access to PCP miss out on CRC screening opportunity [55]. Research has shown that regular care within the medical system and a provider recommendation for screening have been established as the strongest correlates to increases in CRC screening uptake [56, 57]. There are multiple roles that PCP are able to perform including triaging patients who qualify for CRC screening, educating patients on the importance of CRC screening, providing different screening options, educating on bowel preparation or other various tests, assuaging fears patients may have about procedures, and having a risk-benefit discussion with patients regarding the most appropriate screening strategy within the constraints of the healthcare system [58]. This can be particularly useful for patients with low health literacy and patients with no or limited access to technology.

System-Level Interventions

On a population level, two screening approaches have been utilized: (1) opportunistic screening, whereby PCP offers CRC screening to patients either on their request, their risk factors, or their age/comorbidities profile, and (2) organized screening, where screening is offered to all, without any cost. Compared to opportunistic CRC screening commonly practiced in the USA, programmatic approaches such as the

FIT-based programs in the Bowel Cancer Screening Program (BCSP) in England and Kaiser Permanente in Northern California have been shown to be more successful at increasing screening, uptake, and follow-up testing [59–61]. Organized screening programs in France and Italy were shown to have increased screening uptakes with reduced disparities across different SES groups compared to areas with opportunistic screening [62]. Screening methods such as FIT are much easier to implement in a large-scale organized program, are affordable, and are known to increase screening uptake. CRC screening rates in opportunistic screening are negatively impacted by insurance coverage and amount of copay [63].

System-level interventions that can increase awareness and subsequent uptake include free screening programs and mandatory health insurance coverage for screening and diagnostic testing. These free interventions can eliminate financial barriers, particularly for individuals with low socioeconomic status [62]. Other barriers to address on a system level include transportation issues, lack of chaperone to colonoscopy involving sedation, language or literacy barriers in understanding bowel preparation instructions, and homelessness where access to a restroom to complete bowel preparation is not feasible [64]. Furthermore, assuring adequate staffing with patient educators and navigators, financial counselors, and social workers is important to overcome the aforementioned logistical barriers. Their tasks include, for a minimum, sending appointment reminders, scheduling timely CRC screening, and ensuring appropriate following up of both normal and abnormal tests which have been shown to increase CRC screening [65].

Disparities in CRC Screening

CRC disproportionately affects certain racial-ethnic groups and people with low socioeconomic status. Multiple factors contribute to these socioeconomic disparities including differences in access to CRC screening, timely follow-up of abnormal tests, lack of access to high-quality resources, and different lifestyle risk factors including smoking, obesity, sedentary lifestyle, and unhealthy diet including consumption of red meat, processed meat, and alcohol, low consumption of fruits and vegetables, and SES [66, 67]. Compared to people with the highest SES, people with the lowest SES are 40% more likely to be diagnosed with CRC. Even after controlling for risk factors between the two populations, non-Hispanic Blacks have a similar rate of developing CRC as NHW but are less likely to receive high-quality colonoscopy or timely follow-up [68].

Compared to other races/ethnicities, the incidence and mortality rates of CRC are highest among Black adults. From 2013 to 2017, the CRC incidence rates were as follows: 43.6 cases per 100,000 Black adults, 39.0 cases per 100,000 American Indian/Alaska Native adults, 37.8 cases per 100,000 White adults, 33.7 cases per 100,000 Hispanic/Latino adults, and 31.8 cases per 100,000 Asian/Pacific Islander adults [69].

Recent evidence suggests that inequities in access to, utilization of, and quality of CRC screening and treatment, rather than genetic differences, are the primary driver of this health disparity [70]. White and Hispanic/Latino adults, but not Black or Asian/Pacific Islander adults, have exhibited a recent trend of increasing CRC incidence among adults younger than 50 years [71]. Development of systems of care with outreach programs is vital with a particular focus on Black communities and those with lower SES, which have historically had poorer CRC health outcomes [14].

Quality Issues with CRC Screening in the Elderly

Elderly population is more susceptible to overuse of CRC when screening is offered to those above 85 years of age or those with severe comorbid conditions. Several studies have shown that those with severe comorbid conditions are screened approximately as frequently as those without comorbid diseases [72, 73].

These issues are of particular interest in the elderly population on when to stop screening. In practice, clinicians base their decisions regarding screening on age, while a minority continue to provide CRC screening for those with less than 5 years of life expectancy, resulting in underuse or overuse of CRC screening [72, 74]. Previous guidelines suggest screening through age 75, particularly for individuals who are up-to-date on screening and have prior negative screening tests or have a life expectancy of less than 10 years. There is a paucity of data regarding the benefits of continued screening past age 75. Thus, the ACG, USPSTF, American College of Physicians (ACP), and ACS recommended that 75–86-year-olds should have a shared decision with their provider regarding continued screening, weighing risks vs. benefits and factoring in their life expectancy, comorbidities, prior screening history, and their own preferences. The USMSTF, on the other hand, recommends screening up to age 85 years old with no prior screening history, factoring in their comorbidities. There is a growing body of evidence highlighting the need for patient-centered discussion to assess risk vs. benefit of CRC screening and surveillance [75]. CRC screening is no longer recommended past age 86, as the risk of screening from direct visualization test may outweigh the benefits. Furthermore, older patients are also prone to post-polypectomy bleeding and a 30% increase in perforation compared to the younger population [76]. Other factors must also be factored including withholding hypoglycemic agents, antithrombotic, and anticoagulants in this population. Furthermore, bowel preparation could lead to electrolyte derangements, dehydration, and falls among the elderly.

Using a microsimulation model, Hees et al. developed a web-based tool, Colosmart (http://www.frankly.yetes.nl/), to determine the most appropriate age at which to stop CRC screening, factoring in commodities, race, sex, prior screening history, and risk of CRC [77].

Conclusions

There is strong evidence that increasing CRC screening rate will lower CRC incidence and mortality [78]. Despite the availability of multiple screening modalities and numerous public health initiatives, CRC screening options are underused, and approximately one-third of the eligible US population remains unscreened [13]. On the other hand, significant overuse and misuse of resources exist [79]. Overall effectiveness of CRC screening depends not only on the efficacy of the screening modality but also on the education, outreach, and navigation [78]. Elimination of cost sharing across the continuum of screening process is crucial to improve effectiveness of the screening program and reduce disparities. Quality assurance with monitoring and steps to improve the process at each step are imperative regardless of the modality of screening.

Quality assurance programs should also aim to achieve equity in care to eliminate racial and ethnic disparities in CRC screening uptake. Furthermore, with the advances made in technology, artificial intelligence tools may play an important role in improving quality of CRC screening.

References

1. Siegel R, Miller K, Fuchs H, Jemal A. Cancer statistics. CA Cancer J Clin. 2021;71(1):7–33.
2. Siegel RL, Fedewa SA, Anderson WF, et al. Colorectal cancer incidence patterns in the United States, 1974–2013. JNCI J Natl Cancer Inst. 2017;109(8):djw322.
3. Edwards BK, Ward E, Kohler BA, et al. Annual report to the nation on the status of cancer, 1975–2006, featuring colorectal cancer trends and impact of interventions (risk factors, screening, and treatment) to reduce future rates. New York: Wiley Online Library; 2010. p. 544–73.
4. Piscitello A, Edwards DK. Estimating the screening-eligible population size, ages 45–74, at average risk to develop colorectal cancer in the United States. Population estimate after lowering CRC screening start age. Cancer Prev Res. 2020;13(5):443–8.
5. Burke CA, Lieberman D, Feuerstein JD. AGA clinical practice update on approach to the use of noninvasive colorectal cancer screening options: commentary. Gastroenterology. 2022;162(3):952–6.
6. Siegel RL, Miller KD, Goding Sauer A, et al. Colorectal cancer statistics, 2020. CA Cancer J Clin. 2020;70(3):145–64.
7. Patel SG, May FP, Anderson JC, et al. Updates on age to start and stop colorectal cancer screening: recommendations from the US Multi-Society Task Force on Colorectal Cancer. Gastroenterology. 2022;162(1):285–99.
8. Stoffel EM, Murphy CC. Epidemiology and mechanisms of the increasing incidence of colon and rectal cancers in young adults. Gastroenterology. 2020;158(2):341–53.
9. Murphy CC, Sandler RS, Grubber JM, Johnson MR, Fisher DA. Underuse and overuse of colonoscopy for repeat screening and surveillance in the Veterans Health Administration. Clin Gastroenterol Hepatol. 2016;14(3):436–444.e1.
10. Goodwin JS, Singh A, Reddy N, Riall TS, Kuo Y-F. Overuse of screening colonoscopy in the Medicare population. Arch Intern Med. 2011;171(15):1335–43.
11. Dominitz JA, Levin TR. What is organized screening and what is its value? Gastrointest Endosc Clin. 2020;30(3):393–411.

12. Kanth P, Inadomi JM. Screening and prevention of colorectal cancer. BMJ. 2021;374:n1855.
13. Shaukat A, Kahi CJ, Burke CA, Rabeneck L, Sauer BG, Rex DK. ACG clinical guidelines: colorectal cancer screening 2021. Am J Gastroenterol. 2021;116(3):458–79.
14. Davidson KW, Barry MJ, Mangione CM, et al. Screening for colorectal cancer: US Preventive Services Task Force recommendation statement. JAMA. 2021;325(19):1965–77.
15. Goshgarian G, Sorourdi C, May FP, et al. Effect of patient portal messaging before mailing fecal immunochemical test kit on colorectal cancer screening rates: a randomized clinical trial. JAMA Netw Open. 2022;5(2):e2146863.
16. Daskalakis C, Vernon SW, Sifri R, et al. The effects of test preference, test access, and navigation on colorectal cancer screening. Assessing elements of colorectal cancer screening strategies. Cancer Epidemiol Biomarkers Prev. 2014;23(8):1521–8.
17. Solmi F, Von Wagner C, Kobayashi LC, Raine R, Wardle J, Morris S. Decomposing socioeconomic inequality in colorectal cancer screening uptake in England. Soc Sci Med. 2015;134:76–86.
18. Senore C, Inadomi J, Segnan N, Bellisario C, Hassan C. Optimising colorectal cancer screening acceptance: a review. Gut. 2015;64(7):1158–77.
19. Zhu X, Parks PD, Weiser E, et al. National survey of patient factors associated with colorectal cancer screening preferences. Cancer Prev Res. 2021;14(5):603–14.
20. Hawley ST, Volk RJ, Krishnamurthy P, Jibaja-Weiss M, Vernon SW, Kneuper S. Preferences for colorectal cancer screening among racially/ethnically diverse primary care patients. Med Care. 2008;46(9):S10–6.
21. Raine R, Atkin W, von Wagner C, et al. Testing innovative strategies to reduce the social gradient in the uptake of bowel cancer screening: a programme of four qualitatively enhanced randomised controlled trials. Southampton: NIHR Journals Library; 2017.
22. Kerrison RS, McGregor LM, Counsell N, et al. Use of two self-referral reminders and a theory-based leaflet to increase the uptake of flexible sigmoidoscopy in the English bowel scope screening program: results from a randomized controlled trial in London. Ann Behav Med. 2018;52(11):941–51.
23. Mankaney G, Rizk M, Sarvepalli S, et al. Patient-initiated colonoscopy scheduling effectively increases colorectal cancer screening adherence. Dig Dis Sci. 2019;64(9):2497–504.
24. Dougherty MK, Brenner AT, Crockett SD, et al. Evaluation of interventions intended to increase colorectal cancer screening rates in the United States: a systematic review and meta-analysis. JAMA Intern Med. 2018;178(12):1645–58.
25. Imperiale TF, Ransohoff DF, Itzkowitz SH, et al. Multitarget stool DNA testing for colorectal-cancer screening. N Engl J Med. 2014;370(14):1287–97.
26. Berger BM, Kisiel JB, Imperiale TF, et al. Low incidence of aerodigestive cancers in patients with negative results from colonoscopies, regardless of findings from multitarget stool DNA tests. Clin Gastroenterol Hepatol. 2020;18(4):864–71.
27. Cotter TG, Burger KN, Devens ME, et al. Long-term follow-up of patients having false-positive multitarget stool DNA tests after negative screening colonoscopy: the LONG-HAUL cohort study. Long-term outcomes of false-positive multitarget stool DNA. Cancer Epidemiol Biomarkers Prev. 2017;26(4):614–21.
28. Lin JS, Perdue LA, Henrikson NB, Bean SI, Blasi PR. Screening for colorectal cancer: an evidence update for the US Preventive Services Task Force. Rockville, MD: Agency for Healthcare Research and Quality (US); 2021.
29. Lin JS, Perdue LA, Henrikson NB, Bean SI, Blasi PR. Screening for colorectal cancer: updated evidence report and systematic review for the US Preventive Services Task Force. JAMA. 2021;325(19):1978–98.
30. Singh S, Singh PP, Murad MH, Singh H, Samadder JN. Prevalence, risk factors, and outcomes of interval colorectal cancers: a systematic review and meta-analysis. Am J Gastroenterol. 2014;109(9):1375–89.
31. Wang P, Berzin TM, Brown JRG, et al. Real-time automatic detection system increases colonoscopic polyp and adenoma detection rates: a prospective randomised controlled study. Gut. 2019;68(10):1813–9.

32. Barua I, Vinsard DG, Jodal HC, et al. Artificial intelligence for polyp detection during colonoscopy: a systematic review and meta-analysis. Endoscopy. 2021;53(03):277–84.
33. Repici A, Spadaccini M, Antonelli G, et al. Artificial intelligence and colonoscopy experience: lessons from two randomised trials. Gut. 2022;71(4):757–65.
34. Nishihara R, Wu K, Lochhead P, et al. Long-term colorectal-cancer incidence and mortality after lower endoscopy. N Engl J Med. 2013;369(12):1095–105.
35. Berzin TM, Parasa S, Wallace MB, Gross SA, Repici A, Sharma P. Position statement on priorities for artificial intelligence in GI endoscopy: a report by the ASGE Task Force. Gastrointest Endosc. 2020;92(4):951–9.
36. Atkin WS, Edwards R, Kralj-Hans I, et al. Once-only flexible sigmoidoscopy screening in prevention of colorectal cancer: a multicentre randomised controlled trial. Lancet. 2010;375(9726):1624–33.
37. Brenner H, Stock C, Hoffmeister M. Effect of screening sigmoidoscopy and screening colonoscopy on colorectal cancer incidence and mortality: systematic review and meta-analysis of randomised controlled trials and observational studies. BMJ. 2014;348:g2467.
38. Atkin W, Rogers P, Cardwell C, et al. Wide variation in adenoma detection rates at screening flexible sigmoidoscopy. Gastroenterology. 2004;126(5):1247–56.
39. Fracchia M, Senore C, Armaroli P, et al. Assessment of the multiple components of the variability in the adenoma detection rate in sigmoidoscopy screening, and lessons for training. Endoscopy. 2010;42(6):448–55.
40. Rogal SS, Pinsky PF, Schoen RE. Relationship between detection of adenomas by flexible sigmoidoscopy and interval distal colorectal cancer. Clin Gastroenterol Hepatol. 2013;11(1):73–8.
41. Bevan R, Blanks RG, Nickerson C, et al. Factors affecting adenoma detection rate in a national flexible sigmoidoscopy screening programme: a retrospective analysis. Lancet Gastroenterol Hepatol. 2019;4(3):239–47.
42. Levin T, Farraye F, Schoen R, et al. Quality in the technical performance of screening flexible sigmoidoscopy: recommendations of an international multi-society task group. Gut. 2005;54(6):807–13.
43. Zalis ME, Barish MA, Choi JR, et al. CT colonography reporting and data system: a consensus proposal. Radiology. 2005;236(1):3–9.
44. IJspeert J, Nolthenius CT, Kuipers E, et al. CT-colonography vs. colonoscopy for detection of high-risk sessile serrated polyps. Am J Gastroenterol. 2016;111(4):516–22.
45. Church TR, Wandell M, Lofton-Day C, et al. Prospective evaluation of methylated SEPT9 in plasma for detection of asymptomatic colorectal cancer. Gut. 2014;63(2):317–25.
46. Spada C, Pasha SF, Gross SA, et al. Accuracy of first- and second-generation colon capsules in endoscopic detection of colorectal polyps: a systematic review and meta-analysis. Clin Gastroenterol Hepatol. 2016;14(11):1533–1543.e8.
47. Voska M, Zavoral M, Grega T, et al. Accuracy of colon capsule endoscopy for colorectal neoplasia detection in individuals referred for a screening colonoscopy. Gastroenterol Res Pract. 2019;2019:1.
48. Doubeni CA, Fedewa SA, Levin TR, et al. Modifiable failures in the colorectal cancer screening process and their association with risk of death. Gastroenterology. 2019;156(1):63–74.e6.
49. McArdle F, Neuman T, Huang J. Retiree health benefits at the crossroads. Menlo Park, CA: Kaiser Family Foundation; 2014. http://kff.org/report-section/retiree-health-benefits-at-the-crossroadsoverview-of-health-benefits-for-pre-65-and-medicare-eligible-retirees.
50. US Department of Labor UDoHaHS, US Department of the Treasury. FAQs about Affordable Care Act Implementation Part 51, Families First Coronavirus Response Act and Coronavirus Aid, Relief, and Economic Security Act Implementation. https://www.dol.gov/sites/dolgov/files/EBSA/about-ebsa/our-activities/resource-center/faqs/aca-part-51.pdf. Accessed 27 Aug 2022.
51. Inadomi JM, Vijan S, Janz NK, et al. Adherence to colorectal cancer screening: a randomized clinical trial of competing strategies. Arch Intern Med. 2012;172(7):575–82.
52. Bibbins-Domingo K, Grossman DC, Curry SJ, et al. Screening for colorectal cancer: US Preventive Services Task Force recommendation statement. JAMA. 2016;315(23):2564–75.

53. Pilonis ND, Bugajski M, Wieszczy P, et al. Participation in competing strategies for colorectal cancer screening: a randomized health services study (PICCOLINO Study). Gastroenterology. 2021;160(4):1097–105.
54. Melson JE, Imperiale TF, Itzkowitz SH, et al. AGA white paper: roadmap for the future of colorectal cancer screening in the United States. Clin Gastroenterol Hepatol. 2020;18(12):2667–2678.e2.
55. Levin TR, Jamieson L, Burley DA, Reyes J, Oehrli M, Caldwell C. Organized colorectal cancer screening in integrated health care systems. Epidemiol Rev. 2011;33(1):101–10.
56. Laiyemo AO, Adebogun AO, Doubeni CA, et al. Influence of provider discussion and specific recommendation on colorectal cancer screening uptake among US adults. Prev Med. 2014;67:1–5.
57. Vernon SW. Participation in colorectal cancer screening: a review. J Natl Cancer Inst. 1997;89(19):1406–22.
58. Grazzini G, Castiglione G, Isu A, et al. Colorectal cancer screening by fecal occult blood testing: results of a population-based experience. Tumori J. 2000;86(5):384–8.
59. Libby G, Brewster D, McClements P, et al. The impact of population-based faecal occult blood test screening on colorectal cancer mortality: a matched cohort study. Br J Cancer. 2012;107(2):255–9.
60. Zorzi M, Fedeli U, Schievano E, et al. Impact on colorectal cancer mortality of screening programmes based on the faecal immunochemical test. Gut. 2015;64(5):784–90.
61. McClements PL, Madurasinghe V, Thomson CS, et al. Impact of the UK colorectal cancer screening pilot studies on incidence, stage distribution and mortality trends. Cancer Epidemiol. 2012;36(4):e232–42.
62. Eisinger F, Cals L, Calazel-Benque A, et al. Impact of organised programs on colorectal cancer screening. BMC Cancer. 2008;8(1):1–8.
63. Seeff LC, Shapiro JA, Nadel MR. Are we doing enough to screen for colorectal cancer? Findings from the 1999 behavioral risk factor surveillance system. J Fam Pract. 2002;51(9):761.
64. Issaka RB, Bell-Brown A, Snyder C, et al. Perceptions on barriers and facilitators to colonoscopy completion after abnormal fecal immunochemical test results in a safety net system. JAMA Netw Open. 2021;4(8):e2120159.
65. Thompson NJ, Boyko EJ, Dominitz JA, et al. A randomized controlled trial of a clinic-based support staff intervention to increase the rate of fecal occult blood test ordering. Prev Med. 2000;30(3):244–51.
66. Doubeni CA, Major JM, Laiyemo AO, et al. Contribution of behavioral risk factors and obesity to socioeconomic differences in colorectal cancer incidence. J Natl Cancer Inst. 2012;104(18):1353–62.
67. Carethers JM, Doubeni CA. Causes of socioeconomic disparities in colorectal cancer and intervention framework and strategies. Gastroenterology. 2020;158(2):354–67.
68. Fedewa SA, Flanders WD, Ward KC, et al. Racial and ethnic disparities in interval colorectal cancer incidence: a population-based cohort study. Ann Intern Med. 2017;166(12):857–66.
69. Races A, Rates A-A, Rates A-S. SEER cancer statistics review 1975–2017; 2020.
70. Rutter CM, Knudsen AB, Lin JS, Bouskill KE. Black and white differences in colorectal cancer screening and screening outcomes: a narrative review. Cancer Epidemiol Biomarkers Prev. 2021;30(1):3–12.
71. Virostko J, Capasso A, Yankeelov TE, Goodgame B. Recent trends in the age at diagnosis of colorectal cancer in the US National Cancer Data Base, 2004-2015. Cancer. 2019;125(21):3828–35.
72. Walter LC, Lindquist K, Nugent S, et al. Impact of age and comorbidity on colorectal cancer screening among older veterans. Ann Intern Med. 2009;150(7):465–73.
73. Fisher DA, Judd L, Sanford NS. Inappropriate colorectal cancer screening: findings and implications. Am J Gastroenterol. 2005;100(11):2526–30.
74. Kahi CJ, Van Ryn M, Juliar B, Stuart JS, Imperiale TF. Provider recommendations for colorectal cancer screening in elderly veterans. J Gen Intern Med. 2009;24(12):1263–8.

75. Cenin DR, Tinmouth J, Naber SK, et al. Calculation of stop ages for colorectal cancer screening based on comorbidities and screening history. Clin Gastroenterol Hepatol. 2021;19(3):547–55.
76. Day LW, Walter LC, Velayos F. Colorectal cancer screening and surveillance in the elderly patient. Am J Gastroenterol. 2011;106(7):1197–206.
77. Van Hees F, Saini SD, Lansdorp-Vogelaar I, et al. Personalizing colonoscopy screening for elderly individuals based on screening history, cancer risk, and comorbidity status could increase cost effectiveness. Gastroenterology. 2015;149(6):1425–37.
78. Lieberman D, Ladabaum U, Brill JV, et al. Reducing the burden of colorectal cancer: AGA position statements. Gastroenterology. 2022;163(2):520–6.
79. Holden DJ, Harris R, Porterfield DS, et al. Enhancing the use and quality of colorectal cancer screening. Evid Rep Technol Assess. 2010;190:1–195, v.

Chapter 10
Quality in Management of GI Bleeding

Ryan Flanagan and Daniel J. Stein

Table of Quality Measures/Metrics

R. Flanagan (✉)
Division of Gastroenterology, Hepatology and Endoscopy, Brigham and Women's Hospital, Boston, MA, USA

Harvard Medical School, Boston, MA, USA
e-mail: rflanagan1@bwh.harvard.edu

D. J. Stein
Harvard Medical School, Brigham and Women's Hospital, Boston, MA, USA
e-mail: djstein@bwh.harvard.edu

J. D. Feuerstein, D. J. Stein (eds.), *Quality in Gastroenterology*,
https://doi.org/10.1007/978-3-031-58492-3_10

Key Points

- Management of GI bleeding involves a coordination of both procedural and medical aspects.
- Risk stratification of all patients is key to appropriate intervention choice and timing.
- Endoscopy is the mainstay of therapy for most patients, but coordination with radiology and surgery when appropriate is key, especially for patients with rapid bleeding or after failure of endoscopic therapy.

Society Guidelines and Quality Indicators

Clinical care for gastrointestinal (GI) bleeding is informed by several society guidelines, likely owing to the clinical frequency and considerable associated morbidity [1–7]. While there is some variability in recommendations, these generally offer concise and evidence-based approaches. Similar to other guidelines, they are not universally applicable and may not provide sufficient guidance in cases with significant additional clinical considerations. Despite their existence, there remains an ongoing need for explicitly defined quality indicators which are specific and measurable and can be used for ongoing quality improvement of the sort seen in colorectal cancer screening. While there has been a move to develop some of these quality metrics in non-variceal upper GI bleeding, there are far fewer quality indicators in lower GI bleeding, and none for small bowel bleeding [8–10]. Additionally, the quality indicators that do exist for non-variceal upper GI bleeding often have limited evidence, with some guidelines basing up to half (13/26) of the recommendations solely on case series or expert opinion [9]. There are far fewer quality indicators that have been explicitly designed for the purpose of tracking over time for continuous quality improvement. In this chapter, we will highlight the most impactful guideline recommendations, discuss previously suggested quality indicators, and explore additional aspects of quality in the treatment of GI bleeding.

Medical Management of GI Bleeding

There are a variety of considerations in the medical management of GI bleeding which include pre-procedural treatment, management of anticoagulation and coagulopathy, and evidence-based medications for improving outcomes.

General Care for all Patients with GI Bleeding

When a patient presents with GI bleeding, initial evaluation includes assessing vital signs, obtaining secure IV access to allow rapid resuscitation (typically two large-bore intravenous catheters 18 gauge or larger), and alerting the GI consultant or GI bleed team within 1 h if there is clinically significant bleeding [3, 8]. Significant bleeding should be suspected in cases of hemodynamic instability (including positive orthostatic signs in patients with normal vital signs while lying in bed) or ongoing high-volume bleeding that is evident on exam (i.e., high volume of hematemesis, melena, or hematochezia). When clinically significant bleeding is suspected, the care team should initiate plans for rapid transfusion if required and start a multidisciplinary discussion between gastroenterology and where appropriate interventional radiology and surgery about diagnostic and therapeutic strategy to minimize all potential delays in appropriate care. The involvement of a critical care team for evaluation and provision of ICU-level care is also indicated in cases with any clinically significant bleeding.

Hemoglobin/hematocrit values should be interpreted with caution, given that these rarely indicate the severity or duration of bleeding in isolation, compared with the clinical history and physical exam. Hemodynamic resuscitation should be initiated early and guided primarily by hemodynamics. While exact hemoglobin thresholds have been debated, the fundamental balance is between adequate end-organ perfusion and risk of volume overload (manifested by transfusion-associated cardiac overload (TACO) and by increased portal pressures in variceal bleed patients). For most patients, a threshold of >7–8 g/dL has been suggested by evidence showing this restrictive transfusion strategy is associated with lower mortality and rebleeding rates in upper GI bleeding [11]. This threshold has also been used for lower GI bleeding, with recent data showing no difference between restrictive and liberal strategies in this population [12]. In general, patients should not be transfused in the absence of rapid bleeding or a hemoglobin level that is expected to be less than 7–8 g/dL. Higher transfusion thresholds are appropriate for patients with concern for active coronary ischemia.

Management of Anticoagulation, Antiplatelet Agents, and Coagulopathy

The management of anticoagulation and antiplatelet medications, as well as the management of coagulopathy during a GI bleed, is nuanced but can be guided by general principles. Specific management of anticoagulation and antithrombotic medications depends on the severity of the bleeding, the indication for the medication, and the stability of the patient. In general, endoscopy should not be delayed for GI bleeding solely due to anticoagulation or antithrombotic medication. Historically, an INR <2.5 (in reference to vitamin K antagonist use) has been recommended prior to endoscopy if the patient can safely await any delay this may cause, based on research showing endoscopy is generally safe with this INR value [13–15]. However there are multiple controversial clinical implications of using this cutoff including the appropriate methods for achieving this INR, the safety of endoscopy with an

INR >2.5, the correct approach when the INR may not reflect true coagulopathy such as in a patient with advanced liver disease, and the potential benefits of endoscopy on anticoagulation for obscure GI bleeding. Importantly, there is no data directly comparing hemostasis and rebleeding rates between hemostatic methods for patients taking anticoagulation or antiplatelet agents, so choice of hemostatic method should be based on lesion characteristics rather than the presence of anticoagulation or antiplatelet agents.

In the setting of severe life-threatening bleeding, reversal of anticoagulation should be considered, and endoscopy should generally not be delayed. When reversing warfarin, prothrombin complex concentrate (PCC) is preferred over fresh frozen plasma (FFP) due to decreased effects on intravascular volume and increased efficacy of INR reduction [15]. Vitamin K administration should generally be avoided given its latent effect and risk of prolonged subtherapeutic INR once anticoagulation is resumed. Aspirin taken for secondary prevention should be continued during most GI bleeding episodes but, if stopped for severe bleeding, should be restarted on the day of endoscopic hemostasis to prevent cardiovascular events [16]. Clopidogrel should generally not be stopped in a patient who has had percutaneous coronary intervention with stent placement within the prior 30 days, due to the high risk of in-stent thrombosis. When necessary, multidisciplinary discussion between cardiology and gastroenterology can help weigh the cardiovascular risks of stopping anticoagulation or anti-platelets with the risk of bleeding. Reversal of anticoagulation is generally not necessary except for the setting of severe life-threatening bleeding. However, the specific indication for antithrombotic therapy plays an important role in whether holding or reversing a medication is indicated. For instance, atrial fibrillation with a low stroke risk would pose a much lower embolic risk than a patient with a mechanical mitral valve or a left ventricular assist device (LVAD). While the risks and benefits need to be weighed in each case, endoscopy often provides definitive hemostasis; thus significant delays due to coagulopathy would likely be harmful in many cases. After hemostasis is achieved, anticoagulation should be restarted in 7–14 days, as this has been shown in multiple studies to decrease the risk of thromboembolic events, without an increased risk of recurrent GI bleeding [17, 18]. If antiplatelet agents are stopped for a procedure, they should be resumed after hemostasis has been achieved [14].

Similar to management of coagulopathy, management of thrombocytopenia in the periprocedural period has limited direct evidence for specific thresholds and efficacy to reduce bleeding and rebleeding. There is evidence to suggest that patients with GI bleeding and platelet counts as low as 20×10^3/mL can undergo endoscopy safely with high rates of effective hemostasis [19]. Avoiding delays in endoscopy for thrombocytopenia can decrease overall packed RBC and platelet transfusion requirements, as effective hemostasis directly reduces this need. Additional considerations for managing coagulopathy in severe bleeding include ensuring the fibrinogen is 120–150 mg/dL or giving antifibrinolytic agents such as aminocaproic acid or tranexamic acid, though both of these interventions have limited data to support their use [20, 21]. Furthermore, the use of anti-fibrinolytics has not shown any benefit for patients who undergo endoscopic treatment for their bleeding [21].

Evidence-Based Medications for GI Bleeding

Proton Pump Inhibitor

For patients presenting with upper GI bleeding, a proton pump inhibitor (PPI) given intravenously is the standard of care, as it has been shown to reduce the need for endoscopic intervention during the index endoscopy [22]. However, there has not been sufficient evidence from randomized controlled trials to show decreases in patient-specific outcomes such as rebleeding, need for blood transfusion, need for surgery, or mortality. Thus, while PPI treatment is standard of care, the clinical impact of its use is relatively small compared with endoscopic intervention. However, by reducing the need for endoscopic therapy at index endoscopy, PPI therapy decreases healthcare costs and has been shown to be a cost-effective strategy [23]. In patients with ulceration on endoscopy, the recommended duration of PPI therapy should be explicitly stated in the procedure documentation, to avoid long-term PPI therapy, particularly in patients with an identifiable reversible cause such as NSAIDs or *H. pylori* infection. Patients with *H. pylori* usually only need PPI treatment as part of their *H. pylori* treatment, while patients with gastric ulcers from NSAIDs often need 8 weeks of therapy for highest healing rates [24, 25]. Additionally, there should be explicit recommendations for patients with lifelong indication for PPI and for patients without ulceration on endoscopy that the PPI should be stopped if no longer indicated.

Erythromycin

Erythromycin prior to endoscopy for upper GI bleeding has been shown to significantly improve gastric visualization, decrease the need for second-look endoscopy, and decrease length of stay by approximately 2 days [26]. Early consideration of ordering and administering this medication is paramount, as it may not be readily available due its decreasing use in clinical practice for other indications. Delays in medication administration can occur that limit its use prior to urgent endoscopy when it may be most helpful. Erythromycin is also cost-effective by decreasing the need for repeat procedures [27]. Nasogastric lavage does not provide any additional benefit compared with erythromycin, and is not recommended [28]. Metoclopramide has not been found to be efficacious in gastric visualization in limited studies, so routine use is not recommended [29].

Antibiotics, Octreotide, and Nonselective Beta-Blockers for Patients with Cirrhosis

Patients with cirrhosis who present with GI bleeding should receive a third-generation cephalosporin (or equivalent) and octreotide, in addition to standard care for all patients with GI bleeding regardless of ascites presence. Ceftriaxone or an equivalent antibiotic is preferable to a fluoroquinolone, due to the use of fluoroquinolones for prophylaxis and increasing resistance patterns. However, the specific choice of antibiotic should be informed by the patient's prior microbiology results, prior antibiotic courses, contraindications, medication interactions, and local antibiotic resistance patterns. The use of antibiotics in patients with cirrhosis and GI bleeding decreases the rate of rebleeding, bacterial infections (including but not limited to spotaneous bacterial peritonitis (SBP)), and morality [30]. Octreotide has been associated with improved initial control of bleeding and 5-day hemostasis when combined with endoscopic treatment [31]. By itself, octreotide also slightly reduces the need for blood transfusion by about half of a unit on average, though it has not been shown to reduce mortality [32].

All patients with cirrhosis who have esophageal variceal bleeding should have consideration of nonselective beta-blocker (NSBB) therapy after acute bleeding, as this has been shown to decrease the risk of rebleeding as well as death from rebleeding [33]. In addition to usual considerations of beta-blocker use, there are multiple important contraindications for NSBB therapy in cirrhosis specifically. These are related to the degree of decompensation and include hyponatremia, acute kidney injury, decreased systolic blood pressure or mean arterial pressure, diuretic-resistant ascites, or history of spontaneous bacterial peritonitis. In most cases, endoscopic variceal ligation in addition to NSBB therapy is preferred for secondary prophylaxis due to lower rebleeding rates compared to either strategy on its own [34, 35]. While NSBB therapy has high-quality evidence for reduced rebleeding in esophageal hemorrhage, adherence to this practice has been suboptimal, prompting an important consideration as a potential quality metric similar to beta-blockers after acute coronary syndrome [36].

Risk Stratification

Risk stratification in GI bleeding has evolved over time with the introduction of multiple risk scores for bleeding, yet the utility and uptake of these scores into clinical practice has varied. The most validated use for clinical risk scores has been using the Glasgow-Blatchford score (GBS) to determine when a patient has a very low risk for rebleeding and mortality [37]. The GBS is based on the blood urea nitrogen, hemoglobin, pulse rate, systolic blood pressure, presence of melena, syncope, hepatic disease, or cardiac failure and notably can be calculated on initial hospital presentation as it does not include endoscopic findings. Patients with a GBS ≤ 1 are considered to be at very low risk of rebleeding, very unlikely to have an endoscopically treatable lesion, and very low risk for mortality [38]. Thus, as long as discharge is otherwise appropriate for the patient, they can be safely discharged with outpatient follow-up, which can greatly reduce healthcare resource utilization.

Despite society recommendations to utilize the GBS to identify low-risk patients, there are several barriers that have contributed to limited uptake in routine clinical practice. There are both a lack of knowledge that the score exists and a belief that it has limited utility among GI providers as well as other hospital providers [39]. By using the GBS on initial presentation to the emergency department, low-yield endoscopies and potential hospitalizations may be avoided. The Oakland Score is a scoring system to identify patients with lower GI bleeding who are at low risk for experiencing adverse outcomes, and may similarly help in reducing unnecessary hospitalizations, though its role in clinical practice thus far has been limited [40].

Determining whether a patient needs ICU level of care depends on the rapidity of bleeding, hemodynamics, need for urgent endoscopy, and risk of airway compromise, among many other factors. The AIMS65 score was developed to determine in-hospital mortality risk and has been found to be the best performing risk score for predicting ICU level of care in upper GI bleeding [41]. While the score is not routinely used by emergency departments, the underlying components of the score may be helpful to consider when deciding appropriate level of care. Albumin <3 g/dL, INR >1.5, altered mental status, systolic blood pressure <90 mmHg, and age >65 years are all risk factors for needing ICU level of care. Additional considerations for ICU placement are whether an urgent endoscopy for upper GI bleeding will require intubation, the need for multiple units of packed RBC transfusion, the need for vasopressor medications, and other comorbidities that could contribute to higher mortality risk such as cardiopulmonary disease.

Timing of Endoscopy

There have been multiple studies assessing the optimal timing of endoscopy for both upper and lower GI bleeding. While the considerations for timing vary for each individual patient, studies have shown that EGD for non-variceal upper GI bleeding should generally be done within 24 h, as early endoscopy within 6 h of presentation does not improve mortality outcomes, in the absence of persistent hypovolemic shock [42]. While patients who are unstable despite significant blood product transfusion may need earlier intervention, the majority of patients can safely undergo endoscopy within 24 h. Early endoscopy in less than 6 h before presentation may lead to poor visualization and inadequate resuscitation. Though endoscopy is recommended within 24 h, there has been poor adherence to this timing noted in the literature [43]. This threshold could potentially be used as a quality measure that can be tracked and assessed by quality improvement initiatives. While current guidelines recommend endoscopy within 12 h for variceal bleeding, this has not been shown to improve outcomes in a meta-analysis [44]. Thus, there are likely more important prognostic factors than timing of endoscopy such as severity of liver disease, hemodynamic instability at presentation, and concurrent infection that should influence the most appropriate timing for endoscopy in patients with suspected variceal bleeding [45, 46].

Colonoscopy for lower GI bleeding can generally occur more than 24 h after presentation without decreased diagnostic yield, likelihood of hemostatic intervention, or change in mortality risk [47]. As in the case of upper GI bleeding, severity and rate of bleeding should be taken into account along with other patient-related factors to determine optimal procedure timing. Patients with suspected rapid lower GI bleeding may benefit from a rapid colonoscopy prep via nasogastric tube to achieve adequate visualization with urgent colonoscopy. Patients with distal sources of bleeding such as rectal ulcers can have life-threatening bleeding that does not require a full colonoscopy prep, so earlier intervention in these patients with flexible sigmoidoscopy, along with surgical team backup, is prudent.

Endoscopic Management of GI Bleeding

Non-variceal Upper GI Bleeding

Once the patient has an identified source of bleeding, the endoscopist should determine if the lesion has an actively bleeding or non-bleeding blood vessel, as treatment of these lesions has been demonstrated to be very effective at reducing further bleeding [2]. There is not a universal recommendation regarding whether to attempt removing an adherent clot after vigorous lavage. If rebleeding occurs on such a lesion, removal of clot may reveal a treatable vessel during subsequent endoscopy. Injection of epinephrine prior to clot removal could potentially reduce bleeding and improve visualization during clot removal. Lesions with a pigmented spot or a clean base do not benefit from endoscopic therapy, so use of therapy in these cases is generally not recommended.

The specific method for treating a visible vessel or actively bleeding lesion has been a focus in many studies but is likely less important than general principles of hemostasis. Epinephrine can be a useful adjunct in severe bleeding limiting visualization or as a temporizing method if adequate hemostasis cannot be achieved; however it should not be used as the only therapy due to high rebleeding rates [2]. Additionally, epinephrine injected before other therapy may stop bleeding and make it more difficult to accurately apply additional hemostasis or cause local tissue swelling that can make clip placement more challenging. Thus, use of epinephrine should be situation dependent rather than routine.

Bipolar cautery and hemostatic clips have equivalent rates of rebleeding, though additional factors can be helpful in deciding between the two [48]. Bipolar cautery may be more advantageous in large ulcers when clips cannot be placed safely across the ulcer, when it allows for easier targeting of the culprit vessel, or if other hemostatic methods have previously failed for the given lesion. While there has been a suggestion to avoid bipolar therapy and other tissue destructive methods when the INR is >1.5, there is insufficient evidence to suggest a benefit to clips rather than bipolar cautery in this setting [9]. Evidence from the use of electrocautery in surgical practice (e.g., Bovie electrocautery) indicates relative efficacy despite a lack of published data in endoscopy. Argon plasma coagulation (APC) has limited direct comparative evidence to clips and bipolar cautery in the treatment of ulcer bleeding but is generally used for superficial vascular lesions such as gastric antral vascular ectasia (GAVE) and angioectasias.

Hemostatic sprays can be used as an adjunctive treatment in GI bleeding when initial hemostasis cannot be achieved or the treatment area is diffuse (such as a bleeding tumor), or if rebleeding has occurred [49]. Recent data suggests that monotherapy with hemostatic spray may have similar rates of initial hemostasis and rebleeding compared to conventional therapy, though some data has suggested lower 30-day mortality with combination therapy compared to monotherapy [49–52]. If a hemostatic spray is used as monotherapy for initial management of a high-risk lesion, a repeat endoscopy with hemostatic clip placement or bipolar coagulation may be needed for high-risk lesions (Forrest Ia). While a majority of patients will have successful initial hemostasis, there is a variable reported risk of rebleeding with hemostatic spray as both a monotherapy and salvage therapy, with rebleeding rates between 8% and 49% within 7 days of initial intervention [52, 53]. In the case of tumor bleeding, further cancer-directed treatments, IR angiography, surgery, and radiation therapy, should be considered when hemostatic spray is utilized given its short-term durability. Hemostatic spray has a clearly established role in the management of GI bleeding, and this role may expand with further data from real-world practice and additional studies.

The over-the-scope clip (OTSC) is a relatively new device that can be used as an initial treatment for a visible vessel or as salvage treatment. Use of an OTSC can significantly reduce rates of rebleeding, severe complications, and red blood cell transfusion for lesions with high-risk stigmata [54]. In refractory peptic ulcer bleeding, using an OTSC has shown to be more successful than IR-guided therapy at decreasing ICU stay and in-hospital mortality [55]. Clinical success in hemostasis of non-variceal upper GI bleeding has been shown to be higher with OTSC compared to conventional therapies, both as an initial treatment and salvage treatment [56]. Use of the OTSC requires adequate training of the endoscopist since its deployment mechanism differs from traditional hemostatic clips. In the future, the use of an OTSC as an initial therapy in cases where there are significant stigmata of bleeding will likely become routine, as it provides a safe and definitive treatment in these cases.

Variceal Bleeding

Variceal bleeding represents an important subset of GI bleeding, with particularly high morbidity and mortality. While the most common site of varices is the esophagus, patients can also present with gastric varices, rectal varices, or ectopic varices elsewhere in the GI tract. For esophageal varices, endoscopic variceal ligation (EVL) is the preferred method of treatment [57]. When there is active bleeding or high-risk stigmata such as a white fibrin plug, the source of bleeding can be definitively attributed to varices. However, if there is no other source of bleeding in a patient with recent hemorrhage, then EVL should be performed in this setting, as varices are the assumed source. Once EVL has been done for initial bleeding, there should be consideration of an early interval endoscopy for repeat banding, as the majority of recurrent bleeding occurs within 14 days [58]. EVL often leads to post-banding ulcers, and there has been some data to suggest higher risk of rebleeding with more bands placed, so excessive banding should be avoided [58, 59]. Bands should be placed on any varix with active bleeding or high-risk stigmata. Future EVL should occur at regular intervals (e.g., 4–6 weeks) until the varices are eradicated. Sucralfate and PPI use after banding have both been independently shown to decrease the size of post-banding ulcers, but effect on post-banding ulcer bleeding is unclear [60, 61].

Transjugular intrahepatic portosystemic shunt (TIPS) placement should also be considered in the setting of acute variceal bleeding. A randomized controlled trial has found benefit for early TIPS (within 72 h of admission) in certain high-risk patients, defined as Child-Turcotte-Pugh class C with score 10–13 or Child-Turcotte-Pugh class B with active bleeding on endoscopy [62]. Observational data on outcomes after this trial has confirmed the role of early TIPS to decrease rebleeding risk, though not in improving 1-year mortality [63]. TIPS should also be considered as a salvage therapy for any patient with persistent bleeding or severe rebleeding, despite EVL [64]. Other adjunct treatments for esophageal varices, which can provide initial hemostasis and allow more time for definitive therapies, include hemostatic spray and balloon tamponade devices [65, 66].

Gastric varices and ectopic varices have significantly less data given their rarity, but treatment options include tissue adhesive injection (e.g., cyanoacrylate), endoscopic band ligation, TIPS, and balloon-occluded retrograde transvenous obliteration (BRTO) [67]. Treatment depends in part on the type of gastric varix, according to the Sarin classification [68]. GOV1 can be managed similarly to esophageal varices with EVL. For GOV2 and IGV1, otherwise known as cardiofundal varices, there has been a lower risk of rebleeding documented with tissue adhesive injection compared with EVL, so this method is generally preferred. TIPS and BRTO are also definitive treatment options, and interventional radiology should be involved early in cases of gastric variceal bleeding that cannot be controlled with endoscopic methods, given the effectiveness of both procedures.

Small Intestinal Bleeding

While small intestinal bleeding represents only 5–10% of GI bleeding, it can represent a unique diagnostic and management dilemma [69]. Patients with overt signs of bleeding (e.g., melena) should generally undergo video capsule endoscopy (VCE), as this has a high yield (92.3%) in patients with overt bleeding [70]. If the patient is unstable, which is generally rare in small intestine bleeding, then proceeding directly to CT angiography (CTA) and possible embolization may be necessary. Once a lesion has been located by VCE or CTA, a deep enteroscopy should be performed for treatment of the lesion. If deep enteroscopy with push enteroscopy (PE), single-balloon enteroscopy (SBE), or double-balloon enteroscopy (DBE) is nondiagnostic and the patient continues to have bleeding, an intraoperative enteroscopy can be considered in coordination with the surgery team. While the diagnostic yield of VCE, PE, and DBE is similar (35–45%), VCE is less invasive and carries less procedural risk, so generally it should be the first-line diagnostic test [69]. Imaging with CT enterography and MR enterography can be helpful in cases of a suspected mass causing bleeding or Crohn's disease. Non-overt obscure GI bleeding can be more difficult to diagnose, with the diagnostic yield of VCE dropping to 12.9% in this setting [70]. Iron supplementation and serial CBC monitoring may be appropriate for patients without significant bleeding and a negative VCE. Availability of equipment and adequate training are both necessary for SBE and DBE, so if patients require these tests, care should be taken to ensure the patient is at an institution that can perform such procedures.

Lower GI Bleeding

There are multiple clinical differences that make lower GI bleeding distinct from upper GI bleeding, including the time needed for bowel preparation, the likelihood of finding a bleeding source, and the types of lesions encountered. The TYPICAL Index is a prediction tool that can be helpful for determining the likelihood of finding a bleeding source requiring hemostasis, malignant-appearing lesions, or active bleeding [71]. As previously discussed, risk assessment is often more complex than the prediction models for GI bleeding; however the TYPICAL Index could still be helpful in the informed consent process, risk/benefit calculation, and possibly avoiding colonoscopies that might be particularly low yield.

Endoscopic evaluation of lower GI bleeding should generally include a full colonoscopy, including terminal ileum intubation, to ensure complete evaluation for a source of bleeding. Similar to upper GI bleeding, the same endoscopic tools are available for hemostasis including hemostatic clips, APC, bipolar coagulation, and hemostatic spray depending on the lesion found. Similar to upper GI bleeding, endoscopic hemostasis is recommended for patients with high-risk stigmata, including active bleeding, non-bleeding visible vessel, or adherent clot [6]. Patients with hemodynamically significant or rapid bleeding should have CT angiography and potentially IR intervention, since the time needed for bowel preparation could lead to clinical deterioration. As a last resort in severe bleeding refractory to GI and IR intervention, or for patients who have recurrent life-threatening bleeding, surgery with partial or total colectomy could be considered. Diverticular bleeding can be particularly difficult to locate, and if patients have had multiple prior colonoscopies for non-life-threatening bleeding in this setting, close observation and serial CBC monitoring can be considered in lieu of a repeat colonoscopy.

Other Considerations

Nutrition

Patients who present with GI bleeding, like other hospitalized patients, have improved outcomes such as decreased length of hospital stay, when they receive early feeding within 24–48 h of admission [72]. Patients with high-risk stigmata or variceal bleeding may require holding of feeding for 48 h to ensure adequate visualization in the event of a rebleeding, though this has not been rigorously studied [73]. Patients with low-risk stigmata ulcer bleeding or other causes of bleeding such as esophagitis, gastritis, or angioectasias should be fed early after endoscopy. After EVL for varices, the optimal diet has not been established, but often a liquid or soft diet is recommended for the initial 24–48 h after the procedure, to prevent the theoretical risk of band dislodgement.

Procedural Documentation

Accurate and comprehensive procedural documentation is important to ensure appropriate care of patients in the post-procedure period. There are some guidelines available regarding suggested photo documentation and written documentation for procedure reports, but few recommendations specific to GI bleeding exist [74, 75]. All reports should include an accurate description of the bleeding lesion (including appropriate classification such as Forrest classification for ulcers and Sarin classification for gastric varices). The report should clearly indicate whether effective hemostasis has been achieved and, if possible, an estimate of the rebleeding risk. If multiple potential bleeding sources are seen, the endoscopist should make a judgment about the most likely source of bleeding. A recommendation as to when anticoagulation and anti-platelets can be restarted is helpful for the primary inpatient team, acknowledging that the benefits and risks must be weighed in each case. There should be specific diet recommendations with time intervals documented if a regular diet after endoscopy is inappropriate. If medications are recommended for treatment of bleeding such as PPI or octreotide, a specific length of time or date for stopping these medications should be clearly documented, given the potential associated harms of unnecessary PPI use [76]. Finally, the endoscopist should document the need and timing for a repeat endoscopy, if indicated.

References

1. Hwang JH, Fisher DA, Ben-Menachem T, et al. The role of endoscopy in the management of acute non-variceal upper GI bleeding. Gastrointest Endosc. 2012;75:1132–8.
2. Laine L, Barkun AN, Saltzman JR, Martel M, Leontiadis GI. ACG clinical guideline: upper gastrointestinal and ulcer bleeding. Am J Gastroenterol. 2021;116:899–917.
3. Barkun AN, Almadi M, Kuipers EJ, et al. Management of nonvariceal upper gastrointestinal bleeding: guideline recommendations from the international consensus group. Ann Intern Med. 2019;171:805–22.
4. Gralnek IM, Dumonceau JM, Kuipers EJ, et al. Diagnosis and management of nonvariceal upper gastrointestinal hemorrhage: European Society of Gastrointestinal Endoscopy (ESGE) guideline. Endoscopy. 2015;47:a1–a46.

5. Gralnek IM, Stanley AJ, Morris AJ, et al. Endoscopic diagnosis and management of nonvariceal upper gastrointestinal hemorrhage (NVUGIH): European Society of Gastrointestinal Endoscopy (ESGE) guideline—update 2021. Endoscopy. 2021;53:300–32.
6. Strate LL, Gralnek IM. ACG clinical guideline: management of patients with acute lower gastrointestinal bleeding. Am J Gastroenterol. 2016;111:459–74.
7. Oakland K, Chadwick G, East JE, et al. Diagnosis and management of acute lower gastrointestinal bleeding: guidelines from the British Society of Gastroenterology. Gut. 2019. https://doi.org/10.1136/GUTJNL-2018-317807.
8. Cohen J, Safdi MA, Deal SE, et al. Quality indicators for esophagogastroduodenoscopy. Gastrointest Endosc. 2006;63:S10–5.
9. Kanwal F, Barkun A, Gralnek IM, et al. Measuring quality of care in patients with nonvariceal upper gastrointestinal hemorrhage: development of an explicit quality indicator set. Am J Gastroenterol. 2010;105:1710–8.
10. Rex DK, Petrini JL, Baron TH, et al. Quality indicators for colonoscopy. Gastrointest Endosc. 2006;63:S16–28.
11. Odutayo A, Desborough MJR, Trivella M, et al. Restrictive versus liberal blood transfusion for gastrointestinal bleeding: a systematic review and meta-analysis of randomised controlled trials. Lancet Gastroenterol Hepatol. 2017;2:354–60.
12. Kherad O, Restellini S, Martel M, Sey M, Murphy MF, Oakland K, Barkun A, Jairath V. Outcomes following restrictive or liberal red blood cell transfusion in patients with lower gastrointestinal bleeding. Aliment Pharmacol Ther. 2019;49:919–25.
13. Wolf AT, Wasan SK, Saltzman JR. Impact of anticoagulation on rebleeding following endoscopic therapy for nonvariceal upper gastrointestinal hemorrhage. Am J Gastroenterol. 2007;102:290–6.
14. Acosta RD, Abraham NS, Chandrasekhara V, et al. The management of antithrombotic agents for patients undergoing GI endoscopy. Gastrointest Endosc. 2016;83:3–16.
15. Abraham NS, Barkun AN, Sauer BG, Douketis J, Laine L, Noseworthy PA, Telford JJ, Leontiadis GI. American College of Gastroenterology-Canadian Association of Gastroenterology clinical practice guideline: management of anticoagulants and antiplatelets during acute gastrointestinal bleeding and the periendoscopic period. Am J Gastroenterol. 2022;117:542–58.
16. Sung JJY, Lau JYW, Ching JYL, Wu JCY, Lee YT, Chiu PWY, Leung VKS, Wong VWS, Chan FKL. Continuation of low-dose aspirin therapy in peptic ulcer bleeding: a randomized trial. Ann Intern Med. 2010;152:1–9.
17. Zhou Y, Guo Y, Liu D, Feng H, Liu J. Restarting of anticoagulation in patients with atrial fibrillation after major bleeding: a meta-analysis. J Clin Pharm Ther. 2020;45:591–601.
18. Kido K, Scalese MJ. Management of oral anticoagulation therapy after gastrointestinal bleeding: whether to, when to, and how to restart an anticoagulation therapy. Ann Pharmacother. 2017;51:1000–7.
19. Ramos GP, Binder M, Hampel P, et al. Outcomes of endoscopic intervention for overt GI bleeding in severe thrombocytopenia. Gastrointest Endosc. 2018;88:55–61.
20. Tripodi A, Primignani M, Mannucci PM, Caldwell SH. Changing concepts of cirrhotic coagulopathy. Am J Gastroenterol. 2017;112:274–81.
21. Bennett C, Klingenberg SL, Langholz E, Gluud LL. Tranexamic acid for upper gastrointestinal bleeding. Cochrane Database Syst Rev. 2014;2014(11):CD006640. https://doi.org/10.1002/14651858.CD006640.PUB3.
22. Kanno T, Yuan Y, Tse F, Howden CW, Moayyedi P, Leontiadis GI. Proton pump inhibitor treatment initiated prior to endoscopic diagnosis in upper gastrointestinal bleeding. Cochrane Database Syst Rev. 2022. https://doi.org/10.1002/14651858.CD005415.PUB4.
23. Tsoi KKF, Lau JYW, Sung JJY. Cost-effectiveness analysis of high-dose omeprazole infusion before endoscopy for patients with upper-GI bleeding. Gastrointest Endosc. 2008;67:1056–63.
24. Gisbert JP, Pajares JM. Systematic review and meta-analysis: is 1-week proton pump inhibitor-based triple therapy sufficient to heal peptic ulcer? Aliment Pharmacol Ther. 2005;21:795–804.

25. Yeomans ND. New data on healing of nonsteroidal anti-inflammatory drug-associated ulcers and erosions. Omeprazole NSAID Steering Committee. Am J Med. 1998;104(3A):56S–61S. https://doi.org/10.1016/S0002-9343(97)00213-1.
26. Rahman R, Nguyen DL, Sohail U, Almashhrawi AA, Ashraf I, Puli SR, Bechtold ML. Pre-endoscopic erythromycin administration in upper gastrointestinal bleeding: an updated meta-analysis and systematic review. Ann Gastroenterol. 2016;29:312–7.
27. Winstead NS, Wilcox CM. Erythromycin prior to endoscopy for acute upper gastrointestinal haemorrhage: a cost-effectiveness analysis. Aliment Pharmacol Ther. 2007;26:1371–7.
28. Pateron D, Vicaut E, Debuc E, et al. Erythromycin infusion or gastric lavage for upper gastrointestinal bleeding: a multicenter randomized controlled trial. Ann Emerg Med. 2011;57:582–9.
29. Daram SR, Garretson R. Erythromycin is preferable to metoclopramide as a prokinetic in acute upper GI bleeding. Gastrointest Endosc. 2011;74:234.
30. Chavez-Tapia NC, Barrientos-Gutierrez T, Tellez-Avila F, Soares-Weiser K, Mendez-Sanchez N, Gluud C, Uribe M. Meta-analysis: antibiotic prophylaxis for cirrhotic patients with upper gastrointestinal bleeding—an updated Cochrane review. Aliment Pharmacol Ther. 2011;34:509–18.
31. Bañares R, Albillos A, Rincón D, Alonso S, González M, Ruiz-del-Arbol L, Salcedo M, Molinero LM. Endoscopic treatment versus endoscopic plus pharmacologic treatment for acute variceal bleeding: a meta-analysis. Hepatology. 2002;35:609–15.
32. Gøtzsche PC, Hróbjartsson A. Somatostatin analogues for acute bleeding oesophageal varices. Cochrane Database Syst Rev. 2008;2008(3):CD000193. https://doi.org/10.1002/14651858.CD000193.PUB3.
33. Hayes PC, Bouchier I, Davis JM, Lewis JA. Meta-analysis of value of propranolol in prevention of variceal haemorrhage. Lancet. 1990;336:153–6.
34. Puente A, Hernández-Gea V, Graupera I, Roque M, Colomo A, Poca M, Aracil C, Gich I, Guarner C, Villanueva C. Drugs plus ligation to prevent rebleeding in cirrhosis: an updated systematic review. Liver Int. 2014;34:823–33.
35. Thiele M, Krag A, Rohde U, Gluud LL. Meta-analysis: banding ligation and medical interventions for the prevention of rebleeding from oesophageal varices. Aliment Pharmacol Ther. 2012;35:1155–65.
36. Wooller KR, Yelle D, Fisher S, Carrigan I, Kelly E. Adherence to quality indicators and hospital outcomes for patients with decompensated cirrhosis: an observational study. Can Liver J. 2020;3:348–57. https://doi.org/10.3138/canlivj-2020-0003.
37. Blatchford O, Murray WR, Blatchford M. A risk score to predict need for treatment for upper-gastrointestinal haemorrhage. Lancet (London, England). 2000;356:1318–21.
38. Stanley AJ, Laine L, Dalton HR, et al. Comparison of risk scoring systems for patients presenting with upper gastrointestinal bleeding: international multicentre prospective study. BMJ. 2017;356:i6432. https://doi.org/10.1136/BMJ.I6432.
39. Liang PS, Saltzman JR. A national survey on the initial management of upper gastrointestinal bleeding. J Clin Gastroenterol. 2014;48:e93–8.
40. Oakland K, Kothiwale S, Forehand T, Jackson E, Bucknall C, Sey MSL, Singh S, Jairath V, Perlin J. External validation of the Oakland score to assess safe hospital discharge among adult patients with acute lower gastrointestinal bleeding in the US. JAMA Netw Open. 2020;3:e209630.
41. Robertson M, Majumdar A, Boyapati R, Chung W, Worland T, Terbah R, Wei J, Lontos S, Angus P, Vaughan R. Risk stratification in acute upper GI bleeding: comparison of the AIMS65 score with the Glasgow-Blatchford and Rockall scoring systems. Gastrointest Endosc. 2016;83:1151–60.
42. Lau JYW, Yu Y, Tang RSY, et al. Timing of endoscopy for acute upper gastrointestinal bleeding. N Engl J Med. 2020;382:1299–308.
43. Cooper GS, Kou TD, Wong RCK. Use and impact of early endoscopy in elderly patients with peptic ulcer hemorrhage: a population-based analysis. Gastrointest Endosc. 2009;70:229–35.
44. Jung DH, Huh CW, Kim NJ, Kim BW. Optimal endoscopy timing in patients with acute variceal bleeding: a systematic review and meta-analysis. Sci Rep. 2020;101(10):1–7.

45. Rudler M, Bureau C, Carbonell N, et al. Recalibrated MELD and hepatic encephalopathy are prognostic factors in cirrhotic patients with acute variceal bleeding. Liver Int. 2018;38:469–76.
46. Amitrano L, Guardascione MA, Bennato R, Manguso F, Balzano A. MELD score and hepatocellular carcinoma identify patients at different risk of short-term mortality among cirrhotics bleeding from esophageal varices. J Hepatol. 2005;42:820–5.
47. Tsay C, Shung D, Stemmer Frumento K, Laine L. Early colonoscopy does not improve outcomes of patients with lower gastrointestinal bleeding: systematic review of randomized trials. Clin Gastroenterol Hepatol. 2020;18:1696–1703.e2.
48. Laine L, McQuaid KR. Endoscopic therapy for bleeding ulcers: an evidence-based approach based on meta-analyses of randomized controlled trials. Clin Gastroenterol Hepatol. 2009;7:33–47.
49. Hussein M, Alzoubaidi D, Lopez MF, et al. Hemostatic spray powder TC-325 in the primary endoscopic treatment of peptic ulcer-related bleeding: multicenter international registry. Endoscopy. 2021;53:36–43.
50. Sung JJY, Moreea S, Dhaliwal H, et al. Use of topical mineral powder as monotherapy for treatment of active peptic ulcer bleeding. Gastrointest Endosc. 2022;96:28–35.e1.
51. Baracat FI, de Moura DTH, Brunaldi VO, Tranquillini CV, Baracat R, Sakai P, de Moura EGH. Randomized controlled trial of hemostatic powder versus endoscopic clipping for non-variceal upper gastrointestinal bleeding. Surg Endosc. 2020;34:317–24.
52. Lau JYW, Pittayanon R, Kwek A, et al. Comparison of a hemostatic powder and standard treatment in the control of active bleeding from upper nonvariceal lesions. Ann Intern Med. 2021;175:171–8. https://doi.org/10.7326/M21-0975.
53. Cahyadi O, Bauder M, Meier B, Caca K, Schmidt A. Effectiveness of TC-325 (hemospray) for treatment of diffuse or refractory upper gastrointestinal bleeding—a single center experience. Endosc Int Open. 2017;5:E1159.
54. Jensen DM, Kovacs T, Ghassemi KA, Kaneshiro M, Gornbein J. Randomized controlled trial of over-the-scope clip as initial treatment of severe nonvariceal upper gastrointestinal bleeding. Clin Gastroenterol Hepatol. 2021;19(11):2315–2323.e2. https://doi.org/10.1016/J.CGH.2020.08.046.
55. Kuellmer A, Mangold T, Bettinger D, et al. Over-the-scope clip versus transcatheter arterial embolization for refractory peptic ulcer bleeding—a propensity score matched analysis. United Eur Gastroenterol J. 2021;9:1048.
56. Meier B, Wannhoff A, Denzer U, et al. Over-the-scope-clips versus standard treatment in high-risk patients with acute non-variceal upper gastrointestinal bleeding: a randomised controlled trial (STING-2). Gut. 2022;71(7):1251–8. https://doi.org/10.1136/gutjnl-2021-325300.
57. Garcia-Tsao G, Abraldes JG, Berzigotti A, Bosch J. Portal hypertensive bleeding in cirrhosis: risk stratification, diagnosis, and management: 2016 practice guidance by the American Association for the study of liver diseases. Hepatology. 2017;65:310–35.
58. Lee SW, Lee TY, Sen CC. Independent factors associated with recurrent bleeding in cirrhotic patients with esophageal variceal hemorrhage. Dig Dis Sci. 2009;54:1128–34.
59. Xu L, Ji F, Xu QW, Zhang MQ. Risk factors for predicting early variceal rebleeding after endoscopic variceal ligation. World J Gastroenterol. 2011;17:3347.
60. Yang WG, Hou MC, Lin HC, Kuo BIT, Lee FY, Chang FY, Lee SD. Effect of sucralfate granules in suspension on endoscopic variceal sclerotherapy induced ulcer: analysis of the factors determining ulcer healing. J Gastroenterol Hepatol. 1998;13:225–31.
61. Shaheen NJ, Stuart E, Schmitz SM, Mitchell KL, Fried MW, Zacks S, Russo MW, Galanko J, Shrestha R. Pantoprazole reduces the size of postbanding ulcers after variceal band ligation: a randomized, controlled trial. Hepatology. 2005;41:588–94.
62. García-Pagán JC, Caca K, Bureau C, et al. Early use of TIPS in patients with cirrhosis and variceal bleeding. N Engl J Med. 2010;362:2370–9.
63. Rudler M, Cluzel P, Corvec TL, Benosman H, Rousseau G, Poynard T, Thabut D. Early-TIPSS placement prevents rebleeding in high-risk patients with variceal bleeding, without improving survival. Aliment Pharmacol Ther. 2014;40:1074–80.

64. García-Pagán JC, Saffo S, Mandorfer M, Garcia-Tsao G. Where does TIPS fit in the management of patients with cirrhosis? JHEP Rep. 2020;2:100122.
65. Ibrahim M, El-Mikkawy A, Abdel Hamid M, Abdalla H, Lemmers A, Mostafa I, Devière J. Early application of haemostatic powder added to standard management for oesophagogastric variceal bleeding: a randomised trial. Gut. 2019;68:844–53.
66. Panés J, Terés J, Bosch J, Rodés J. Efficacy of balloon tamponade in treatment of bleeding gastric and esophageal varices—results in 151 consecutive episodes. Dig Dis Sci. 1988;33:454–9.
67. Vine LJ, Subhani M, Acevedo JG. Update on management of gastric varices. World J Hepatol. 2019;11:250.
68. Sarin SK, Lahoti D, Saxena SP, Murthy NS, Makwana UK. Prevalence, classification and natural history of gastric varices: a long-term follow-up study in 568 portal hypertension patients. Hepatology. 1992;16:1343–9.
69. Gunjan D, Sharma V, Rana SS, Bhasin DK. Small bowel bleeding: a comprehensive review. Gastroenterol Rep. 2014;2:262.
70. Baptista V, Marya N, Singh A, Rupawala A, Gondal B, Cave D. Continuing challenges in the diagnosis and management of obscure gastrointestinal bleeding. World J Gastrointest Pathophysiol. 2014;5:523.
71. Chung W, Rich H, Wands J. A predictive model for the diagnostic and therapeutic yield of colonoscopy performed for lower gastrointestinal bleeding. J Clin Gastroenterol. 2022;56:154–60.
72. Zhang H, Wang Y, Sun S, Huang X, Tu G, Wang J, Lin Y, Xia H, Yuan Y, Yao S. Early enteral nutrition versus delayed enteral nutrition in patients with gastrointestinal bleeding: a PRISMA-compliant meta-analysis. Medicine (Baltimore). 2019;98(11):e14864. https://doi.org/10.1097/MD.0000000000014864.
73. Hébuterne X, Vanbiervliet G. Feeding the patients with upper gastrointestinal bleeding. Curr Opin Clin Nutr Metab Care. 2011;14:197–201.
74. Bjorkman D, Popp J. Communication from the ASGE Quality Assurance in Endoscopy Committee Defining and measuring quality in endoscopy. Gastrointest Endosc. 2015. https://doi.org/10.1016/j.gie.2014.07.052.
75. Marques S, Bispo M, Pimentel-Nunes P, Chagas C, Dinis-Ribeiro M. Image documentation in gastrointestinal endoscopy: review of recommendations. GE Port J Gastroenterol. 2017;24:269.
76. Brisebois S, Merati A, Giliberto JP. Proton pump inhibitors: review of reported risks and controversies. Laryngoscope Investig Otolaryngol. 2018;3:457.

Chapter 11
Quality in GERD and Barrett's Esophagus

Suqing Li, Mandip Rai, and Jeffrey D. Mosko

Table of Quality Measures/Metrics

S. Li
Division of Gastroenterology and Hepatology, Department of Medicine, University of Calgary, Calgary, AB, Canada

Division of Gastroenterology and Hepatology, Department of Medicine, The Center for Advanced Therapeutic Endoscopy and Endoscopic Oncology, St. Michael's Hospital, Toronto, ON, Canada

M. Rai
Division of Gastroenterology and Hepatology, Department of Medicine, The Center for Advanced Therapeutic Endoscopy and Endoscopic Oncology, St. Michael's Hospital, Toronto, ON, Canada

Division of Gastroenterology, Queen's University, Kingston, ON, Canada

J. D. Mosko (✉)
Division of Gastroenterology and Hepatology, Department of Medicine, The Center for Advanced Therapeutic Endoscopy and Endoscopic Oncology, St. Michael's Hospital, Toronto, ON, Canada
e-mail: Jeff.mosko@unityhealth.to

J. D. Feuerstein, D. J. Stein (eds.), *Quality in Gastroenterology*,
https://doi.org/10.1007/978-3-031-58492-3_11

Key Points

- All patients with GERD must be assessed for the presence of alarm symptoms and, if present, undergo objective testing.
- PPI therapy remains the first-line medical therapy for patients with GERD and must be regularly reviewed and titrated to the lowest effective dose in the absence of indications for indefinite therapy (severe esophagitis and/or Barrett's esophagus).
- In patients with BE-associated neoplasia, the goal of endoscopic treatment should be the complete eradication of the BE segment in addition to any dysplastic lesions.
- The rate at which CE-IM is achieved by 18 months in patients with Barrett's-related dysplasia and intramucosal cancer referred for EET (endoscopic eradication therapy) should be monitored (recommended threshold = 70%).

GERD

Introduction

Gastroesophageal reflux (GERD) is a common condition affecting 20% of the population in Western countries [1, 2]. Its burden to the medical system is high, representing the third most common reason for office or emergency department visits in the United States [3]. The Montreal Consensus describes the condition as when "reflux of gastric contents causes complications and/or symptoms troublesome for the patient" [2, 4, 5]. Typical symptoms of GERD include heartburn and regurgitation but it may present with a variety of other symptoms (see Table 11.1) [2]. Therefore, rather than a single uniform disorder, GERD is better conceptualized as a disorder with multiple clinical phenotypes [6, 7].

With the complexity of diagnosing and assessing GERD, there are increasing concerns about the inappropriate usage of diagnostic tests and medications such as proton pump inhibitors (PPIs) [8–11]. Ultimately, GERD can significantly impact patient quality of life (QoL) and, in some patients, may result in complications such as Barrett's

Table 11.1 Typical and atypical symptoms/presentations of GERD

Typical symptoms	
	Heartburn
	Regurgitation
	Water brash
Atypical symptoms/presentations	
	Chest pain
	Nausea/vomiting
	Excessive belching
	Dysphagia
	Globus
	Respiratory symptoms (chronic cough, wheeze, exacerbation of asthma)
	ENT symptoms (rhinosinusitis, hoarseness, laryngitis)

esophagus (BE), a precursor lesion to esophageal adenocarcinoma [12]. Thus, careful assessment and management of GERD is crucial to optimize patient outcomes and manage healthcare resources. This section will present a concise, evidence-based, practical approach to quality standards in the diagnosis and management of GERD.

Diagnosis and Evaluation

General Approach

Key Quality Measures

- The diagnosis of GERD can be made clinically on the presence of typical clinical symptoms.
- All patients presenting with GERD should be assessed for the presence of alarm symptoms.
- Objective testing, including endoscopy, should only be used in cases of diagnostic uncertainty, presence of alarm symptoms, and/or refractory symptoms.

In most patients, GERD is a clinical diagnosis and can be established based on the presence of typical symptoms [13]. As per the Montreal Consensus, patients presenting with cardinal symptoms of heartburn and regurgitation, occurring with enough frequency/severity to impact QoL, are presumed to have a diagnosis of GERD and can be started on empiric PPI therapy [5]. Most guidelines endorse the pragmatic approach of treating those with typical symptoms empirically with an 8-week trial of once-daily PPI therapy [4, 14]. Responsiveness to PPI can then be utilized to support the diagnosis [4, 15].

Objective testing, including upper endoscopy and ambulatory reflux monitoring, should be reserved for patients who have had an incomplete response to an initial empiric trial of PPI therapy and/or those with alarm symptoms (Table 11.2) [4]. The presence of LA grade C or D esophagitis (see Fig. 11.1), a peptic esophageal stricture, and/or long-segment Barrett's esophagus (>3 cm) on endoscopy is definitive evidence for the diagnosis of GERD [4, 15]. However, most patients with typical reflux symptoms will have a normal endoscopy, with only 30% having evidence of erosive esophagitis and 10% with BE [16, 17]. When performing upper endoscopy to assess for evidence of GERD, one can increase the sensitivity of the examination

Table 11.2 GERD alarm symptoms

Alarm symptoms
• Dysphagia • Odynophagia • Weight loss • Anemia • Gastrointestinal bleeding • Vomiting

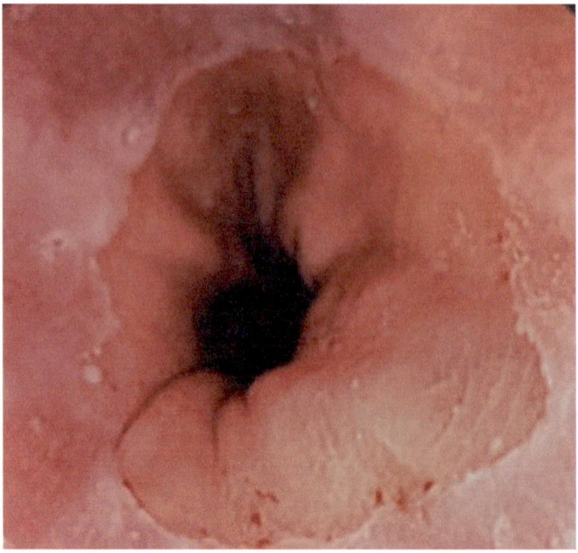

Fig. 11.1 Normal gastroesophageal junction (GEJ)

by discontinuing PPI therapy for at least 2 weeks prior [4, 15]. In those for whom the diagnosis remains unclear after an endoscopic evaluation, referral for ambulatory reflux monitoring should be considered [4]. Similarly, patients should hold their PPI therapy for at least 7 days prior [4].

In practice, upper endoscopy is overutilized, with up to 40% of upper endoscopies being performed for GERD without an appropriate indication [9]. There are multiple reasons for this, including concerns of medicolegal liability, financial incentives, and patient expectations. Ultimately, the inappropriate use of endoscopy may subject patients to rare but serious procedural risks, unnecessary downstream testing, and a significant cost burden for both patients and healthcare systems [18]. Thus, we strongly recommend ensuring appropriate indications are reviewed prior to the provision of endoscopy as well as monitoring for inappropriate usage on a system-based level.

Extraesophageal Symptoms

Key Quality Measures

- In patients with atypical extraesophageal symptoms, evaluation for non-GERD-related causes should be undertaken *before* objective testing for GERD.
- PPI therapy should only be started for individuals with an objective diagnosis of GERD in the setting of atypical/extraesophageal symptoms.

As discussed above, GERD can present with atypical extraesophageal symptoms. In the absence of typical GERD symptoms, evaluation for non-GERD-related causes should precede objective testing for GERD as our current diagnostic tools struggle to pinpoint GERD as a cause of extraesophageal symptoms [4, 19]. In patients with both typical symptoms and extraesophageal symptoms, it is recommended to initiate an 8–12-week trial of PPI therapy [4].

PPI therapy should not be started empirically in cases where patients lack typical symptoms until a diagnosis of GERD has been confirmed by endoscopy and/or ambulatory reflux monitoring [4]. Prior studies have shown that the cost of the evaluation and management of patients with suspected extraesophageal reflux is almost five times that of those with typical GERD, with most of the cost associated with the recurrent and/or prolonged use of PPI therapy. Furthermore, only 54% of patients had improvement in symptoms in this cohort [20]. As such, judicious testing and limiting the use of PPI therapy only to individuals with an objective diagnosis of GERD in the setting of atypical extraesophageal symptoms is recommended.

Refractory GERD

Key Quality Measures

- Patients with presumed refractory GERD should first have their non-pharmacologic and pharmacologic therapy reviewed and optimized.
- In patients with presumed refractory GERD who have not undergone objective testing, ambulatory reflux monitoring should be performed *off* PPI therapy.
- Ambulatory reflux monitoring should be performed *on* PPI therapy in patients with presumed refractory GERD with prior objective evidence of GERD to confirm presence of ongoing reflux despite medical therapy.

A proportion of patients (17–32%) will have ongoing symptoms of GERD despite PPI therapy [21]. Patients in whom GERD symptoms are persistent despite an 8–12-week trial of BID PPI therapy are considered to have "refractory GERD," although the exact definition is not well defined [4]. Before establishing a diagnosis of refractory GERD, patients should first have their non-pharmacologic and acid suppression therapy optimized, and a thorough history and physical examination are important. In such patients, there are likely multiple contributing factors beyond persistent abnormal acid reflux including reflux hypersensitivity, other esophageal disorders (i.e., achalasia and eosinophilic esophagitis), non-esophageal disorders, and functional disorders [4].

In patients with a presumed diagnosis of refractory GERD who have not had prior objective testing, an upper endoscopy should be performed, followed by ambulatory reflux monitoring off PPIs to confirm the diagnosis of GERD [4, 15]. In those who already have objective evidence of GERD, ambulatory pH monitoring should be performed while on optimized PPI therapy to establish the presence of ongoing reflux despite maximal therapy [4, 15]. In patients with a confirmed diagnosis of refractory GERD, further management generally involves an escalation of medical therapy and/or surgical/endoscopic interventions described below.

Management and Monitoring

Key Quality Measures

- All patients with GERD should be counselled on lifestyle measures and the optimal method of taking PPIs.
- PPI therapy should be prescribed as the first-line medical therapy in patients with a diagnosis of GERD; non-PPI medical reflux therapies should only be trialed as an adjunct to PPI therapy.
- PPI therapy should be regularly reviewed and titrated to the lowest effective dose.
- Patients with a history of severe esophagitis and/or Barrett's esophagus should remain on PPI therapy indefinitely.
- In patients with confirmed PPI-refractory GERD, surgical anti-reflux interventions should be considered.

The management of GERD includes lifestyle modification, medical therapy, and endoscopic/surgical therapy in select patients. All patients should receive counselling on diet and lifestyle modifications [4, 9, 14]. However, most patients require medical therapy, with PPIs being the first line due to their established efficacy [4].

In patients with typical GERD symptoms, an empiric trial of once-daily PPI lasting at least 8 weeks allows for the maximal effect of the therapy to be achieved [4, 14]. Initial management of ongoing symptoms involves increasing the PPI dose to twice per day. Patients must be counselled on the most effective way to take PPI therapy. PPIs should be taken 30–60 min before their first and last meal of the day (in cases of BID dosing) as they only bind to proton pumps actively secreting acid [22]. The exception is delayed-release formulations such as dexlansoprazole, in which pH control does not appear to be impacted by meal timing [23]. Although multiple formulations of PPIs exist with differences in relative acid suppression potency, there is limited evidence showing significant differences in symptom control and healing of erosive esophagitis in practice [24, 25]. While there is little evidence supporting switching between different PPIs, societal guidelines advise a single switch can be trialed where appropriate [4].

Overuse of PPI therapy is common in practice. Thus, to ensure quality care, it is essential that clinicians review the indications for PPI therapy for any particular patient and that therapy is titrated to symptom response with the goal of patients taking the lowest effective dose [9]. Patients prescribed PPI therapy should have their symptoms and therapy reviewed within 12 weeks of initiating therapy and at least once every 12 months thereafter [11]. Trials of discontinuation of PPI should be undertaken in patients without an objective indication for maintenance therapy. On-demand ("pill-in-pocket") regimens of PPIs can be effective for symptom control in those with nonerosive disease [26]. PPI therapy should be discontinued in those who are found to have no evidence of GERD on ambulatory reflux monitoring [4].

In patients with a history of severe esophagitis (LA grade C/D) and/or a diagnosis of Barrett's esophagus, clinicians must reinforce that indefinite PPI therapy is indicated to prevent future complications [4]. Additionally, in patients with a history of severe esophagitis (LA grade C/D), repeat upper endoscopy should be performed after an 8–12-week course of PPI therapy to exclude underlying Barrett's esophagus [11].

There has been significant concern surrounding the potential adverse effects of PPI use. Although there have been many reports of various adverse effects of long-term PPI use from observational studies, high-quality studies have only demonstrated a slightly increased risk of intestinal infections [4, 27]. It is important that clinicians regularly counsel and follow up with patients on the risks and benefits of PPI therapy to ensure optimal adherence.

H2 receptor antagonists (H2RA) are not as effective as PPI therapy and can be limited by tachyphylaxis [28]. Nevertheless, they can be utilized on an as-needed basis and/or as adjunctive therapy in cases of incomplete PPI response [29]. We recommend adding an H2RA to BID PPI dosing before bed for bothersome nocturnal symptoms. Baclofen is an additional adjunctive measure that can be given with ongoing objective evidence of reflux despite optimized PPI therapy [30]. Baclofen exerts its effects by reducing transient lower esophageal sphincter relaxations, one of the primary pathophysiological mechanisms for GERD [30]. The use of sucralfate has limited evidence for GERD and is used primarily for symptomatic GERD in pregnancy [31].

Surgical and/or endoscopic anti-reflux interventions should only be considered in those with true medication-refractory reflux and patients with severe esophagitis who prefer not to remain on lifelong PPI therapy [4, 14]. Available options include surgical fundoplication, magnetic sphincter augmentation, Roux-en-Y gastric bypass, and newer endoscopic anti-reflux devices [4]. Patients most likely to respond to surgical intervention are those with typical GERD symptoms [32]. In patients with objectively confirmed PPI-refractory reflux, laparoscopic surgical anti-reflux therapy has been found to be more effective than medical therapy [33]. Therefore, a thorough systematic evaluation to objectively establish GERD as the cause of symptoms must be conducted, including obtaining high-resolution manometry to rule out concomitant motility disorders before surgical anti-reflux therapy is considered [4].

Barrett's Esophagus

Introduction

Barrett's esophagus (BE) is a condition that is associated with chronic GERD [34]. The normal esophagus is lined by squamous epithelium. In response to chronic GERD, this normal lining is changed to specialized columnar epithelium with goblet cells [35]. BE has been found in 10–15% of patients with chronic GERD [36]. This is significant as BE is a precursor to esophageal adenocarcinoma. Patients with BE have a 10–55-fold increased risk of esophageal adenocarcinoma compared to the general population [37]. Optimal diagnosis and management of BE are integral to the prevention of progression to esophageal adenocarcinoma, a cancer that has been rapidly increasing in incidence in Western countries [36].

The American Gastroenterological Association (AGA), the American College of Gastroenterology (ACG), and the American Society for Gastrointestinal Endoscopy (ASGE) have published recommended quality indicators for the diagnosis and management of BE which will be highlighted in this chapter at the beginning of each section [38, 39]. This section will focus on a concise, evidence-based, practical approach to establishing quality standards in the diagnosis and management of Barrett's esophagus.

Diagnosis

Key Quality Measures

- For patients in whom BE is being considered, the squamocolumnar junction, the gastroesophageal junction, and the location of the diaphragmatic hiatus (if there is a hiatal hernia present) should be recorded on upper endoscopy.
- If BE is suspected on endoscopy, the endoscopist should document the extent of suspected BE using the Prague criteria.
- For patients in whom a diagnosis of dysplasia has been made, the rate at which the reading is made by a GI pathologist or confirmed by a second pathologist before endoscopic eradication therapy (EET) is initiated should be documented (recommended threshold = 90%).

BE develops when the normal esophageal lining is replaced by specialized columnar epithelium with intestinal-type goblet cells. The presence of intestinal metaplasia on histopathology is required by many societal guidelines [40]. As such, an endoscopic evaluation with confirmed histopathology is considered the gold standard.

A high-quality examination is integral to the diagnosis of BE, detecting dysplasia, making decisions around endoscopic eradication, and thus preventing esophageal adenocarcinoma. The first step involves visualization and assessment of the gastroesophageal junction (GEJ). This is best done by locating the proximal end of the gastric folds in a partially inflated esophagus. It is important to evaluate the GEJ with partial inflation as full insufflation flattens the gastric folds and can lead to misclassification of a hiatal hernia as columnar epithelium. In patients without BE, the squamocolumnar junction, also referred to as the Z line, coincides with the GEJ (Fig. 11.1). In BE, the proximal level of the Z line no longer coincides with the GEJ [41]. The columnar-lined mucosa now occupying the esophageal mucosa appears salmon-colored. At least 1 cm of columnar-lined mucosa is required to make a diagnosis of BE [40, 42]. In patients with an irregular Z line (less than 1 cm of columnar epithelium), we recommended against routine biopsies. These patients, however, can still have dysplasia/neoplasia arising at the GEJ, and therefore a thorough endoscopic examination is required with targeted biopsies of visible abnormalities.

The Prague classification is used to reporting the length of BE [41]. As shown in Fig. 11.2, this involves identifying three landmarks. These are the top of the gastric

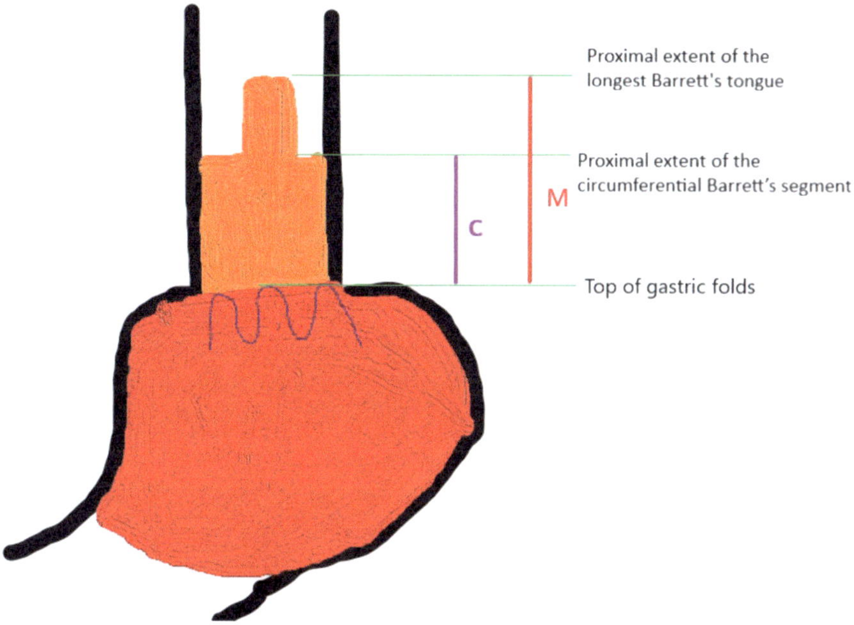

Fig. 11.2 Prague classification

folds, the proximal extent of the circumferential Barrett's segment (labelled as the "C"), and the proximal extent of the longest Barrett's tongue (labelled as the "M").

Dysplasia Detection

Key Quality Measures

- If a patient with known BE undergoes surveillance endoscopy, systematic biopsies should be taken every 1–2 cm from four quadrants throughout the extent of the endoscopically involved segment.
- The rate at which the presence or absence of visible lesions is reported in patients with BE referred for EET (recommended threshold = 90%).
- The rate at which the BE segment is inspected using high-definition white-light endoscopy (HD-WLE) (recommended threshold = 95%).

Once BE has been identified, a careful endoscopic examination is required to identify changes concerning for dysplasia. To do this, any mucous, bubbles, and/or retained secretions should be washed away. First, an examination with HD-WLE is performed (Fig. 11.3). We then utilize digital chromoendoscopy to further examine the mucosal surface and vascular pattern (narrowband imaging (NBI), Olympus; i-scan, Pentax; blue-light imaging (BLI), Fujinon). Magnifying endoscopy can assist with the characterization of the mucosal surface and vascular pattern in an

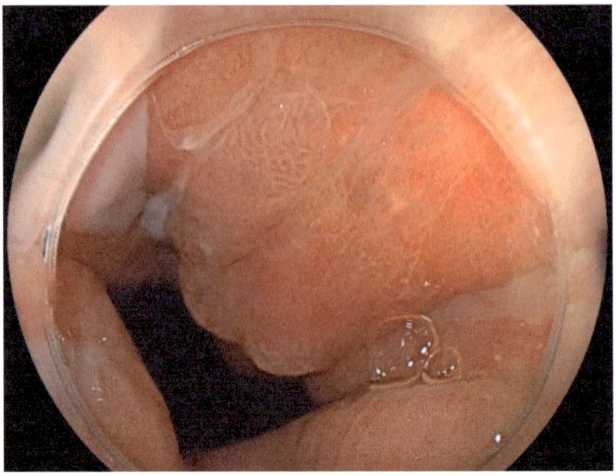

Fig. 11.3 Visible lesion seen on white-light endoscopy in BE

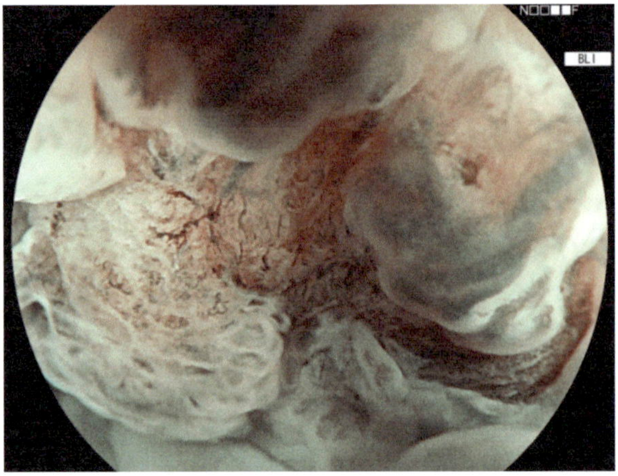

Fig. 11.4 Magnifying electronic chromoendoscopy with Fujinon (BLI) showing dysplasia within Barrett's esophagus

effort to differentiate between dysplastic and non-dysplastic epithelium (Fig. 11.4). Any areas that are raised and/or possess irregular surface/vascular pattern should be identified, closely examined, well-documented, and biopsied.

Acetic acid chromoendoscopy is a simple technique thought to improve dysplasia detection. This involves spraying dilute acetic acid through the scope onto Barrett's mucosa. Concentrations utilized in the literature have varied, but 2–3% is most commonly used [43]. This initially leads to whitening of the BE mucosa. Areas with High-Grade Dysplasia (HGD) or esophageal adenocarcinoma will proceed to lose this whitening faster than non-dysplastic BE (focal, early loss of acetowhitening). A meta-analysis of studies assessing the diagnostic accuracy of acetic acid for detection of Barrett's-associated neoplasia (HGD or early cancer) found the pooled sensitivity and specificity were 0.92 (95% CI 0.83–0.97) and 0.96 (95% CI 0.85–0.99) [43].

Longer inspection time has been shown to increase detection of HGD and esophageal adenocarcinoma in Barrett's esophagus [44]. Gupta et al. found a direct correlation between the amount of time spent examining per centimeter of BE and the detection of HGD and early esophageal adenocarcinoma [44]. Endoscopists who spent longer than 1 min per centimeter of BE detected more suspicious lesions (54.2% vs 13.3%, $P = 0.04$) with a trend toward higher detection of HGD/early esophageal adenocarcinoma (40.2% versus 6.7%, $P = 0.06$).

With the improvement in optical diagnosis of dysplasia in Barrett's esophagus, the majority of dysplasia should now come from targeted biopsies. However, it is still considered the standard of care to perform Seattle protocol biopsies [45]. This involves taking four-quadrant biopsies every 1–2 cm for circumferential BE and one biopsy per cm in tongues of BE.

Management

Key Quality Measures

- In patients with dysplastic BE or early esophageal adenocarcinoma, a diagnostic endoscopic resection should be performed on any raised or suspicious areas.
- Centers offering endoscopic eradication therapy (EET) require expertise in optical diagnosis, mucosal resection, and mucosal ablation techniques.
- The rate at which a discussion of the risks, benefits, and alternatives to EET is undertaken before a course of treatment is initiated (recommended threshold = 99%).
- In patients with BE-associated neoplasia, the goal of endoscopic treatment should be the complete eradication of the BE segment in addition to any dysplastic lesions.
- The rate at which CE-IM is achieved by 18 months in patients with Barrett's-related dysplasia and intramucosal cancer referred for EET (recommended threshold = 70%).
- The rate at which adverse events are tracked and documented in individuals after EET (recommended threshold = 90%).

Barrett's-associated dysplasia requires eradication to prevent esophageal adenocarcinoma. This is best performed endoscopically at high-volume centers with expertise in advanced imaging, different BE treatment modalities (radiofrequency ablation, cryoablation, endoscopic mucosal resection, endoscopic submucosal dissection, etc.), access to expert GI pathologists, and multidisciplinary teams that include surgeons and oncologists. This approach has been shown to improve patient outcomes while decreasing time to complete eradication of the BE (CE-IM) [46].

Endoscopic therapy is the established first-line therapy for all patients with visible lesions and/or dysplasia on biopsies. This minimally invasive approach is appropriate based on the very low risk of lymph node metastasis in BE-associated dysplasia and intramucosal cancer (IMC) [47]. Esophagectomy, by comparison, is associated with a high morbidity and mortality rate [48].

All visible and raised lesions must be resected endoscopically. Traditional resection is via endoscopic mucosal resection (EMR). Endoscopic submucosal dissection (ESD) is recommended for lesions requiring en bloc resection, with concern for superficial submucosal invasion and/or with significant fibrosis/scarring where EMR would be difficult.

All patients with HGD or IMC should undergo endoscopic eradication therapy. In patients with low-grade dysplasia (LGD), this should be confirmed by a second pathologist with expertise in GI pathology. These patients should also be referred to an expert center for consideration of endoscopic eradication therapy to prevent progression to HGD or IMC.

Endoscopic eradication therapy involves the resection of all visible dysplasia followed by ablation of the remainder of Barrett's mucosa. The goals are both complete eradication of dysplasia (CE-D) and intestinal metaplasia (CE-IM).

Patients with cancers extending in the superficial submucosa (SM1) can still be managed with endoscopic eradication therapy as the risk of lymph node metastasis remains low. Those with cancer invading deeper in the submucosa and beyond (SM2 or greater) should be referred for esophagectomy [49].

All patients with BE should be on at least once a day proton pump inhibitor therapy unless contraindicated.

Surveillance

Key Quality Measures

- If systematic surveillance biopsies performed in a patient known to have BE show no evidence of dysplasia, follow-up endoscopy should be performed no sooner than 3–5 years.
- Among patients who achieve CE-IM, the rate at which a recommendation for endoscopic surveillance at a defined interval is documented (recommended threshold = 90%).
- During endoscopic surveillance after EET, the rate at which biopsies of any visible mucosal abnormalities are performed (recommended threshold = 95%).
- The rate at which an anti-reflux regimen is recommended after EET (recommended threshold = 90%).

Patients with histologic changes that are indefinite for dysplasia can be challenging to manage as the literature does support endoscopic eradication therapy. If changes indefinite for dysplasia are confirmed by a second GI pathologist, the patient should be treated with twice daily proton pump inhibitor therapy, and a repeat endoscopy should be performed in 6 months. If no dysplasia is found on repeat assessment, then further surveillance can be performed in 3–5 years. However, if dysplasia is found (LGD or HGD), patients should be referred for endoscopic eradication therapy. If changes indefinite for dysplasia persist, patients should undergo repeat endoscopy every 6–12 months as these changes have been shown to be a risk factor to progression to LGD [50].

Once patients with dysplastic Barrett's achieve CE-IM, they should undergo surveillance based on their most advanced pathology. Patients with prior LGD require surveillance at 1 year and then every 2 years. Patients with HGD and early cancer (after curative endoscopic treatment) require surveillance at 3 months, 6 months, 12 months, and then yearly thereafter.

References

1. El-Serag HB, Sweet S, Winchester CC, Dent J. Update on the epidemiology of gastro-oesophageal reflux disease: a systematic review. Gut. 2014;63(6):871–80.
2. Nirwan JS, Hasan SS, Babar ZU, Conway BR, Ghori MU. Global prevalence and risk factors of gastro-oesophageal reflux disease (GORD): systematic review with meta-analysis. Sci Rep. 2020;10(1):5814.
3. Peery AF, Crockett SD, Murphy CC, Jensen ET, Kim HP, Egberg MD, et al. Burden and cost of gastrointestinal, liver, and pancreatic diseases in the United States: update 2021. Gastroenterology. 2022;162(2):621–44.
4. Katz PO, Dunbar KB, Schnoll-Sussman FH, Greer KB, Yadlapati R, Spechler SJ. ACG clinical guideline for the diagnosis and management of gastroesophageal reflux disease. Am J Gastroenterol. 2022;117(1):27–56.
5. Vakil N, van Zanten SV, Kahrilas P, Dent J, Jones R. The Montreal definition and classification of gastroesophageal reflux disease: a global evidence-based consensus. Am J Gastroenterol. 2006;101(8):1900–20; quiz 43.
6. Katzka DA, Pandolfino JE, Kahrilas PJ. Phenotypes of gastroesophageal reflux disease: where Rome, Lyon, and Montreal meet. Clin Gastroenterol Hepatol. 2020;18(4):767–76.
7. Ribolsi M, Giordano A, Guarino MPL, Tullio A, Cicala M. New classifications of gastro-esophageal reflux disease: an improvement for patient management? Expert Rev Gastroenterol Hepatol. 2019;13(8):761–9.
8. Allen JI. Endoscopy for gastroesophageal reflux disease: choose wisely. Ann Intern Med. 2012;157(11):827–8.
9. Yadlapati R, Dakhoul L, Pandolfino JE, Keswani RN. The quality of care for gastroesophageal reflux disease. Dig Dis Sci. 2017;62(3):569–76.
10. Desai M, Sharma P. What quality metrics should we apply in Barrett's esophagus? Am J Gastroenterol. 2019;114(8):1197–8.
11. Yadlapati R, Gawron AJ, Bilimoria K, Keswani RN, Dunbar KB, Kahrilas PJ, et al. Development of quality measures for the care of patients with gastroesophageal reflux disease. Clin Gastroenterol Hepatol. 2015;13(5):874–83.e2.
12. Eloubeidi MA, Provenzale D. Health-related quality of life and severity of symptoms in patients with Barrett's esophagus and gastroesophageal reflux disease patients without Barrett's esophagus. Am J Gastroenterol. 2000;95(8):1881–7.
13. Young A, Kumar MA, Thota PN. GERD: a practical approach. Cleve Clin J Med. 2020;87(4):223–30.
14. Hunt R, Armstrong D, Katelaris P, Afihene M, Bane A, Bhatia S, et al. World gastroenterology organisation global guidelines: GERD global perspective on gastroesophageal reflux disease. J Clin Gastroenterol. 2017;51(6):467–78.

15. Gyawali CP, Kahrilas PJ, Savarino E, Zerbib F, Mion F, Smout A, et al. Modern diagnosis of GERD: the Lyon consensus. Gut. 2018;67(7):1351–62.
16. Poh CH, Gasiorowska A, Navarro-Rodriguez T, Willis MR, Hargadon D, Noelck N, et al. Upper GI tract findings in patients with heartburn in whom proton pump inhibitor treatment failed versus those not receiving antireflux treatment. Gastrointest Endosc. 2010;71(1):28–34.
17. Sharma P. Review article: prevalence of Barrett's oesophagus and metaplasia at the gastro-oesophageal junction. Aliment Pharmacol Ther. 2004;20(s5):48–54.
18. Upper Endoscopy for Gastroesophageal Reflux Disease. Best practice advice from the clinical guidelines Committee of the American College of physicians. Ann Intern Med. 2012;157(11):808–16.
19. Vaezi MF, Katzka D, Zerbib F. Extraesophageal symptoms and diseases attributed to GERD: where is the pendulum swinging now? Clin Gastroenterol Hepatol. 2018;16(7):1018–29.
20. Francis DO, Rymer JA, Slaughter JC, Choksi Y, Jiramongkolchai P, Ogbeide E, et al. High economic burden of caring for patients with suspected extraesophageal reflux. Am J Gastroenterol. 2013;108(6):905–11.
21. El-Serag H, Becher A, Jones R. Systematic review: persistent reflux symptoms on proton pump inhibitor therapy in primary care and community studies. Aliment Pharmacol Ther. 2010;32(6):720–37.
22. Hatlebakk JG, Berstad A. Pharmacokinetic optimisation in the treatment of gastro-oesophageal reflux disease. Clin Pharmacokinet. 1996;31(5):386–406.
23. Lee RD, Mulford D, Wu J, Atkinson SN. The effect of time-of-day dosing on the pharmacokinetics and pharmacodynamics of dexlansoprazole MR: evidence for dosing flexibility with a dual delayed release proton pump inhibitor. Aliment Pharmacol Ther. 2010;31(9):1001–11.
24. Graham DY, Tansel A. Interchangeable use of proton pump inhibitors based on relative potency. Clin Gastroenterol Hepatol. 2018;16(6):800–8.e7.
25. Ip S, Bonis P, Tatsioni A, Raman G, Chew P, Kupelnick B, et al. AHRQ comparative effectiveness reviews. Comparative effectiveness of management strategies for gastroesophageal reflux disease. Rockville: Agency for Healthcare Research and Quality; 2005.
26. Lind T, Havelund T, Lundell L, Glise H, Lauritsen K, Pedersen SA, et al. On demand therapy with omeprazole for the long-term management of patients with heartburn without oesophagitis--a placebo-controlled randomized trial. Aliment Pharmacol Ther 1999;13(7):907–914.
27. Moayyedi P, Eikelboom JW, Bosch J, Connolly SJ, Dyal L, Shestakovska O, et al. Safety of proton pump inhibitors based on a large, multi-year, randomized trial of patients receiving rivaroxaban or aspirin. Gastroenterology. 2019;157(3):682–91.e2.
28. Khan M, Santana J, Donnellan C, Preston C, Moayyedi P. Medical treatments in the short term management of reflux oesophagitis. Cochrane Database Syst Rev. 2007;2007(2):CD006036.
29. Peghini PL, Katz PO, Castell DO. Ranitidine controls nocturnal gastric acid breakthrough on omeprazole: a controlled study in normal subjects. Gastroenterology. 1998;115(6):1335–9.
30. Grossi L, Spezzaferro M, Sacco LF, Marzio L. Effect of baclofen on oesophageal motility and transient lower oesophageal sphincter relaxations in GORD patients: a 48-h manometric study. Neurogastroenterol Motil. 2008;20(7):760–6.
31. Richter JE. Review article: the management of heartburn in pregnancy. Aliment Pharmacol Ther. 2005;22(9):749–57.
32. Oelschlager BK, Quiroga E, Parra JD, Cahill M, Polissar N, Pellegrini CA. Long-term outcomes after laparoscopic antireflux surgery. Am J Gastroenterol. 2008;103(2):280–7; quiz 8.
33. Spechler SJ, Hunter JG, Jones KM, Lee R, Smith BR, Mashimo H, et al. Randomized trial of medical versus surgical treatment for refractory heartburn. N Engl J Med. 2019;381(16):1513–23.
34. Winters C Jr, Spurling TJ, Chobanian SJ, Curtis DJ, Esposito RL, Hacker JF 3rd, et al. Barrett's esophagus. A prevalent, occult complication of gastroesophageal reflux disease. Gastroenterology. 1987;92(1):118–24.
35. Barrett NR. Chronic peptic ulcer of the oesophagus and 'oesophagitis'. Br J Surg. 1950;38(150):175–82.

36. Thrift AP. Global burden and epidemiology of Barrett oesophagus and oesophageal cancer. Nat Rev Gastroenterol Hepatol. 2021;18(6):432–43.
37. Cook MB, Coburn SB, Lam JR, Taylor PR, Schneider JL, Corley DA. Cancer incidence and mortality risks in a large US Barrett's oesophagus cohort. Gut. 2018;67(3):418–529.
38. Sharma P, Katzka DA, Gupta N, Ajani J, Buttar N, Chak A, et al. Quality indicators for the management of Barrett's esophagus, dysplasia, and esophageal adenocarcinoma: international consensus recommendations from the American Gastroenterological Association symposium. Gastroenterology. 2015;149(6):1599–606.
39. Wani S, Muthusamy VR, Shaheen NJ, Yadlapati R, Wilson R, Abrams JA, et al. Development of quality indicators for endoscopic eradication therapies in Barrett's esophagus: the TREAT-BE (treatment with resection and endoscopic ablation techniques for Barrett's esophagus) consortium. Am J Gastroenterol. 2017;112(7):1032–48.
40. Shaheen NJ, Falk GW, Iyer PG, Souza RF, Yadlapati RH, Sauer BG, et al. Diagnosis and management of Barrett's esophagus: an updated ACG guideline. Am Coll Gastroenterol. 2022;117(4):559.
41. Sharma P, Dent J, Armstrong D, Bergman JJGHM, Gossner L, Hoshihara Y, et al. The development and validation of an endoscopic grading system for Barrett's esophagus: the Prague C & M Criteria. Gastroenterology. 2006;131(5):1392–9.
42. Fitzgerald RC, di Pietro M, Ragunath K, Ang Y, Kang JY, Watson P, et al. British Society of Gastroenterology guidelines on the diagnosis and management of Barrett's oesophagus. Gut. 2014;63(1):7–42.
43. Coletta M, Sami SS, Nachiappan A, Fraquelli M, Casazza G, Ragunath K. Acetic acid chromoendoscopy for the diagnosis of early neoplasia and specialized intestinal metaplasia in Barrett's esophagus: a meta-analysis. Gastrointest Endosc. 2016;83(1):57–67.e1.
44. Gupta N, Gaddam S, Wani SB, Bansal A, Rastogi A, Sharma P. Longer inspection time is associated with increased detection of high-grade dysplasia and esophageal adenocarcinoma in Barrett's esophagus. Gastrointest Endosc. 2012;76(3):531–8.
45. Levine DS, Blount PL, Rudolph RE, Reid BJ. Safety of a systematic endoscopic biopsy protocol in patients with Barrett's esophagus. Am J Gastroenterol. 2000;95(5):1152–7.
46. Fudman DI, Lightdale CJ, Poneros JM, Ginsberg GG, Falk GW, Demarshall M, et al. Positive correlation between endoscopist radiofrequency ablation volume and response rates in Barrett's esophagus. Gastrointest Endosc. 2014;80(1):71–7.
47. Dunbar KB, Spechler SJ. The risk of lymph-node metastases in patients with high-grade dysplasia or intramucosal carcinoma in Barrett's esophagus: a systematic review. Am J Gastroenterol. 2012;107(6):850–62; quiz 63.
48. Wani S, Qumseya B, Sultan S, Agrawal D, Chandrasekhara V, Harnke B, et al. Endoscopic eradication therapy for patients with Barrett's esophagus-associated dysplasia and intramucosal cancer. Gastrointest Endosc. 2018;87(4):907–31.e9.
49. Manner H, Pech O, Heldmann Y, May A, Pauthner M, Lorenz D, et al. The frequency of lymph node metastasis in early-stage adenocarcinoma of the esophagus with incipient submucosal invasion (pT1b sm1) depending on histological risk patterns. Surg Endosc. 2015;29(7):1888–96.
50. Henn AJ, Song KY, Gravely AA, Mesa H, Sultan S, Shaheen NJ, et al. Persistent indefinite for dysplasia in Barrett's esophagus is a risk factor for dysplastic progression to low-grade dysplasia. Dis Esophagus. 2020;33(9)

Chapter 12
Quality in Inflammatory Bowel Disease

Daniela Fluxa, Maryam Alahmad, and Francis A. Farraye

Table of Quality Measures/Metrics

D. Fluxa · F. A. Farraye (✉)
Department of Gastroenterology, Mayo Clinic in Florida, Jacksonville, FL, USA
e-mail: fluxacardenas.daniela@mayo.edu; farraye.francis@mayo.edu

M. Alahmad
Department of Gastroenterology, Sheikh Shakhbout Medical City in Partnership with Mayo Clinic College of Medicine Abu Dhabi, Abu Dhabi, UAE
e-mail: maalahmad@ssmc.ae

J. D. Feuerstein, D. J. Stein (eds.), *Quality in Gastroenterology*,
https://doi.org/10.1007/978-3-031-58492-3_12

Key Points

- Inflammatory bowel disease has all the attributes that make this disease suitable for quality care improvement such as disease chronicity, complex medical algorithms, variability of care, medication-and disease-related complications, as well as high personal and societal costs of the disease.
- Variation of care is a surrogate for poor-quality care and may translate in overuse, underuse, and misuse of healthcare resources.
- Quality measurements are quantifiable features of care that can be used to assess care quality in an unbiased manner and include structure, process, and outcome measures.
- Multiple organizations have created initiatives to define quality of care and ultimately improve the quality of care delivered, while others have created learning health systems as a modality to improve quality of care.
- IBD Specialty Medical Home at the University of Pittsburgh Medical Center (UPMC) and Project Sonar have shown that IBD patients can receive comprehensive health care resulting in decreased use of healthcare services and improvement in patient-focused outcomes.

Introduction

Inflammatory bowel diseases (IBD), including ulcerative colitis (UC), Crohn's disease (CD), and indeterminate colitis, are chronic immune-mediated intestinal diseases which are often debilitating and expensive to treat [1–3]. Patients affected by these conditions may experience a significant reduction in their quality of life in terms of lost productivity in school and/or work, complications related to the disease or medications, emergency department visits and hospitalization, and surgical interventions among others [4–6]. This translates in a significant burden for both the patient and their families, not only from a health perspective but also a socioeconomic standpoint [4].

In the year 2000, the Institute of Medicine published *To Err Is Human: Building a Safer Health System* [7], alerting the healthcare community of several serious deficiencies in the healthcare system in the United States. It was a call to action to begin making changes in the healthcare system to improve quality of care delivered to patients. Some of the key points included the following: [1] Half of adverse events were caused by errors that could have been prevented [2]. 44,000–98,000 people die annually from healthcare errors [3]. Healthcare errors cost $17–29 billion/year, among others [7]. In 2001, a follow-up report *Crossing the Quality Chasm: A New Health System for the twenty-first Century* [8] proposed efforts to improve six deficient dimensions in order to meet patient needs. These included safety, effectiveness, patient-centeredness, timeliness, efficiency, and equity [8].

One of the biggest challenges in IBD care is the heterogeneity in clinical practice, with variations in diagnostic testing, treatment, and monitoring as well as preventive health measures [9]. As the treatment options for IBD expand, it is anticipated that this variability will increase. For these reasons, measures to quantify and assess quality have gained significant interest through the years with the goal of improving patient care. Quality improvement is influenced by the perspective of stakeholders who engaged in the development of quality improvement and include providers, patients, and third-party payers [10]. Different stakeholders may preferentially value distinct aspects of care, but ideally, all perspectives should be taken into account in the quality improvement process [10].

Why Should We Care About Quality?

There are several reasons why providers and patients alike should care about quality for patients living with IBD. Most importantly, improvement in the quality of care translates into better patient outcomes, with improvement of patient's quality of life, decrease in economic burden, decreased complication rates related to both the disease and medications, and decreased emergency department visits and/or hospitalization, among others [2]. Additionally, quality of care measures aims to ensure all patients are offered a uniform and basic minimum level of care. Moreover, there is a transition taking place in the existing healthcare system from a fee-for-service paradigm to a performance-based model [11]. In IBD specifically, the creation of quality measures and their incorporation into federal programs are shifting Medicare reimbursement from a volume-based to a value-based structure [12].

Why Do We Need Quality in IBD?

There are several factors that make IBD care suitable for quality improvement, such as substantial variability in care, potential prevention of progressive disease, medication-related complications, and overall cost burden of the disease to patients and society [3].

Increased Cost of Care

CD and UC flares place a significant financial strain on the healthcare system, both in terms of direct and indirect costs. Despite having the lowest prevalence of all the GI disorders, IBD is one of the five most costly GI conditions [13]. It has been estimated that IBD's annual disease-related direct costs in the United States reached $6.3 billion in the early 2000s [14]. Although treatment costs make up a significant amount of IBD costs, ineffective medicines, poor adherence, and subpar care have caused estimates of the total cost burden to range from $14.6 billion to $31.6 billion in 2014 [6]. The "Cost of IBD Initiative" was introduced by the Crohn's & Colitis Foundation in 2016 with the aim of better understanding IBD treatment costs at both the system and patient levels. In this study, researchers were able to determine that the average annual healthcare costs for individuals with IBD were around $23,000 compared to $7000 for people without IBD and that individuals with IBD typically had higher out-of-pocket expenses and ongoing indirect costs associated with managing their condition [15]. A recent study demonstrated that annual indirect costs due to total work impairment were higher in patients with increased disease activity for both patients with CD ($7169/patient/year for patients in remission and up to $29,524/patient/year in patients with moderate to severe active disease). In patients with UC, the costs were $4348/patient/year for patient on remission and up to $24,283/patient/year in patients with moderate to severe active disease [16].

Variability in Care

Variability in care is a surrogate for inferior care and has been considered an indicator of poor quality in health care as this may lead to underuse, overuse, or misuse of healthcare resources leading to waste and gaps in quality [4, 5, 10]. More importantly, variability in care may be associated with poor outcomes.

Identifying Variation in Care

Identifying variation in care is an initial step in quality improvement.

Overuse

Overuse occurs when excessive or unnecessary care is provided, leading to increased healthcare cost or harm which may potentially exceed its benefit [6, 17]. Overuse may not only cause inefficiency but may also place patient at a higher risk of adverse events [6]. For example, a patient with colonic CD who reports persistent symptoms including diarrhea and abdominal pain and in whom the dose of anti-TNF is intensified despite a normal drug level, colonoscopy, and pathology represents an example of overuse. In this case, the increased dose of anti-TNF is not providing any benefit for the patient as the patient is already in endoscopic remission and in fact could place the patient at higher risk for adverse effects. Additionally, this would also increase health cost utilization with no added benefit.

Underuse

Underuse represents the failure to provide services that would lead to a favorable outcome in the patient [17], such as utilization of appropriate therapeutic agents or healthcare maintenance services, that will help keep the patient healthy and decrease the risk of disease progression as well as disease complications [6, 17]. A patient with IBD, who receives six course of prednisone per year, would represent an example of underuse if the patient had never been offered a steroid-sparing therapy or bone density scan (DEXA) to evaluate for osteopenia/osteoporosis because of prolonged steroid use. Therefore, underuse may lead to significant morbidity in patients with IBD.

Misuse

Misuse occurs when an appropriate intervention has been taken but an avoidable complication occurs, and the patient does not obtain complete benefit from this intervention [17]. Preventable complications from both surgery and medication use may lead to misuse issues [17]. A patient with Crohn's disease who develops pancreatitis after receiving treatment with azathioprine despite the fact he had reported a prior episode of pancreatitis while taking 6-mercaptopurine is an example of misuse.

Defining and Measuring Quality

Quality measures or indicators are measurable items that allow to objectively assess and quantify quality of care [4, 10]. Quality measures can be evaluated based on care structure, process, or outcomes [10]. Measuring quality is not an easy task and a significant challenge to the implementation of quality improvement in IBD care; however, this is essential for any quality initiative [10].

Main Domains of Standards in Quality of Care in Patients with IBD: Quality Measures

Structure of Care

Structural measures relate to the resources available in the healthcare system and organization such as staffing and availability of health services [2, 4, 6]. Examples of these measures include electronic medical records, accreditation status, nurse/medical assistant availability, examination room numbers and turnover, hospital volume, and teaching status staff deployment and qualifications [6, 18].

Process of Care

Process measures are activities that are executed for, on behalf of, or by a patient [6] and include measures for diagnosis, treatment, referral, and preventive care [4, 10]. Examples include scheduling of surveillance colonoscopy, yearly influenza vaccination rates, and medication refill rates [6]. These measures are easy to quantify and may influence outcomes [6].

Outcomes of Care

What happens to the patient because of the care received defines outcome measures [6, 18, 19]. Examples include disease activity/remission rates, surgical and hospitalization rates, steroid exposure, admission length of stay, as well as patient-reported outcomes and quality of life [6, 18, 19]. Outcomes of care are what matter most to patients and should ideally improve as high-quality processes are implemented [4]; however, outcome measures are more difficult to measure as they usually take a longer time to assess [10].

Additionally, process and outcome measures for quality improvement in patients with IBD are important for numerous reasons, such as [5]:

1. Comprehending where deficiencies in quality care exist and helping direct and prioritize quality improvement efforts.
2. Establishing goals for performance competency in IBD care.
3. Creating physician-established measures in anticipation of mandated quality improvement development by third-party payers.
4. Defining outcome measures for future quality of care initiatives.
5. Improving patient care.

A systemic review performed by Fiorino and colleagues [19] reviewed the current evidence available in relation to standards of quality of care in IBD and proposed a core set of minimal standards required to manage IBD by identifying these three main domains (structural, process, outcomes) as shown in Fig. 12.1 [19].

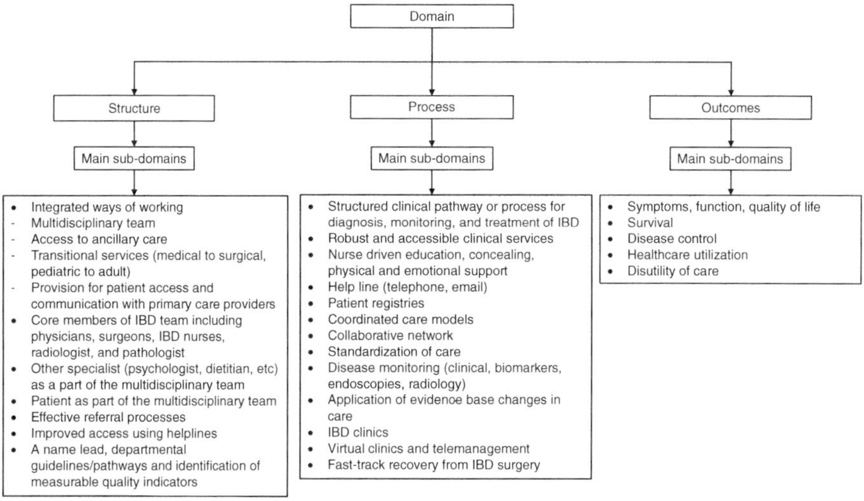

Fig. 12.1 Core list of minimal requirements for managing IBD proposed by Fiorino et al. [19]. (Adapted from Fiorino et al. [19])

Quality Initiatives for Patients with IBD

Multiple initiatives have been taken by different organizations to define quality care in patients with IBD, including the International Consortium for Health Outcomes Measurement (ICHOM) outcome measures, American Gastroenterological Association (AGA) Physician Quality Reporting System (PQRS) performance measures, and the Crohn's & Colitis Foundation's process and outcome measures [4]. Others have centered their efforts on the development of learning health systems including ImproveCareNow and IBD Qorus [4]. Other models that have emerged include specialty patient-centered IBD medical homes, which were designed to enhance patient experience, improve healthcare quality, and decrease healthcare costs [20]. Some examples of specialty medical home are the IBD Medical Home at the University of Pittsburgh Medical Center (UPMC) and Project Sonar [4].

ICHOM

The ICHOM has gathered global teams including healthcare professionals, patient advocates, and researchers from different continents around the globe to define outcome measures for different diseases and specific patient populations. This consortium has published over 40 sets of patient-centered outcome measures to date which aim to transform health care by providing informed decision-making, quality improvement, and reducing costs [21]. Among these 40 sets of patient-centered outcome measures, a specific set has been created for IBD which includes outcomes that are prioritized by patients affected by this condition (Table 12.1) [22].

Table 12.1 ICHOM Standard Set for Inflammatory Bowel Disease [36]

Outcomes	
Symptoms, function, and quality of life	Change in bowel symptoms Pain and discomfort Normal activities Energy and fatigue Weight
Disutility of care	Complications of interventions Steroid use
Healthcare utilization	Hospitalization and emergency visits
Survival and disease control	Anemia Disease activity and remission Colorectal cancer Overall and cause-specific survival

Table 12.2 AGA Physician Performance Measure Set for patient with IBD. (Adapted from Walker et al. [23])

IBD assessment
IBD type, anatomical location, and activity
Preventative care
Corticosteroid-sparing therapy
Corticosteroid-related iatrogenic injury—Bone loss assessment
Influenza immunization
Pneumococcal immunization
Tobacco user—Screening and cessation intervention
Treatment
Testing for latent TB before initiating anti-TNF therapy
Hepatitis B virus-documented assessment prior to initiating anti-TNF therapy
Inpatient measures
Clostridium difficile infection testing
Venous thromboembolism prophylaxis

AGA

In 2011, the AGA developed quality process measures for patients with IBD (Table 12.2) [23] that were intended to be used for Physician Quality Reporting System (PQRS) in the United States [24]. These process measures have been used by Medicare and have mainly been employed for financial incentives or to avoid financial penalties [12]. Currently, the AGA is committed in supporting gastroenterologists in providing high-quality care and has recently developed three quality measures that have completed the public comment period and has been approved by the AGA Quality Committee to progress into the alpha testing phase. These measures include (1) thiopurine methyltransferase testing and documentation in all patients prior to starting azathioprine or 6-mercaptopurine, (2) postoperative monitoring for Crohn's disease recurrence 6–12 months after surgical resection, and (3) percentage of patients diagnosed with mild to moderate pan-ulcerative colitis treated with high or standard dose mesalamine or diazo-bonded ASA, instead of low dose mesalamine, sulfasalazine or no treatment [25]. Additionally, the AGA maintains a range of performance measures that are available for public reporting in the Quality Payment Program and are updated on an annual basis by the AGA. To date, the performance measure for IBD includes assessment of hepatitis B virus status prior to initiation of anti-tumor necrosis factor therapy [25].

Crohn's & Colitis Foundation

The Crohn's & Colitis Foundation has developed a quality intervention program by outlining process and outcome quality indicators for the care of adult IBD patients based on expert opinion and extensive literature review by using the RAND Appropriateness Panel methodology [10]. In 2013, a set of ten process and ten outcome indicators were published by the Crohn's & Colitis Foundation (Tables 12.3 and 12.4).

Table 12.3 Crohn's & Colitis Foundation Top 10 Quality Process Indicators [10]. (Adapted from Melmed et al. [10])

Treatment
Documented tuberculosis risk assessment using either tuberculin skin testing or interferon gamma release assay prior to anti-TNF therapy initiation
Risk assessment and documentation of hepatitis B virus prior to anti-TNF therapy initiation
Appropriate-dosed corticosteroid-sparing agent or operation should be considered for IBD patients who require at least 10 mg of prednisone (or equivalent) for ≥16 weeks
Flexible sigmoidoscopy with biopsy and surgical consultation should be obtained to exclude cytomegalovirus in patients with severe UC who do not improve on intravenous corticosteroids within 3 days of treatment
Clostridium difficile infection should be ruled out if acute flare of IBD is suspected
TPMT testing prior to starting therapy with 6-mercaptopurine/azathioprine
Surveillance
Consider either proctocolectomy or surveillance within 6 months in patients with UC and flat low-grade dysplasia
Perform a surveillance colonoscopy every 1–3 years in patient with extensive ulcerative colitis or colonic Crohn's disease who has had disease for >8–10 years. **If* a patient with UC has co-existing primary sclerosing cholangitis of any duration, surveillance colonoscopy should be performed annually
Health maintenance
Vaccination education for patients on immunosuppressive therapy including (a) annual inactivated influenza, (b) pneumococcal vaccination with a 5-year booster, (c) avoidance of live virus vaccines
Smoking cessation recommendation and treatment or referral in patients with CD who are active smokers at least on annual basis

Abbreviations: *CD* Crohn's disease, *TNF* tumor necrosis factor, *TPMT* thiopurine S-methyltransferase, *UC* ulcerative colitis

Table 12.4 Crohn's & Colitis Foundation Top Ten Outcome Indicators [10]. (Adapted from Melmed et al. [10])

Corticosteroid use (a) Proportion of patients with steroid-free clinical remission for a 12-month period (b) Proportion of patients currently taking prednisone (excluding those who received a diagnosis within the past 112 days)
Days per month and year lost from school or work due to IBD
Days of hospitalization per year secondary to IBD
Emergency room visits per year for IBD
Malnutrition
Anemia
Proportion of patients with normal disease-targeted health-related quality of life
Proportion of patients with narcotic analgesics usage
Proportion of patients with nocturnal bowel movements or leakage
Proportion of patients with incontinence in the past month

These measures were created under a rigorous methodology derived from physician, nurse, and patient input with the aim of providing metrics for quality improvement to provide optimal care for patients with IBD. These measures are not used for accountability or economic incentives, in contrast to AGA measures [4, 10].

Despite the release of the AGA performance measures and the Crohn's and Colitis Foundation quality indicators, multiple studies show that goal-directed interventions are necessary to increase adherence of these measures [26–28].

ImproveCareNow

ImproveCareNow is a learning health system that aims to improve IBD care in the pediatric population. Multiple centers in the United States of America, United Kingdom, and Qatar participate in this network, with over 900 participating pediatric gastroenterologists and 27,000 patients. Clinical data, patient-reported outcomes, and best practices are shared by both physicians and patients to improve pediatric IBD care [4]. Shared learning is possible by comparing process and outcome indicators across the different sites [10]. Initiative at ImproveCareNow sites has demonstrated improvement in patient outcomes such as clinical remission and decreased corticosteroid use [29]. This indicates that collaborative quality improvement efforts are effective in identifying variation in care and enable improvement [10].

Crohn's & Colitis Foundation IBD Qorus

Another learning health system which focuses on adult patients with IBD is the Crohn's & Colitis Foundation's IBD Qorus program, in which goals are to define, measure, and improve quality of care in this patient population and designed to facilitate data sharing among physicians and patients [4]. One of the main goals of IBD Qorus has been to improve unplanned visits to the emergency department and hospital by creating an Urgent Care Best Practices Toolkit [30]. Following the implementation of these interventions and data analysis, improvements were observed in a number of areas, such as the decrease in patients' need for opioids, hospital stays, and urgent care as well as $2500 annual cost savings per patient [31]. Other initiatives by the IBD Qorus program include the IBD Qorus Value Compass which aims to identify causes for variation in quality of care and describe metrics for high-quality care; treat-to-target initiative, a therapeutic approach that balances the patient's own quality-of-life objectives with a remission-based therapy goal; and development of clinical care pathways for treatment of anemia and malnutrition [32].

IBD Patient-Centered Care: Moving from Subspecialty Centers to Subspecialty Homes

A patient-centered medical home, which was first described in 1967, is a system of care that is centered on the patient and in which comprehensive primary care is delivered by a multidisciplinary team that is coordinated, accessible, and oriented on quality, safety, and outcomes [4]. Clinicians that treat patients with IBD understand that they need specialized and individualized care given that a subset of these patients are heavy users of medical services and experience greater rates of unexpected care, such as frequent trips to the emergency room or more diagnostic testing, as much as with other chronic conditions [33]. The IBD Medical Home at the University of Pittsburgh Medical Center (UPMC) is an illustration of a specialty medical home at an academic medical center in which providers aimed to offer patient-centered, interdisciplinary coordinated care led by a gastroenterologist with a multidisciplinary team composed by psychiatrists, nutritionists, social workers, advanced practice providers, and nurse care coordinators [34]. Studies have demonstrated that it is possible to implement a patient-centered specialized medical home for patients with IBD and doing so leads to a considerable decrease in unplanned treatment, an improvement in disease activity, and increased quality of life [20]. Project Sonar is another illustration of a specialty-specific medical home for IBD. Project Sonar is a community-based registry and disease management program created by a joint venture between Illinois Gastroenterology Group and Blue Cross and Blue Shield of Illinois to enhance clinical and financial outcomes in IBD [35]. This project integrates clinical data, patient-reported outcomes, and healthcare claims/resource utilization data and demonstrated value-based improvement in care for patients with CD in a community-based context with reduction in hospital admissions and emergency department visits by over 50% [35].

IBD Specialty Medical Home has demonstrated that IBD patients can receive comprehensive health care through this model, which uses matched incentives with a payer partner and incorporates multidisciplinary care and which leads to considerable decrease in the use of healthcare services as well as an improvement in patient-focused outcomes [34]. Despite specialty medical home appearing to be cost-saving due to reduced resource use over time, it does require upfront staff expenditures [1].

Conclusion

The care provided to patients with IBD varies widely and is likely related to the range of IBD phenotypes, complexity of medical algorithms, and variety of guidelines available as well as the growing medical knowledge in IBD. Delivering consistent, high-quality care is necessary in order to enhance patient outcomes, and therefore multiple opportunities exist to improve quality of care delivered to patients with IBD. Over the past 20 years, there has been significant progress in the creation of quality indicators for IBD care across numerous organizations. However, adherence to these quality measures is still lacking. The development of specialized IBD centers and learning health systems have further contributed to quality improvement with improved patient outcomes.

Disclosures Daniela Fluxa, Maryam Alahmed, and Francis A. Farraye have no relevant disclosures.

References

1. Melmed GY, Oliver B, Hou JK, Lum D, Singh S, Crate D, et al. Quality of care program reduces unplanned health care utilization in patients with inflammatory bowel disease. Am J Gastroenterol. 2021;116(12):2410–8.
2. Ye BD, Travis S. Improving the quality of care for inflammatory bowel disease. Intest Res. 2019;17(1):45–53.
3. Berry SK, Melmed GY. Quality indicators in IBD. Intest Res. 2018;16(1):43–7. https://doi.org/10.5217/ir.2018.16.1.43.
4. Berry SK, Siegel CA, Melmed GY. Quality improvement initiatives in inflammatory bowel disease. Curr Gastroenterol Rep. 2017;19(8):41.
5. Melmed GY, Siegel CA, Spiegel BM, Allen JI, Cima R, Colombel JF, et al. Quality indicators for inflammatory bowel disease: development of process and outcome measures. Inflamm Bowel Dis. 2013;19(3):662–8.
6. Egberg MD, Gulati AS, Gellad ZF, Melmed GY, Kappelman MD. Improving quality in the care of patients with inflammatory bowel diseases. Inflamm Bowel Dis. 2018;24(8):1660–9.
7. Kohn LT, Corrigan JM, Donaldson MS, editors. To err is human: building a safer health system. Washington, DC: National Academy Press; 2000.
8. Institute of Medicine (US) Committee on Quality of Health Care in America. Crossing the quality Chasm: a new health system for the 21st century. Washington, DC: National Academies Press; 2001.
9. Strohl M, Gonczi L, Kurt Z, Bessissow T, Lakatos PL. Quality of care in inflammatory bowel diseases: what is the best way to better outcomes? World J Gastroenterol. 2018;24(22):2363–72.

10. Melmed GY, Siegel CA. Quality improvement in inflammatory bowel disease. Gastroenterol Hepatol. 2013;9(5):286–92.
11. Shah R, Hou JK. Approaches to improve quality of care in inflammatory bowel diseases. World J Gastroenterol. 2014;20(28):9281–5.
12. Siegel CA, Allen JI, Melmed GY. Translating improved quality of care into an improved quality of life for patients with inflammatory bowel disease. Clin Gastroenterol Hepatol. 2013;11(8):908–12.
13. Mehta F. Economic implications of inflammatory bowel disease and its management. Am J Manag Care. 2016;22(3 Suppl):s51–60.
14. Kappelman MD, Rifas-Shiman SL, Porter CQ, Ollendorf DA, Sandler RS, Galanko JA, et al. Direct health care costs of Crohn's disease and ulcerative colitis in US children and adults. Gastroenterology. 2008;135(6):1907–13.
15. Park KT, Ehrlich OG, Allen JI, Meadows P, Szigethy EM, Henrichsen K, et al. The cost of inflammatory bowel disease: an initiative from the Crohn's & colitis foundation. Inflamm Bowel Dis. 2020;26(1):1–10.
16. Ding Z, Muser E, Izanec J, Lukanova R, Kershaw J, Roughley A. Work-related productivity loss and associated indirect costs in patients with Crohn's disease or ulcerative colitis in the United States. Crohns Colitis. 2022;360(6):1–12.
17. Chassin MR, Galvin RW. He urgent need to improve health care quality. Institute of Medicine National Roundtable on health care quality. JAMA. 1998;280(11):1000–5.
18. Kappelman MD, Palmer L, Boyle BM, Rubin DT. Quality of care in inflammatory bowel disease: a review and discussion. Inflamm Bowel Dis. 2010;16(1):125–33.
19. Fiorino G, Allocca M, Chaparro M, Coenen S, Fidalgo C, Younge L, et al. 'Quality of care' standards in inflammatory bowel disease: a systematic review. J Crohns Colitis. 2019;13(1):127–37.
20. Regueiro M, Click B, Anderson A, Shrank W, Kogan J, McAnallen S, et al. Reduced unplanned care and disease activity and increased quality of life after patient enrollment in an inflammatory bowel disease medical home. Clin Gastroenterol Hepatol. 2018;16(11):1777–85.
21. ICHOM—International Consortium for Health Outcomes Measurement-Our Mission [Internet]. [Internet]. https://www.ichom.org/mission/. [cited 2022 Sep 9]. https://www.ichom.org/mission/.
22. ICHOM International Consortium for Health Outcomes Measurement. [cited 2022 Sept 10]. ICHOM—International Consortium for Health Outcomes Measurement [Internet]. [Internet]. [cited 2022 Sep 9]. http://www.ichom.org/medical-conditions/inflammatorybowel-disease/.
23. Walker T, Christophi GP. Quality improvement indicators in inflammatory bowel disease. Adv Res Gastroentero Hepatol. 2017;5(3):555667.
24. Ahmed S, Siegel CA, Melmed GY. Implementing quality measures for inflammatory bowel disease. Curr Gastroenterol Rep. 2015;17(4):14.
25. AGA. Quality and Performance Measures [Internet]. https://gastro.org/practice-resources/quality-and-performance-measures/. [cited 2022 Sep 9]. https://gastro.org/practice-resources/quality-and-performance-measures/.
26. Feuerstein JD, Castillo NE, Siddique SS, Lewandowski JJ, Geissler K, Martinez-Vazquez M, et al. Poor documentation of inflammatory bowel disease quality measures in academic, community, and private practice. Clin Gastroenterol Hepatol. 2016;14:421–8.
27. Parker S, White LC, Spangler C, Rosenblum J, Sweeney S, Homan E, et al. A quality improvement project significantly increased the vaccination rate for immunosuppressed patients with IBD. Inflamm Bowel Dis. 2013;19(9):1809–14.
28. Tkacz J, Brady BL, Meyer R, Lofland JH, Ruetsch C, Coelho-Prabhu N. An assessment of the AGA and CCFA quality indicators in a sample of patients diagnosed with inflammatory bowel disease. J Manag Care Spec Pharm. 2015;21(11):1064. www.amcp.org.
29. Crandall WV, Margolis PA, Kappelman MD, King EC, Pratt JM, Boyle BM, et al. Improved outcomes in a quality improvement collaborative for pediatric inflammatory bowel disease. Pediatrics. 2012;129(4):e1030–41.

30. IBD Qorus. Urgent Care Best Practices Toolkit [Internet]. https://www.crohnscolitisfoundation.org/urgentcare. [cited 2022 Sep 9]. https://www.crohnscolitisfoundation.org/urgentcare.
31. Almario CV, Kogan L, van Deen WK, Scott FI, Singh S, Hou JK, et al. Health economic impact of a multicenter quality-of-care initiative for reducing unplanned healthcare utilization among patients with inflammatory bowel disease. Am J Gastroenterol. 2021;116(12):2459–64.
32. IBD Qorus. Improvement Initiatives & Impact [Internet]. [cited 2022 Sep 10]. https://www.crohnscolitisfoundation.org/research/ibd-qorus/improvement-initiatives.
33. Regueiro MD, McAnallen SE, Greer JB, Perkins SE, Ramalingam S, Szigethy E. The inflammatory bowel disease specialty medical home: a new model of patient-centered care. Inflamm Bowel Dis. 2016;22(8):1971–80.
34. Click B, Regueiro M. The inflammatory bowel disease medical home: from patients to populations. Inflamm Bowel Dis. 2019;25(12):1881–5.
35. Kosinski L, Brill JV, Sorensen M, Baum C, Turpin R, Landsman P. 824 Project sonar: reduction in cost of Care in an Attributed Cohort of patients with Crohn's disease. Gastroenterology. 2016;150(4):S173.
36. ICHOM—International Consortium for Health Outcomes Measurement [Internet]. ICHOM International Consortium for Health Outcomes Measurement. [cited September 10, 2022]. http://www.ichom.org/medical-conditions/inflammatorybowel-disease/.

Chapter 13
Quality in Upper Gastrointestinal Motility Disorders

Mayssan Muftah and Jennifer X. Cai

Table of Quality Measures/Metrics

M. Muftah · J. X. Cai (✉)
Brigham and Women's Hospital, Boston, MA, USA

Harvard Medical School, Boston, MA, USA
e-mail: mmuftah@bwh.harvard.edu; jxcai@bwh.harvard.edu

J. D. Feuerstein, D. J. Stein (eds.), *Quality in Gastroenterology*,
https://doi.org/10.1007/978-3-031-58492-3_13

Key Points

- High-resolution manometry and Chicago Classification v4.0 should be used in the evaluation of esophageal motility disorders.
- Scintigraphic gastric emptying study is the gold standard for diagnosis of gastroparesis.
- Functional disorders of the upper gastrointestinal tract are diagnosed using Rome IV criteria.

Introduction

Upper gastrointestinal (UGI) motility disorders are commonly encountered in gastroenterology. However, evaluation and management of these disorders may not be consistent across clinical practices. The level of evidence regarding the diagnosis and treatment of motility disorders varies. Achalasia is the only motility disorder with published quality metrics [1], with varying levels of adherence across multiple medical centers [2]. Other neurogastroenterologic disorders have standard recommendations for diagnosis and treatment based on society guidelines [3–5] and expert consensus. The purpose of this chapter is to describe clinical standards in evaluating and managing upper gastrointestinal motility disorders and to outline quality metrics when employing diagnostic tests and treatments. We will specifically discuss esophageal motility disorders as outlined in the Chicago Classification v4.0 [6] (CCv4.0) as well as standard of care for gastroparesis. We will also touch on the management of esophageal and gastric functional disorders as they are often part of the differential when evaluating patients with UGI symptoms and may overlap with motility disorders.

Motility Disorders of the Esophagus

Achalasia

Achalasia is an esophageal motility disorder characterized by impaired lower esophageal sphincter (LES) relaxation and absent peristalsis in the esophageal body. The diagnosis is rare, with a prevalence of 1.8–12.6 per 100,000 persons per year [3]. It occurs primarily in adults between the ages of 30 and 60 and affects men and women equally. The pathophysiologic mechanism is not entirely known but is believed to be due to a loss of inhibitory neurons in the myenteric plexus, leading to an excess of excitatory activity preventing appropriate LES relaxation [7]. Below we outline standards in diagnosis and management.

Diagnosis

Before motility testing is considered, an esophagogastroduodenoscopy (EGD) with a thorough examination of the esophagus, esophagogastric junction (EGJ), and cardia should be done to rule out luminal and mechanical causes of obstruction, particularly in older patients with risk factors for malignancy. There may be findings on endoscopy that can be suggestive of achalasia, including a puckered or hypertonic LES, retention of food contents or saliva in the esophagus, and esophageal dilation. However, these findings tend to be identified in the latter stages of disease (when therapeutic interventions may not be as effective), and EGD is not sensitive or specific enough to preclude further diagnostic evaluation for achalasia.

High-resolution manometry (HRM) is the gold standard diagnostic test for evaluating achalasia. Per the Chicago Classification, the diagnosis is made in the setting of an elevated integrated relaxation pressure (IRP) in the primary position during the exam (can be upright or supine) with 100% absent peristalsis (defined as swallows with failed peristalsis or premature contractions) [6]. HRM with esophageal pressure topography outperforms conventional manometry with conventional line tracing with regard to diagnostic accuracy and reproducibility among providers [8, 9]. Given its superiority, HRM has supplanted conventional manometry as standard of care.

HRM is the only diagnostic test that allows for classification into one of the three subtypes (per the CCv4.0)—type I, 100% failed peristalsis without pan-esophageal pressurization (PEP); type II, 100% failed peristalsis with PEP in 20% or more swallows; and type III, 100% failed peristalsis with spasm in 20% or more swallows (can also have PEP) [6]. Subtyping patients is critical in evaluating patients with achalasia as it has implications for prognosis and selection of therapy [10–14]. However, while inter-rater agreement for the diagnosis of achalasia is good [8] to very good [15], it is more variable with regard to achalasia subtyping, particularly when distinguishing type I and II achalasia [15]. This is partly due to disagreements in classifying patients with PEPs with ≥30 mmHg isobaric contours limited to small segments of the distal esophagus. This may represent a phenotype of patients progressing from type II to type I achalasia with a longer disease duration; however, more studies are needed to determine this. There is otherwise very good inter-rater agreement when diagnosing patients with type III achalasia [15]. Other important considerations are that (1) HRM testing should ideally be done while off opiate medications, as type III achalasia has been associated with opiate use [16], and (2) the cutoff of spasm in 20% or more of swallows for identifying type III achalasia is arbitrary [6]. More studies are needed to determine what the optimal cutoff is and what the clinical implications of higher versus lower percentages of spasm are.

Other tests that are used in the evaluation of patients with suspected achalasia include barium esophagram and impedance planimetry using the functional luminal imaging probe (FLIP). The role of a barium esophagram is twofold. First, a routine barium esophagram can rule out structural abnormalities causing an obstruction at the EGJ, particularly if there is a persistent concern for an obstructing lesion despite an unremarkable EGD. Second, to assess esophageal emptying, a timed study should be obtained. A timed barium esophagram (TBE) is performed by having a patient drink 100–200 mL of low-density barium followed by upright frontal spot films of the esophagus at 1, 2, and 5 min. Esophageal retention is assessed by measuring the height and width of the barium columns at each time point [17]. A study assessing the accuracy of TBE in distinguishing achalasia from esophagogastric junction outflow obstruction (EGJOO) or nonobstructive dysphagia found that a column ≥5 cm at 1 min had a sensitivity of 94% and specificity of 71% and a column ≥2 cm at 5 min had a sensitivity of 85% and specificity of 86% [18]. Another study suggests that the degree of esophageal stasis on TBE varies among achalasia subtypes, with type I and II achalasia having higher rates (88% and 84%) of esophageal stasis with columns ≥5 cm at 5 min compared to type III achalasia (24%) and EGJOO (8%) [19]. Additionally, a 13 mm barium tablet can be added to the study to assess esophageal retention of solids. This additional component can increase the sensitivity and diagnostic accuracy for achalasia [18].

TBE with a barium tablet provides complementary information to HRM, which is particularly helpful in patients with equivocal findings on HRM (those with borderline elevated IRP in upright and supine positions) and those who cannot tolerate manometry testing. Establishing a baseline assessment of esophageal stasis is also necessary to (1) assess response to therapies at the LES and (2) evaluate patients with recurrent symptoms after therapy. Despite some conflicting data, TBE is recommended as a first-line test in evaluating continued or recurrent symptoms after definitive achalasia treatment [3].

FLIP has emerged as an adjunctive diagnostic tool that evaluates secondary peristalsis and mechanical properties of the esophagus. It uses impedance planimetry to obtain measurements of cross-sectional area (CSA) and pressure following volume-controlled distention of the esophagus. The ratio of CSA to pressure gives a measure of distensibility, which evaluates for obstruction at the EGJ. A distensibility less than 2 mm^2/mmHg with EGJ diameter less than 12 mm when the balloon is distended to 60 and 70 mL is considered abnormal and strongly suggestive of obstructive physiology at the EGJ. FLIP topography also assesses contractile patterns in the esophageal body. FLIP can be particularly helpful in patients with equivocal findings on HRM and TBE or patients who cannot tolerate HRM. One study found that specific phenotypes on FLIP correlate well with manometry findings— (1) having absent or impaired contractile response with reduced EGJ opening was highly correlated with a diagnosis of achalasia on HRM, while (2) having a normal contractile response with a normal EGJ opening was strongly correlated with normal HRM findings per the Chicago Classification [20]. However, findings on FLIP do not accurately subtype achalasia patients; specifically, it cannot distinguish between type I and II achalasia. Generally, the use of FLIP in evaluating patients with suspected achalasia is evolving, and it should not be used in lieu of other standard diagnostic tests.

Management

Achalasia is a chronic, incurable disease, and treatment is achieved primarily by using therapies targeted at the LES. For patients who are operative candidates, one of the three definitive therapies should be offered: pneumatic dilation (PD), laparoscopic Heller myotomy (LHM), or peroral endoscopic myotomy (POEM). For type I and II achalasia, studies suggest equivalent outcomes among the three therapies [3, 21–26]. For type III achalasia, POEM has been shown to have better outcomes as the myotomy can be extended into the esophageal body to treat spastic segments causing obstructive symptoms [3, 11].

PD is typically performed using a polyethylene Rigiflex balloon. The balloons come in three sizes—3.0 cm, 3.5 cm, and 4.0 cm—and dilations are performed in a serial fashion (every 4 to 6 weeks) until symptom resolution, starting with the 3.0 cm balloon. The risk of perforation is approximately 1.9% [27, 28]. There is no standard procedure regarding the type of sedation to use, whether to use fluoroscopy, duration of dilation (15–60 s or longer), or post-dilation recovery. Given the growing use of endoscopy following dilation to assess for tear or perforation, data suggests a post-procedure barium swallow is not needed to assess for a leak in the absence of concerning symptoms [29].

During LHM, division of the LES muscle fibers is achieved without disruption of the esophageal mucosa. Given the incidence of gastroesophageal reflux disease (GERD) following a myotomy, it is now standard to perform a fundoplication at the same time to reduce the risk. One meta-analysis found that the rate of GERD without a fundoplication is 31.5% compared to 8.8% with fundoplication [30]. Studies comparing Dor (anterior) versus Toupet (posterior) fundoplication show that both techniques have comparable outcomes, so either approach can be used at the time of LHM [31, 32].

POEM is an endoscopic procedure that has emerged over the past 10–15 years [33]. A myotomy is performed endoscopically by creating a submucosal tunnel to access the circular muscle fibers of the LES and then cutting them. Success rates are high (90% or greater) [34, 35]; however, this procedure is associated with the highest risk of GERD. This risk is likely because a myotomy is done without subsequent fundoplication. Current studies have conflicting data as to whether the length of the myotomy plays a role. Rates of GERD are quoted at 39–58% in the literature [36–42], and up to a quarter of patients with objective findings of reflux (identified by abnormal ambulatory pH testing and/or post-procedural diagnoses of erosive esophagitis) may not have symptoms [36]. There are no standard recommendations regarding screening for GERD post-POEM; however, there have been some suggestions for performing an EGD every 1–2 years for the first 5 years following the procedure, even in the absence of symptoms. Research regarding modification of the procedural technique is ongoing to reduce the risk of GERD post-procedurally.

For patients who need additional therapy for persistent or recurrent symptoms, any of the three definitive therapies can be offered. A PD can be done following a myotomy and vice versa. For patients who do not respond to any of the above options, specifically those in the latter stages of disease with severely dilated and/or sigmoid esophagus, an esophagectomy can be considered.

For patients who are not operative candidates, endoscopic botulinum toxin injection should be offered. This is performed by delivering 100 U of botulinum toxin in 0.5–1 mL aliquots using a sclerotherapy needle at the EGJ. Immediate success rates are high. However, the therapeutic effects wane over time, and subsequent injections may not be as efficacious [3]. Some patients may be referred for definitive therapy at the LES after botulinum toxin injection has already been performed. Studies suggest that prior botulinum toxin injection may impact subsequent surgical myotomy outcomes, with higher rates of postoperative dysphagia or perforation [43, 44]. However, this increased risk has not been observed in patients undergoing POEM [45, 46]. Overall, data are conflicting regarding the impact of botulinum toxin injection on myotomy outcomes, and current recommendations state that any of the definitive therapies can be considered following botulinum toxin injection [3].

Oral pharmacologic therapy is the least effective treatment for achalasia. It should only be reserved for patients who are not surgical candidates, cannot undergo endoscopic therapy, or do not respond to botulinum toxin injection [3]. Oral medications are associated with systemic side effects and require frequent dosing given the short duration of action. The most common medications include calcium channel blockers (CCBs) and nitrates.

Assessment of Patients Post-Therapy

The goal of therapy in achalasia is to improve esophageal emptying and decrease bolus retention. This has traditionally been done via symptom assessment using the Eckardt score (ES), which has four components. It assesses symptoms of dysphagia, regurgitation, chest pain, and weight loss, each on a scale of 0–3. A total score > 3 is considered abnormal. However, there was no formal validation of this scoring system before its widespread use in clinical and research settings [3]. One study found that the ES has only fair reliability and validity, and the dysphagia component of the score is the most meaningful with regard to assessing symptom improvement post-therapy [47]. Another study found that the ES does not correlate with bolus retention as demonstrated on barium esophagram. In patients with symptom resolution following PD, 30% had <50% improvement in column height on post-procedure TBE. These patients were more likely to have symptom recurrence and need for additional therapy [48].

TBE is better at assessing esophageal emptying and treatment efficacy than patient-reported scores [3, 48, 49]. However, there are currently no recommendations for obtaining TBE or other testing to assess treatment response in the absence of persistent or recurrent symptoms. For symptomatic patients, a TBE with tablet should be obtained to compare pre- and posttreatment column height [3]. Additional therapy should be considered in patients with column >5 cm at 5 min [3, 50].

HRM may also be considered in assessing patients with persistent or recurrent symptoms. One study found that the resolution of achalasia pattern on HRM correlated with improved esophageal emptying and symptom scores. Additionally, patients with a normal IRP could still have bolus retention, while the opposite (abnormal IRP with esophageal emptying) never occurred [50].

There is emerging data regarding the use of FLIP in the post-therapy assessment of achalasia. Increasingly, FLIP is being utilized at the time of surgical and endoscopic myotomy, with data suggesting that intra-procedural EGJ distensibility and CSA correlate with symptomatic outcomes [51–53]. One study also found that distensibility continued to increase in patients post-myotomy on follow-up EGD (median 15 months after the procedure) [54]. Currently, there is limited data on the use of FLIP to assess patients with persistent or recurrent symptoms, and it is unknown how post-therapy measures of distensibility correlate with findings on TBE. Because of this, FLIP should not be used in lieu of TBE or HRM for post-therapy evaluation.

Esophagogastric Junction Outflow Obstruction

Esophagogastric junction outflow obstruction (EGJOO) is characterized by impaired LES relaxation and intact peristalsis in the esophageal body. Previously, EGJOO was felt to be an early manifestation of achalasia. However, studies have found that less than 10% of patients progress to an achalasia phenotype [55–57]. While the pathophysiology of achalasia is relatively well-defined, the causes of EGJOO are heterogeneous [55, 58] Under the prior iteration of Chicago Classification v3.0, it was estimated that 3–21% of patients referred for HRM were diagnosed with EGJOO. With changes in diagnostic criteria in the current CCv4.0 [6], published in 2020, the incidence of EGJOO has significantly decreased [58, 59]. In this section, we outline current standards in diagnosis and management.

Diagnosis

EGJOO was traditionally defined by an elevated median IRP with intact peristalsis in any position on HRM. However, this criterion led to the overdiagnosis of clinically insignificant EGJOO and excessive use of invasive therapeutic interventions [55]. An elevated IRP may occur due to study artifact, coiling of the manometry catheter, as well as anatomic abnormalities. Prone positioning, typically the primary position for manometry testing, can be susceptible to cardiac compression pressure artifact, which may also increase the IRP. Furthermore, an elevated IRP can be associated with certain medications (e.g., opiates and anticholinergic medications) [60] and high body mass index (BMI).

Under CCv4.0, HRM must demonstrate an elevated median IRP in supine and upright positions as well as increased intrabolus pressure. Additionally, an EGJOO diagnosis is still considered inconclusive until additional confirmatory testing with either TBE (with tablet) or FLIP is performed. While conclusive EGJOO will have signs of esophageal retention on TBE, it is not as profound as that seen with achalasia. Many patients will pass liquid barium at 5 min and may have retention of the barium tablet alone [18, 19]. On FLIP, patients may have a low distensibility and reduced diameter at the EGJ [57, 61]. Lastly, positive test results should be associated with obstructive symptoms—specifically dysphagia and/or noncardiac chest pain [6, 55]. Findings of EGJOO on manometry with nonobstructive esophageal symptoms (including reflux) are more likely to be unrelated or incidental.

Prior to motility testing, a thorough history and EGD should be performed to rule out secondary causes of outflow obstruction [62] as luminal strictures, hiatal hernia, extra-luminal compression, and postsurgical anatomy can lead to manometric patterns consistent with EGJOO [55, 56]. Unless there is a strong clinical suspicion for malignancy, further evaluation with cross-sectional imaging and/or endoscopic ultrasound rarely add to the diagnostic workup and are often unremarkable [63, 64].

In patients with symptoms and but inconclusive findings on standard diagnostic testing, further evaluation using a rapid drink challenge (RDC), solid test meal (STM), and pharmacologic provocation during HRM may elicit findings suggestive of outflow obstruction [55, 59, 65].

Management

Unlike achalasia, the optimal treatment strategy for EGJOO is unclear. Most studies on patient outcomes were performed prior to changes in the diagnostic criteria, where a majority of patients had spontaneous resolution of symptoms with expectant management [58, 66–68]. A study by Carlson et al. found that patients with conclusive EGJOO (confirmed on FLIP) had a higher rate of good outcomes (defined as ES < 3) with achalasia-like therapies compared to other treatments. Conversely, patients with normal findings on FLIP despite having an EGJOO pattern on HRM were more likely to have a good outcome with nonachalasia-type therapies [57].

Generally, a more conservative treatment strategy should be employed when managing patients with EGJOO. Even in patients with conclusive EGJOO, the disease course is generally not as severe as that seen in achalasia. There may also be a functional component to obstructive symptoms, as objective evidence of esophageal retention may not be as profound [55, 69]. Still, in certain patient subgroups, it is reasonable to consider LES-directed therapy. Treatment response has been primarily assessed using patient-reported symptom scores such as the ES; however there is minimal literature to support how to best evaluate patients with EGJOO following therapy.

Botulinum toxin injection is a suitable option in patients who are nonoperative candidates or when trying to avoid an irreversible intervention (particularly in patients with unclear or mild symptoms). Response rates for EGJOO are around 50–60%, and some studies suggest that the effects may be longer lasting than that seen in achalasia [70, 71]. For patients who are operative candidates, PD, POEM, or LHM can be considered. While there is limited data demonstrating the efficacy of these interventions in EGJOO [55, 58, 69] and it may be reasonable to favor PD over myotomy to avoid long-term complications related to GERD and postsurgical anatomy, there are no comparative studies in this population.

Distal Esophageal Spasm

Distal esophageal spasm (DES) is characterized by spastic or premature contractions in the distal esophageal body [6]. Primary DES is rare, and the exact cause is unknown. The hypothesized pathophysiologic mechanism is related to an imbalance between nitrogenic inhibition and cholinergic excitation in the myenteric plexus of the esophagus [72, 73].

Diagnosis

Patients who present with symptoms concerning for DES including dysphagia and/or chest pain should undergo an upper endoscopy to rule out structural causes prior to motility testing. It is important to evaluate for erosive esophagitis and Barrett's esophagus when GERD-induced esophageal spasm is suspected as certain medications used to treat esophageal spasticity may worsen underlying reflux symptoms.

Manometric DES requires the presence of premature contractions in at least 20% of swallows on HRM. A premature contraction is defined by a distal latency (DL) less than 4.5 s with a distal contractile integral (DCI) of 450 mmHg·s·cm or more [6]. A clinical diagnosis of DES should also be accompanied by esophageal symptoms of dysphagia and/or chest pain, as manometric DES can be seen in patients with clinically unrelated symptoms [74]. Manometric DES without obstructive symptoms may be the result of GERD, a medication effect, or incidental.

The presence of at least 20% premature contractions but with DCI less than 450 mmHg·s·cm is inconclusive for DES. Inconclusive or borderline findings/symptoms warrant further evaluation. This can be done with provocative maneuvers on HRM using RDC, STM, or multiple rapid swallows (MRS). A repeat HRM in 6–12 months can also be considered to see if findings persist or if symptoms have evolved. Barium esophagram or FLIP can be performed to identify findings that would be supportive of a DES diagnosis. Barium esophagram may reveal corkscrew or rosary bead esophagus and/or tertiary contractions [72, 74]. A spastic reactive contractile response may be seen on FLIP topography; however, one study found that only 27% of patients with DES on HRM had this pattern on FLIP [75]. TBE and FLIP may also be helpful in assessing esophageal retention and EGJ distensibility in patients with borderline median IRP on HRM, which is particularly important in distinguishing DES from type III achalasia.

Some studies have suggested that DES and type III achalasia occur along a disease spectrum. While both DES and spastic achalasia are characterized by premature propagation of contractions and diminished DL, insufficient LES relaxation is only a feature of the latter [74]. The progression from DES to type III achalasia is rare, ranging from 8 to 14% of patients [76, 77].

Management

The management approach for DES includes an initial evaluation and treatment for GERD. In those with reflux, acid suppression therapy may be sufficient to treat esophageal spasm. In patients without typical reflux symptoms or objective evidence of GERD on endoscopy, an empiric proton pump inhibitor (PPI) trial or pH testing driven reflux therapy can be considered [74]. Otherwise, first-line pharmacologic therapy with smooth muscle relaxants including nitrites, phosphodiesterase (PDE) inhibitors, peppermint oil, and CCBs should be employed [72, 78]. Endoscopic intervention may be considered for patients who are refractory to medical therapy. This is limited to botulinum toxin injection in the distal esophagus and myotomy that extends into the distal esophagus. Botulinum toxin injection has been shown to be effective in treating symptoms in a randomized trial [79]; however patients often have more frequent relapses and require re-treatment. POEM with an extended myotomy has been shown to be effective with clinical success rates of 84–100% [80–82], although studies are limited by small sample sizes and lack of comparison to other therapies. An extended surgical myotomy may be considered, but this can be technically challenging with variable success rates [83] and is typically reserved for situations where POEM is not available. Pneumatic dilation has shown negligible success in treating DES [72]. Overall, further studies are needed to find the optimal treatment strategy for DES.

Assessment of treatment response is primarily symptom-based. There is no standard regarding the use of HRM to assess treatment response, particularly since it is unclear what manometric finding would indicate treatment success [74].

Hypercontractile Esophagus

Hypercontractile esophagus (HE) is characterized by normally propagated peristaltic contractions with excessive contractile vigor in the esophageal body, specifically in the absence of esophageal obstruction (as obstructive lesions can trigger a hypercontractile response) [84]. HE has a prevalence of 2–4% among patients referred for motility testing. It affects women more than men and has a mean age at diagnosis of 65.2 years [85]. HE has been associated with GERD [86], opiate use [16], elevated BMI [87], and eosinophilic esophagitis [84, 85]. The pathophysiologic mechanism is hypothesized to be related to excessive cholinergic activity in the myenteric plexus of the esophagus [72, 85].

Diagnosis

Similar to DES, HE requires a specific manometric pattern and clinically relevant symptoms, specifically dysphagia and/or chest pain. The manometric pattern of HE on HRM requires 20% or more hypercontractile swallows having

DCI > 8000 mmHg·s·cm. There is disagreement among experts about whether the LES should be included in the measurement of the DCI. In circumstances where 20% or more of swallows do not have DCI > 8000 mmHg·s·cm but vigorous contractions involving the LES are visualized, it is reasonable to include the LES in DCI calculations. Otherwise, for patients with inconclusive findings on HRM but high clinical suspicion, increased intrabolus pressure may also support a diagnosis of HE. Further evaluation with RDC, MRS, or pharmacologic provocation may also give diagnostic clarity.

There are three manometric subtypes of HE described in the literature— (1) single-peaked esophageal body contractions, (2) multi-peaked esophageal body contractions (also known as jackhammer esophagus), and (3) vigorous LES after-contractions. However, subtyping patients has no clinical utility currently [84]. Since jackhammer esophagus refers to a specific manometric subtype, the term should not be used interchangeably with HE. There is also no utility to distinguishing LES-dependent versus LES-independent HE as this has no impact on management or long-term outcomes [88].

Even in the presence of hypercontractile swallows, a manometric diagnosis of HE can only be made if the criteria for achalasia and DES are not met [84]. An upper endoscopy should be performed prior to HRM, as esophageal obstruction can lead to compensatory hypercontractile swallows.

TBE and FLIP have limited roles in the diagnostic evaluation of HE. A routine (non-timed) barium esophagram may aid in evaluating esophageal anatomy, particularly if there is an ongoing concern for mechanical obstruction despite an unremarkable EGD. However, there are no findings on TBE that are specific to HE. FLIP may be helpful in evaluating the EGJ if there is a concern for EGJOO with inconclusive findings on HRM. Otherwise, findings on FLIP topography do not correlate with HRM and can range from normal to absent to spastic/reactive contractile response [89].

Management

The data on therapies for HE is limited, primarily consisting of retrospective studies without a control arm. Many patients with HE improve with expectant management [66, 84, 85, 88]; however for those who have severe symptoms or do not improve, the treatment approach is similar to that of DES. Pharmacologic therapies such as smooth muscle relaxants are typically first-line although they have limited efficacy due to inadequate symptom response or relapse after discontinuation. There are also reports of neuromodulator use with some success particularly when chest pain is the predominant symptom. While there is an association between GERD and HE, acid suppression is usually ineffective in treating HE symptoms [85, 86, 90].

For patients who are refractory to medical therapy, endoscopic intervention for HE can be considered. The use of botulinum toxin injection, PD, and POEM have been reported in the literature. A crossover trial randomized 22 patients with DES or HE to endoscopic botulinum toxin or saline injection at the EGJ. Patients who underwent botulinum toxin injection had a 50% symptom response rate at 1 month compared to 10% in the sham group; however, response rates for botulinum toxin dropped to 30% at 1 year [79]. In a randomized controlled trial of patients with hypercontractile motility disorders, response rates (defined by ES) of botulinum toxin were 15% at 3 months versus 20% in the sham arm [91]. The data regarding PD is extremely limited; one study cited a relapse of symptoms in over half of patients [90]. POEM with an extended myotomy has been shown to be effective and is reasonable to consider in patients with severe and/or refractory symptoms, although success rates (72%) [82] appear to be lower than those in achalasia and DES [85, 89].

Absent Contractility

Absent contractility is an esophageal hypomotility disorder characterized by absent peristalsis in the esophageal body without impaired LES relaxation (i.e., with normal median IRP) [6, 92]. It affects more women than men and is typically diagnosed between 40 and 60 years of age [93–95]. There is minimal data on the overall prevalence among patients undergoing motility testing, though it is likely approximately 3% [93, 94]. Absent contractility is associated with GERD and rheumatologic conditions, most notably scleroderma, although associations with rheumatoid arthritis and lupus have also been reported [95]. In one study, the prevalence of absent contractility among GERD patients undergoing motility testing prior to anti-reflux surgery was 3.2% [96]. The prevalence among patients with systemic sclerosis is 40–60% [95, 97, 98]. However, most cases are idiopathic, and a diagnosis of absent contractility does not necessarily indicate a workup for autoimmune conditions [92]. The pathophysiologic mechanism is unknown. In patients with scleroderma, it is hypothesized that collagen deposits, vascular derangement, and autoimmune-mediated injury disrupt neural pathways in the esophagus [99]. In this section, we outline current standards in diagnosis and management.

Diagnosis

Absent contractility requires 100% failed swallows (all swallows with DCI < 100 mmHg·s·cm) and a normal median IRP on HRM. This manometric finding is almost always abnormal, as the prevalence in healthy volunteers is 0.4% [100]. Inconclusive findings on HRM are encountered when the median IRP is borderline, raising concern for type I achalasia. Distinguishing these two disorders is important as it has implications for therapy. Provocative maneuvers on HRM may identify patients with impaired LES relaxation despite normal/borderline median IRP. RDC may reveal latent EGJ obstruction manifesting as esophageal pressurization or increase in trans-EGJ pressure gradients [92]. TBE and FLIP are also helpful in further evaluating the EGJ, assessing for signs of bolus retention and impaired EGJ distensibility.

Patients often present with reflux symptoms (heartburn and regurgitation) and/or dysphagia. The presence of reflux symptoms may be due to comorbid GERD. The prevalence of GERD in patients with absent contractility is 62–64% [94, 101]. GERD patients with absent contractility have significantly higher esophageal acid burden [101] and are more likely to be refractory to PPI. Because of this, ambulatory pH testing may also have a role in evaluating patients with absent contractility.

Management

There are currently no pharmacologic therapies that can restore esophageal peristalsis in patients with absent contractility. Specifically, conventional prokinetic agents such as metoclopramide and domperidone do not improve esophageal hypomotility. There have been limited studies on 5-HT_4 agonists, including prucalopride and buspirone, showing little to no benefit [92, 102]. Hence, management of absent contractility comprises lifestyle modifications and treatment of GERD and its complications. For patients who have GERD refractory to PPI, anti-reflux surgery may be considered, although there is controversy as to whether a fundoplication can be performed with absent contractility due to the risk of prolonged postoperative dysphagia. Several studies have since demonstrated that a partial fundoplication is effective in these patients without increased risk of postoperative dysphagia compared to patients without esophageal hypomotility [103–105].

Ineffective Esophageal Motility

Ineffective esophageal motility (IEM) is an esophageal hypomotility disorder characterized by ineffective swallows. IEM has a similar epidemiologic profile to that of absent contractility [106, 107]. Prior to recent changes in diagnostic criteria, the prevalence of IEM among patients undergoing motility testing was approximately 30% [108, 109]. With the more stringent criteria of CCv4.0, the true prevalence is thought to be two-thirds of that, although data is limited [107]. IEM is associated with GERD, smooth muscle disorders, and medications (including PDE inhibitors and CCBs). The average acid exposure time (AET) in IEM patients diagnosed using the new criteria is higher than in those diagnosed using the old criteria [92, 107, 110]. The pathophysiologic mechanism of IEM is unclear, but it is likely due to a combination of central and peripheral neural dysfunction and primary or secondary muscle dysfunction which can be caused by GERD and smooth muscle disorders, among other conditions [111].

Diagnosis

There have been several changes to the diagnostic criteria of IEM with CCv4.0. This was done to increase specificity for clinically relevant IEM, as it can be seen in asymptomatic patients on HRM. The prevalence of IEM in healthy volunteers decreased from 11–17% to 10% with the changes in diagnostic criteria [92, 100].

IEM is diagnosed by the presence of more than 70% ineffective swallows or at least 50% failed swallows. Ineffective swallows include weak (DCI 100–450 mmHg·s·cm), failed (DCI < 100 mmHg·s·cm), and fragmented swallows (peristaltic break >5 cm with normal DCI). There are several notable changes from CCv3.0, including (1) a change in threshold from 50% to 70% ineffective swallows and (2) recategorizing fragmented swallows under the umbrella of ineffective swallows, thereby eliminating fragmented peristalsis as a separate diagnosis [92]. Patients with 50–70% ineffective swallows are now considered inconclusive for IEM. In patients where there is ongoing clinical suspicion, further evaluation with provocative maneuvers may be helpful. Specifically, the absence of contractile reserve on MRS may support a diagnosis of IEM. However, it is important to note that absent contractile reserve can be seen in up to 35% of patients with IEM, 26% of patients with inconclusive IEM, and 22% of healthy volunteers [101, 112]. Otherwise, there is minimal role for TBE and FLIP in evaluating these patients unless there is concern for concurrent EGJOO.

Patients with clinically relevant IEM often present with reflux symptoms and/or dysphagia. Ambulatory pH testing may play a role in evaluating patients with PPI-refractory symptoms and those being considered for anti-reflux surgery.

Management

For patients with incidental findings of IEM (i.e., asymptomatic or unrelated symptoms), no specific therapy is needed. In patients with a clinically relevant presentation, management is similar to that of absent contractility where treatment focuses primarily on treating concomitant GERD and its complications. For patients with GERD refractory to PPI, surgical fundoplication can be considered. There is debate as to whether a partial fundoplication (Dor or Toupet) should be done to reduce the risk of postoperative dysphagia; however, studies have shown similar outcomes in IEM patients that undergo partial or Nissen fundoplication [113–116]. There is recent data that patients with absent contractile reserve on MRS are more likely to have postoperative dysphagia. Further studies are needed to determine if contractile reserve should be used to determine which IEM patients would benefit from a partial versus Nissen fundoplication [112].

Otherwise, lifestyle recommendations such as eating upright, chewing carefully, and taking small bites can help with symptoms of dysphagia. Some studies have evaluated the use of diaphragmatic breathing and transcutaneous neuromodulation, demonstrating improvements in contractile vigor [92, 117], although the durability of these results and how they translate to patient symptoms are unknown. Lastly, it is important to consider a functional component of patient symptoms that may improve with neuromodulators [118].

Other Functional Disorders of the Esophagus

There are other functional disorders of the esophagus as outlined by the Rome IV criteria [119]. Patients that present with esophageal symptoms and have unremarkable findings on upper endoscopy, HRM, and pH impedance testing likely meet criteria for an underlying functional disorder. Specifically, eosinophilic esophagitis, pathologic GERD, and a major esophageal motility disorder (i.e., achalasia, distal esophageal spasm, hypercontractile esophagus, and absent contractility) need to be excluded. Diagnosis of a functional esophageal disorder is made based on the presenting symptom, and these include globus, functional dysphagia, functional chest pain, functional heartburn, and reflux hypersensitivity. Management typically entails the use of behavioral therapies and neuromodulators. The addition of PPIs may help in the management of reflux hypersensitivity, as symptoms are still induced by reflux events in the absence of pathologic GERD. Functional heartburn and reflux hypersensitivity can be distinguished based on the symptom association index on pH impedance testing [120].

Disorders of the Stomach

Gastroparesis

Gastroparesis (GP) is a motility disorder of the stomach characterized by UGI symptoms with objective evidence of delayed gastric emptying in the absence of a mechanical gastric outlet obstruction [4]. Symptoms of GP include early satiety, fullness, nausea, vomiting, upper abdominal pain, bloating, and/or weight loss in severe cases [121]. Based on studies from the United States and the United Kingdom, the estimated prevalence is 13.8–267.7 per 100,000 adults, and the incidence is estimated to be 1.9–6.3 per 100,000 person-years [122]. GP is more common in women than men and the age at presentation ranges from 45 to 60 years of age [122]. Diabetic and idiopathic GP are the most common subtypes. Other causes of GP include postsurgical etiology, viral illness (including Epstein-Barr virus, cytomegalovirus, norovirus), neurologic conditions (such as Parkinson's disease, amyloidosis, dysautonomia), autoimmune disease, paraneoplastic syndrome, connective tissue diseases (such as systemic sclerosis or systemic lupus erythematosus), and ischemic injury. GP can also be seen as a result of medications that impact gastric motility, such as opioids, antibiotics, antiarrhythmics, and tricyclic antidepressants, among others [121]. The pathophysiology of GP is not completely understood and varies depending on the cause. Delayed emptying in GP may be due to a combination of antral hypomotility and pyloric dysfunction, often with concurrent impairment in gastric accommodation [121, 123]. Below we review the current standards in diagnosis and management.

Diagnosis

Prior to evaluating gastric emptying, an EGD should be performed to rule out mechanical gastric outlet obstruction. If there is a persistent concern despite unremarkable findings on EGD, cross-sectional imaging or endoscopic ultrasound may assist in further evaluation. At the time of endoscopy, the presence of retained food is not diagnostic of GP. One study found that retained food on endoscopy has a positive predictive value of 55% for delayed gastric emptying. Comorbid diabetes mellitus and use of acid suppressants, cardiovascular medications, or opioids were associated with retained food, independent of the presence of delayed emptying [124].

The gold standard to evaluate for delayed gastric emptying is the scintigraphic gastric emptying (SGE) test. The standard protocol is to assess the emptying of a solid meal (usually a low-fat egg white meal) over at least 3 h. If more than 90% of the meal is not emptied at 3 h, the test should be extended to 4 h [4]. A recent meta-analysis found that delayed gastric emptying identified on 3–4-h assessments was found to correlate with UGI symptoms of nausea, vomiting, early satiety, and fullness. This correlation was not seen in patients found to have delayed emptying on assessments less than 3 h [125]. Radiopaque markers should not be used in lieu of a solid meal. They are not as sensitive in identifying GP and delayed emptying of radiopaque markers does not correlate with patient symptoms. Lastly, medications that impair gastric emptying should be discontinued 48 h before the test [4]. Delayed gastric emptying is defined as gastric retention of greater than 10% of the solid meal at 4 h [126].

Alternatives to SGE include wireless motility capsule (WMC) or stable isotope (^{13}C-spirulina) breath test. Evaluation with WMC entails ingestion of a solid nondigestible pill. Changes in pH indicate transit from the stomach to the duodenum. When compared to SGE, WMC has a sensitivity of 59–86% and a specificity of 64–81% for the diagnosis of GP [127]. The advantages of WMC are that measures of gastric contractile amplitude can be obtained and a concurrent assessment of small bowel and colonic transit can be done. However, SGE may be more accurate in assessing gastric emptying as there are inherent pathophysiologic differences between emptying homogenized solid food and a nondigestible pill [4].

Evaluation with a stable isotope breath test entails ingestion of ^{13}C-spirulina followed by the measurement of expiratory $^{13}CO_2$ concentration at 45, 150, and 180 min. A study comparing breath testing to SGE found that breath testing had a sensitivity of 89% when setting the specificity at 80% (AUC 0.89) [128]. Advantages of breath testing include no radiation exposure and approval for use in children [4].

FLIP may play a role in characterizing pyloric function, particularly if pylorus-directed therapies are considered. It has been shown that smaller pyloric diameter and reduced distensibility correlate with delayed gastric emptying [129, 130]; however, there are no established normative values for diameter and distensibility at the pylorus (unlike the LES). Currently, FLIP primarily has a role in assessing changes after gastric peroral endoscopic myotomy (G-POEM), which may help determine if an adequate myotomy has been performed [131].

Other tests to evaluate gastric emptying and GP include mapping electrogastrography, gastroduodenal manometry, full-thickness gastric biopsies, and single-photon emission computed tomography (SPECT). Currently, these tests are primarily reserved for research purposes.

Once a diagnosis of GP has been obtained, identifying the etiology may inform the management approach (e.g., glycemic control in patients with diabetes) as well as prognostication. For patients with an underlying condition that can cause GP, no further evaluation is needed. For patients without an underlying condition, further evaluation with laboratory testing may help in identifying a cause.

GP and functional dyspepsia (FD) often overlap and are felt to be on a disease spectrum of gastric dysfunction. A prospective study following patients with GP (confirmed on SGE) and FD (diagnosed per Rome III criteria) found that presenting symptoms, symptom severity, and baseline characteristics did not differ between the groups. Full-thickness biopsies also did not reveal any histologic differences. Additionally, one study revealed that 42% of patients with GP were reclassified to FD and 37% with FD were reclassified to GP after 48 weeks of follow-up [132]. This may be partly due to limitations or lability of SGE in evaluating gastric emptying. Despite significant similarities, it may be important to distinguish the two diagnoses given implications for management particularly when considering endoscopic or surgical interventions and prognosis which tends to be more favorable in FD [4].

Management

The treatment for gastroparesis entails the use of dietary modification, pharmacologic therapy, nutritional support, and endoscopic or surgical procedures for refractory cases. Management is best tailored to treat predominant symptoms, rather than using a standard approach for all patients [5]. Dietary recommendations, however, should be recommended universally and include a small particle diet. Randomized trials have demonstrated that a small particle diet improves symptoms and gastric emptying in patients with diabetic gastroparesis [133, 134].

For patients not responsive to dietary modification, medications can be used to improve symptoms and gastric emptying. Prokinetic agents are the mainstay of therapy and have been shown to improve symptoms of early satiety, nausea, and vomiting. However, symptom response is heterogeneous and may depend on the underlying cause of gastroparesis. Patients with idiopathic, diabetic, post-viral, or Parkinson's disease-associated gastroparesis tend to have more favorable responses to prokinetic agents [4]. The medications with the most evidence are metoclopramide and domperidone. However, metoclopramide is only approved for use for less than 12 weeks and domperidone has limited availability in the United States [4].

Metoclopramide is a dopamine receptor antagonist that also exhibits partial 5-HT_4 agonism; thus it has both prokinetic and antiemetic properties [123, 135]. Multiple clinical trials have found that metoclopramide improves symptoms and gastric emptying in patients with GP [136–140]. However, these trials were limited to 3–4 weeks of follow-up. It is recommended to use a maximum dose of 10 mg with meals and before sleep for 12 weeks or less. It is primarily used in oral forms; however intravenous [141] and intranasal [142, 143] formulations are also available. There is a black box warning regarding the risk of tardive dyskinesia; however, the risk is lower than previously thought (less than 1%) [144]. Lastly, metoclopramide is not recommended for use in patients 65 years or older.

Domperidone is another dopaminergic antagonist with prokinetic and antiemetic properties. Multiple randomized trials have found that domperidone is effective in improving symptoms and gastric emptying in patients with GP [139, 145, 146]. It is only available through a program administered by the Food and Drug Administration (FDA), severely limiting access to this medication in the United States [4]. Unlike metoclopramide, domperidone does not cross the blood-brain barrier, lowering the risk of extrapyramidal side effects. However, it has a similar risk of QTc interval prolongation [121]. Typically, doses of 10–20 mg with meals and before sleep are used.

Other prokinetic agents include erythromycin (motilin agonist), 5-HT_4 agonists, and relamorelin (ghrelin receptor agonist). Erythromycin is effective in reducing symptoms and improving gastric emptying [140]; however, it exhibits tachyphylaxis and should only be used for 1–4 weeks. 5-HT_4 agonists, such as prucalopride, have been shown to improve gastric emptying, although the effect on symptoms is unclear [4]. Lastly, relamorelin improved symptoms and gastric emptying in phase 2 clinical trials [147, 148]. However, further evidence is needed regarding its efficacy before approval in clinical practice.

Other medications, including antiemetics and neuromodulators, may improve symptoms, but do not impact gastric emptying. Recent guidelines recommended against the use of neuromodulators [4] due to a randomized trial showing no change in global GP symptoms when comparing nortriptyline to placebo in patients with idiopathic GP. However, there was an improvement in pain in the nortriptyline group [149]. Also, as noted above, GP overlaps with and may be on the same spectrum as FD, where neuromodulators are a mainstay of therapy. Further research is needed to examine the role of neuromodulators in GP, but they are reasonable to consider in patients with pain-predominant symptoms [5].

For patients with weight loss, malnutrition, and/or ongoing symptoms despite medical therapy, nutritional support should be considered. The goal of nutritional support is not to eliminate oral intake but rather used as a bridge to reinstating or improving oral intake, which has been shown to improve morbidity and mortality in patients with GP [4]. Enteral nutrition is preferred to parenteral nutrition. To prevent exacerbation of symptoms, jejunal feeds are preferred. Feeds can be delivered using a direct jejunostomy tube, a gastrostomy tube with a jejunal extension, or a gastrojejunostomy tube. The advantage of having the gastric component is to allow for venting if GP symptoms persist despite getting jejunal feeds. Parenteral nutrition is reserved for cases in which enteral feeds are not tolerated. Exclusive long-term parenteral nutrition is feasible if needed, with 68% survival at 15 years in one study [150].

Patients with symptoms refractory to medical or nutritional therapies may be candidates for endoscopic intervention or gastric electrical stimulation (GES) [5]. The only endoscopic intervention recommended in the treatment of GP is G-POEM. This entails a full-thickness pyloromyotomy extending into the antrum [151]. Multiple open-label trials have shown that G-POEM is effective in treating symptoms and improving gastric emptying in GP [151–161]. A recent randomized trial comparing G-POEM to a sham procedure in severe GP demonstrated a significant treatment success rate of 71% versus 22%; however enrollment was stopped after only 41 patients due to significant results and risk of general anesthesia in the sham group [162]. Intrapyloric botulinum toxin injection has been shown to not be effective in treating gastroparesis symptoms in multiple placebo-controlled trials [163].

GES consists of a neurostimulator that is placed in the abdominal wall with electrodes that are implanted in the muscularis propria of the stomach via laparoscopy or laparotomy [164]. A number of trials have shown that GES improves vomiting in patients with GP [164–168]. There are mixed results regarding other GP symptoms, quality of life, and gastric emptying [169, 170]. GES is approved as a humanitarian use device by the FDA for medically refractory diabetic or idiopathic GP.

There are surgical interventions available for the management of gastroparesis; however, they have limited evidence and are not routinely recommended. These include pyloroplasty, partial gastrectomy, or sleeve gastrectomy. During a surgical pyloroplasty, a longitudinal full-thickness incision is performed across the pylorus, which is then closed transversely. This has been shown to be effective in treating symptoms and improving gastric emptying. However, when compared to G-POEM, surgical pyloroplasty has a much higher risk of adverse events, with a morbidity rate of 6.8% [171, 172]. Complications include postoperative leaks and need for subsequent surgical intervention such as subtotal gastrectomy or feeding tube placement for nutrition.

In addition to GP-specific therapies, treatment of the underlying cause may improve symptoms and gastric emptying. Specifically, in patients with diabetes, optimal glucose control reduces the risk of future exacerbation of gastroparesis [4]. Data suggests that acute hyperglycemia impairs gastric emptying and exacerbates GP symptoms [173], while glycemic control improves symptoms, meal tolerance, and quality of life [174].

Supragastric Belching

Supragastric belching is a functional disorder of excessive belching that is characterized by air that enters into the esophagus and is then rapidly expelled. The air does not reach the stomach, hence the term "supragastric" belch. Previously this was thought to be due to aerophagia, or excessive swallowing of air. However, studies using high-resolution impedance manometry (HRIM) have shown that this is in fact driven by two learned behaviors: (1) air can be forcibly pushed into the esophagus through contraction of the muscles of the pharynx, palate, and tongue, and (2) air can be sucked into the esophagus by generating negative intrathoracic pressure, most likely facilitated by inhalation against a closed glottis and relaxation of the UES. Neither mechanism is associated with a peristaltic contraction in the esophageal body [175, 176].

While commonly encountered in clinical practice, the true prevalence of supragastric belching is unknown. One study reports a prevalence of 3.4% in patients referred for motility and impedance testing. There was a relatively equal distribution between males and females and the mean age at diagnosis was 48 years [177]. Supragastric belching can be seen in association with GERD or hypomotility disorders of the esophagus [178].

Diagnosis

A diagnosis of excessive belching can be made clinically using the Rome IV criteria: (1) bothersome (i.e., severe enough to impact usual activities) belching more than 3 days a week and (2) symptoms must be present for the preceding 3 months with symptom onset at least 6 months prior to diagnosis. Use of HRIM can distinguish supragastric from gastric belching which may impact management. Clinically, patients with supragastric belching tend to have observable frequent and repetitive belching [119, 175, 176].

Management

There is very limited data on treatment options for supragastric belching. Generally, behavioral therapies are first-line and patients may benefit from a referral to gastropsychology or behavioral medicine. Potential therapies include biofeedback, hypnosis, and cognitive behavioral therapy (CBT) [179, 180]. The most investigated medical therapy for supragastric belching is baclofen. One uncontrolled study showed that it was effective in reducing belching events with mild side effects such as sleepiness and difficulty to concentrate [181]. However, a subsequent randomized trial demonstrated that it was no different from placebo in treating supragastric belching [182].

Rumination Syndrome

Rumination syndrome is a functional disorder characterized by effortless regurgitation during or soon after eating. This is followed by rechewing, reswallowing, or spitting out of regurgitated food [183, 184]. Epidemiologic data is limited, so the true prevalence is unknown. Studies suggest a prevalence of 0.2–2% in adults [185–188] and a prevalence of 4.7–11.5% [189–192] in children. The prevalence increases in special populations, such as those with fibromyalgia, eating disorders, or developmental delay [183, 193]. The pathophysiology of rumination is not well understood. It is thought to be a learned behavior where the abdominal wall is contracted to generate increased intra-abdominal pressure and negative intrathoracic pressure, resulting in an esophagogastric pressure gradient that allows for rumination [184]. Typically, patients will have normal gastric accommodation and emptying [183].

Diagnosis

Using the Rome IV criteria, a diagnosis of rumination syndrome can be made based on clinical history alone [184]: (1) persistent or recurrent regurgitation of recently ingested food into the mouth with subsequent spitting or remastication and swallowing and (2) regurgitation not preceded by retching. Symptoms must be present for the preceding 3 months with symptom onset at least 6 months prior to diagnosis. Other supportive findings include the following: (1) there is effortless regurgitation without nausea, (2) regurgitant contains recognizable food, and (3) process ceases when regurgitant becomes acidic [119]. The presence of nocturnal regurgitation, dysphagia, nausea, or symptoms occurring in the absence of meals makes rumination syndrome less likely, but does not exclude the diagnosis [183]. Patients may describe associated halitosis, dental caries, and weight loss, although electrolyte disturbances and malnutrition are uncommon [183, 194, 195].

Patients often describe regurgitation 10–15 min after eating which can persist for up to 1–2 h. Episodes do not have to occur with every meal, and there may be certain meals that are more likely to trigger symptoms than others. It is important to recognize that patients may describe regurgitation as vomiting or reflux, and discerning this is important in avoiding excessive testing. While not necessary, patients often get an EGD or barium esophagram to rule out a mechanical cause of vomiting or regurgitation [183].

If the diagnosis of rumination syndrome is unclear or if patients are not improving as expected with treatment, further evaluation should be done with postprandial HRIM. There is no standardized protocol and typically only specialized motility centers perform this testing. Patients are advised to bring a meal that triggers their symptoms in order to ensure potential rumination events are captured. HRIM allows for detection of increased pressurization in the stomach with the return of ingested material into the proximal esophagus. Gastroduodenal manometry and abdominal wall electromyography (EMG) can also be used to diagnose rumination syndrome; however, availability is even more limited than HRIM.

Management

First-line therapy in the management of rumination syndrome is diaphragmatic breathing. This can be taught in the office or can be done in conjunction with a referral to behavioral medicine or GI psychology. Patients are instructed to place a hand on the abdomen and on the chest with the goal to have the abdomen move with inhalation and exhalation while the chest remains still. This should be done slowly, with six to eight respirations per minute. Diaphragmatic breathing should be done for at least 15 min after each meal to prevent subsequent rumination [183, 184]. The technique works by competing with habitual abdominal wall contraction after meals through relaxation of the abdominal wall [184]. A randomized clinical trial demonstrated that diaphragmatic breathing was effective in reducing regurgitation events by 74% [196]. EMG-guided biofeedback is another option that can be considered upfront, used in conjunction with diaphragmatic breathing [196, 197], or in patients who are unable to perform diaphragmatic breathing on their own. It is unclear if diaphragmatic breathing with biofeedback is superior to diaphragmatic breathing alone as there are no comparative trials. Additionally, access to biofeedback is very limited and may not be an option for many patients. For patients who do not respond to diaphragmatic breathing (with or without biofeedback), other behavioral therapies such as CBT can be considered [184].

Patients with refractory symptoms may be candidates for medical therapy. Besides diaphragmatic breathing, baclofen is the only other therapy for rumination syndrome that is supported by randomized controlled trial data. A small crossover trial showed baclofen was effective in reducing regurgitation events and improving symptoms [182]. Other medications for rumination reported in the literature include neuromodulators, PPIs, histamine receptor blockers, prokinetic agents, and antiemetics, although there is limited data to suggest these medications are effective [184].

Surgical intervention should generally be avoided in rumination syndrome [184]. A case series of five patients with rumination demonstrated symptom improvement following fundoplication [198]; however, other studies have reported patients with rumination syndrome who have had prior fundoplications [199]. At this time, there is not sufficient evidence to support the use of fundoplication in this population [183].

Other Functional Disorders of the Stomach

There are other functional disorders of the stomach as outlined by the Rome IV criteria [119]. These include FD, excessive gastric belching, and nausea and vomiting disorders (including chronic nausea and vomiting syndrome, cyclic vomiting, and cannabinoid hyperemesis). Other than excessive gastric belching, an EGD is required to rule out luminal causes of symptoms before a diagnosis can be made, although the yield of EGD is low in patients under the age of 50 years. Management options include neuromodulators, PPIs, histamine receptor blockers, prokinetic agents, and antiemetics. Testing and treatment for *H. pylori* should be done in patients with dyspeptic symptoms (i.e., fullness, early satiety, epigastric pain) [200]. Behavioral therapies may also play a role in management.

Conclusion

Above, we have outlined current standards in the diagnosis and management of UGI motility and functional disorders, with important quality metrics listed in Table 13.1. In general, an EGD should be used to rule out luminal pathology prior to the evaluation of a motility disorder. Gold standard tests, including HRM for esophageal disorders and SGE for GP, should be used to evaluate UGI motility, and these should

Table 13.1 Quality metrics in upper gastrointestinal motility disorders

Esophageal disorders
• All patients with esophageal symptoms should undergo EGD with biopsies prior to consideration of manometry for evaluation of a motility disorder
• HRM should be used for evaluation of motility disorders over conventional manometry
• Chicago classification v4.0 should be used in the diagnosis of esophageal motility disorders using a standardized language
• A diagnosis of achalasia should prompt classification into one of the three subtypes
• Patients with achalasia who are candidates for surgery should be managed with LES-directed therapy (PD, POEM, or LHM) over other therapies
• Patients with achalasia who are not candidates for surgery should be managed with botulinum toxin injection of the LES over medical therapy
• TBE should be used to evaluate for continued or recurrent symptoms following definitive achalasia treatment
• An IRP should be evaluated in upright and supine positions when performing HRM and must be elevated in both positions to be consistent with EGJOO
• Evaluation with barium esophagram or FLIP is needed to make a conclusive diagnosis of EGJOO
• The presence of dysphagia and/or chest pain is needed for the conclusive diagnosis of DES and HE
• Workup with EGD with esophageal biopsies and HRM should be done to exclude luminal pathology, EoE, and major motility disorders before diagnosing functional disorders of the esophagus (according to the Rome IV criteria)
Gastric disorders
• Prior to evaluation for gastroparesis, an EGD should be performed to rule out a mechanical obstruction
• SGE with solid meal for a duration of at least 3 h is the gold standard test to evaluate for delayed gastric emptying
• A small particle diet should be recommended to all patients with gastroparesis.
• Diaphragmatic breathing with or without biofeedback is first-line therapy for patients with rumination syndrome
• An EGD should be done to rule out luminal causes of disease before the diagnosis of a functional gastric disorder (according to the Rome IV criteria) can be made

EGD esophagogastroduodenoscopy, *HRM* high-resolution manometry, *LES* lower esophageal sphincter, *PD* pneumatic dilation, *POEM* peroral endoscopic myotomy, *LHM* laparoscopic Heller myotomy, *TBE* timed barium esophagram, *IRP* integrated relaxation pressure, *EGJOO* esophagogastric junction outflow obstruction, *DES* distal esophageal spasm, *HE* hypercontractile esophagus, *FLIP* functional luminal imaging probe, *EoE* eosinophilic esophagitis, *SGE* scintigraphic gastric emptying be done while off medications that may lead to false positive results. Once a diagnosis is made, evidence-based therapy should be employed, including LES-directed therapy in patients with achalasia and a small particle diet with prokinetic agents for GP. For patients with unrevealing diagnostic testing, it is important to consider an underlying functional disorder. Future research on motility-specific quality metrics may provide further guidance on how to best approach patients with neurogastroenterologic disorders.

References

1. Kamal AN, Kathpalia P, Otaki F, Bredenoord AJ, Castell DO, Clarke JO, Falk GW, Fass R, Prakash Gyawali C, Kahrilas PJ, Katz PO, Katzka DA, Pandolfino JE, Penagini R, Richter JE, Roman S, Savarino E, Triadafilopoulos G, Vaezi MF, Vela MF, Leiman DA. Development of quality indicators for the diagnosis and management of achalasia. Neurogastroenterol Motil. 2021;33(10):e14118. https://doi.org/10.1111/nmo.14118. PubMed PMID: 33720448; PMCID: PMC9380030
2. Romanoff E, Zhuo J, Huang AC, Amador D, Otaki F, Kamal AN, Kathpalia P, Leiman DA. Achalasia quality indicator adherence. Dig Dis Sci. 2023;68(2):389–95. https://doi.org/10.1007/s10620-022-07658-7. Epub 20221202. PubMed PMID: 36459295.
3. Vaezi MF, Pandolfino JE, Yadlapati RH, Greer KB, Kavitt RT. ACG clinical guidelines: diagnosis and management of Achalasia. J Am Coll Gastroenterol. 2020;115(9):1393.
4. Camilleri M, Kuo B, Nguyen L, Vaughn VM, Petrey J, Greer K, Yadlapati R, Abell TL. ACG clinical guideline: gastroparesis. J Am Coll Gastroenterol. 2022;117(8):1197–220. https://doi.org/10.14309/ajg.0000000000001874. PubMed PMID: 00000434-202208000-00015.
5. Lacy BE, Tack J, Gyawali CP. AGA clinical practice update on management of medically refractory gastroparesis: expert review. Clin Gastroenterol Hepatol. 2022;20(3):491–500. https://doi.org/10.1016/j.cgh.2021.10.038. PubMed PMID: 34757197. Epub 20211029.
6. Yadlapati R, Kahrilas PJ, Fox MR, Bredenoord AJ, Prakash Gyawali C, Roman S, Babaei A, Mittal RK, Rommel N, Savarino E, Sifrim D, Smout A, Vaezi MF, Zerbib F, Akiyama J, Bhatia S, Bor S, Carlson DA, Chen JW, Cisternas D, Cock C, Coss-Adame E, de Bortoli N, Defilippi C, Fass R, Ghoshal UC, Gonlachanvit S, Hani A, Hebbard GS, Wook Jung K, Katz P, Katzka DA, Khan A, Kohn GP, Lazarescu A, Lengliner J, Mittal SK, Omari T, Park MI, Penagini R, Pohl D, Richter JE, Serra J, Sweis R, Tack J, Tatum RP, Tutuian R, Vela MF, Wong RK, Wu JC, Xiao Y, Pandolfino JE. Esophageal motility disorders on high-resolution manometry: Chicago classification version 4.0(©). Neurogastroenterol Motil. 2021;33(1):e14058. https://doi.org/10.1111/nmo.14058. PubMed PMID: 33373111; PMCID: PMC8034247.
7. Singaram C, Sengupta A, Sweet MA, Sugarbaker DJ, Goyal RK. Nitrinergic and peptidergic innervation of the human oesophagus. Gut. 1994;35(12):1690–6. https://doi.org/10.1136/gut.35.12.1690. PubMed PMID: 7530228; PMCID: PMC1375254.
8. Carlson DA, Ravi K, Kahrilas PJ, Gyawali CP, Bredenoord AJ, Castell DO, Spechler SJ, Halland M, Kanuri N, Katzka DA, Leggett CL, Roman S, Saenz JB, Sayuk GS, Wong AC, Yadlapati R, Ciolino JD, Fox MR, Pandolfino JE. Diagnosis of esophageal motility disorders: esophageal pressure topography vs. conventional line tracing. Am J Gastroenterol. 2015;110(7):967–77; quiz 78. https://doi.org/10.1038/ajg.2015.159. PubMed PMID: 26032151; PMCID: PMC4587659. Epub 20150602.
9. Roman S, Huot L, Zerbib F, Bruley Des Varannes S, Gourcerol G, Coffin B, Ropert A, Roux A, Mion F. High-resolution manometry improves the diagnosis of esophageal motility disorders in patients with dysphagia: a randomized multicenter study. Am J Gastroenterol. 2016;111(3):372–80. https://doi.org/10.1038/ajg.2016.1. Epub 20160202. PubMed PMID: 26832656.

10. Pandolfino JE, Kwiatek MA, Nealis T, Bulsiewicz W, Post J, Kahrilas PJ. Achalasia: a new clinically relevant classification by high-resolution manometry. Gastroenterology. 2008;135(5):1526–33. https://doi.org/10.1053/j.gastro.2008.07.022. Epub 20080722. PubMed PMID: 18722376; PMCID: PMC2894987.
11. Andolfi C, Fisichella PM. Meta-analysis of clinical outcome after treatment for achalasia based on manometric subtypes. Br J Surg. 2019;106(4):332–41. https://doi.org/10.1002/bjs.11049. Epub 20190128. PubMed PMID: 30690706.
12. Pratap N, Kalapala R, Darisetty S, Joshi N, Ramchandani M, Banerjee R, Lakhtakia S, Gupta R, Tandan M, Rao GV, Reddy DN. Achalasia cardia subtyping by high-resolution manometry predicts the therapeutic outcome of pneumatic balloon dilatation. J Neurogastroenterol Motil. 2011;17(1):48–53. https://doi.org/10.5056/jnm.2011.17.1.48. Epub 20110126. PubMed PMID: 21369491; PMCID: PMC3042218.
13. Rohof WO, Salvador R, Annese V, Bruley Des Varannes S, Chaussade S, Costantini M, Elizalde JI, Gaudric M, Smout AJ, Tack J, Busch OR, Zaninotto G, Boeckxstaens GE. Outcomes of treatment for achalasia depend on manometric subtype. Gastroenterology. 2013;144(4):718–25; quiz e13–4. https://doi.org/10.1053/j.gastro.2012.12.027. Epub 20121228. PubMed PMID: 23277105.
14. Ou YH, Nie XM, Li LF, Wei ZJ, Jiang B. High-resolution manometric subtypes as a predictive factor for the treatment of achalasia: a meta-analysis and systematic review. J Dig Dis. 2016;17(4):222–35. https://doi.org/10.1111/1751-2980.12327. PubMed PMID: 26860986.
15. Hernandez JC, Ratuapli SK, Burdick GE, Dibaise JK, Crowell MD. Interrater and intrarater agreement of the chicago classification of achalasia subtypes using high-resolution esophageal manometry. Am J Gastroenterol. 2012;107(2):207–14. https://doi.org/10.1038/ajg.2011.353. Epub 20111018. PubMed PMID: 22008895.
16. Snyder DL, Crowell MD, Horsley-Silva J, Ravi K, Lacy BE, Vela MF. Opioid-induced esophageal dysfunction: differential effects of type and dose. Am J Gastroenterol. 2019;114(9):1464–9. https://doi.org/10.14309/ajg.0000000000000369. PubMed PMID: 31403963.
17. de Oliveira JM, Birgisson S, Doinoff C, Einstein D, Herts B, Davros W, Obuchowski N, Koehler RE, Richter J, Baker ME. Timed barium swallow: a simple technique for evaluating esophageal emptying in patients with achalasia. AJR Am J Roentgenol. 1997;169(2):473–9. https://doi.org/10.2214/ajr.169.2.9242756. PubMed PMID: 9242756.
18. Blonski W, Kumar A, Feldman J, Richter JE. Timed Barium swallow: diagnostic role and predictive value in untreated achalasia, esophagogastric junction outflow obstruction, and non-achalasia dysphagia. Am J Gastroenterol. 2018;113(2):196–203. https://doi.org/10.1038/ajg.2017.370. Epub 20171219. PubMed PMID: 29257145.
19. Sanagapalli S, Plumb A, Sweis R. Timed barium swallow: esophageal stasis varies markedly across subtypes of esophagogastric junction obstruction. Neurogastroenterol Motil. 2022;34(3):e14322. https://doi.org/10.1111/nmo.14322. Epub 20220124. PubMed PMID: 35072303
20. Carlson DA, Gyawali CP, Khan A, Yadlapati R, Chen J, Chokshi RV, Clarke JO, Garza JM, Jain AS, Katz P, Konda V, Lynch K, Schnoll-Sussman FH, Spechler SJ, Vela MF, Prescott JE, Baumann AJ, Donnan EN, Kou W, Kahrilas PJ, Pandolfino JE. Classifying esophageal motility by FLIP Panometry: a study of 722 subjects with manometry. Am J Gastroenterol. 2021;116(12):2357–66. https://doi.org/10.14309/ajg.0000000000001532. PubMed PMID: 34668487; PMCID: PMC8825704.
21. Moonen A, Annese V, Belmans A, Bredenoord AJ, Bruley Des Varannes S, Costantini M, Dousset B, Elizalde JI, Fumagalli U, Gaudric M, Merla A, Smout AJ, Tack J, Zaninotto G, Busch OR, Boeckxstaens GE. Long-term results of the European achalasia trial: a multicentre randomised controlled trial comparing pneumatic dilation versus laparoscopic Heller myotomy. Gut. 2016;65(5):732–9. https://doi.org/10.1136/gutjnl-2015-310602. Epub 20151127. PubMed PMID: 26614104.

22. Chrystoja CC, Darling GE, Diamant NE, Kortan PP, Tomlinson GA, Deitel W, Laporte A, Takata J, Urbach DR. Achalasia-specific quality of life after pneumatic dilation or laparoscopic heller myotomy with partial fundoplication: a multicenter, randomized clinical trial. Am J Gastroenterol. 2016;111(11):1536–45. https://doi.org/10.1038/ajg.2016.402. Epub 20160913. PubMed PMID: 27619832.
23. Sanaka MR, Hayat U, Thota PN, Jegadeesan R, Ray M, Gabbard SL, Wadhwa N, Lopez R, Baker ME, Murthy S, Raja S. Efficacy of peroral endoscopic myotomy vs other achalasia treatments in improving esophageal function. World J Gastroenterol. 2016;22(20):4918–25. https://doi.org/10.3748/wjg.v22.i20.4918. PubMed PMID: 27239118; PMCID: PMC4873884.
24. Boeckxstaens GE, Annese V, Des Varannes SB, Chaussade S, Costantini M, Cuttitta A, Elizalde JI, Fumagalli U, Gaudric M, Rohof WO, Smout AJ, Tack J, Zwinderman AH, Zaninotto G, Busch OR. Pneumatic dilation versus laparoscopic Heller's myotomy for idiopathic achalasia. N Engl J Med. 2011;364(19):1807–16. https://doi.org/10.1056/NEJMoa1010502. PubMed PMID: 21561346.
25. Werner YB, Hakanson B, Martinek J, Repici A, von Rahden BHA, Bredenoord AJ, Bisschops R, Messmann H, Vollberg MC, Noder T, Kersten JF, Mann O, Izbicki J, Pazdro A, Fumagalli U, Rosati R, Germer CT, Schijven MP, Emmermann A, von Renteln D, Fockens P, Boeckxstaens G, Rösch T. Endoscopic or surgical myotomy in patients with idiopathic achalasia. N Engl J Med. 2019;381(23):2219–29. https://doi.org/10.1056/NEJMoa1905380. PubMed PMID: 31800987.
26. Schlottmann F, Luckett DJ, Fine J, Shaheen NJ, Patti MG. Laparoscopic Heller myotomy versus peroral endoscopic myotomy (POEM) for achalasia: a systematic review and meta-analysis. Ann Surg. 2018;267(3):451–60. https://doi.org/10.1097/sla.0000000000002311. PubMed PMID: 28549006.
27. Vela MF, Richter JE, Khandwala F, Blackstone EH, Wachsberger D, Baker ME, Rice TW. The long-term efficacy of pneumatic dilatation and Heller myotomy for the treatment of achalasia. Clin Gastroenterol Hepatol. 2006;4(5):580–7. https://doi.org/10.1016/s1542-3565(05)00986-9. PubMed PMID: 16630776.
28. Eckardt VF, Kanzler G, Westermeier T. Complications and their impact after pneumatic dilation for achalasia: prospective long-term follow-up study. Gastrointest Endosc. 1997;45(5):349–53. https://doi.org/10.1016/s0016-5107(97)70142-1. PubMed PMID: 9165313.
29. Zori AG, Kirtane TS, Gupte AR, Chauhan SS, Draganov PV, Forsmark CE, Wagh MS. Utility of clinical suspicion and endoscopic re-examination for detection of esophagogastric perforation after pneumatic dilation for achalasia. Endoscopy. 2016;48(2):128–33. https://doi.org/10.1055/s-0034-1392860. Epub 20150921. PubMed PMID: 26394248.
30. Campos GM, Vittinghoff E, Rabl C, Takata M, Gadenstätter M, Lin F, Ciovica R. Endoscopic and surgical treatments for achalasia: a systematic review and meta-analysis. Ann Surg. 2009;249(1):45–57. https://doi.org/10.1097/SLA.0b013e31818e43ab. PubMed PMID: 19106675.
31. Kurian AA, Bhayani N, Sharata A, Reavis K, Dunst CM, Swanström LL. Partial anterior vs partial posterior fundoplication following transabdominal esophagocardiomyotomy for achalasia of the esophagus: meta-regression of objective postoperative gastroesophageal reflux and dysphagia. JAMA Surg. 2013;148(1):85–90. https://doi.org/10.1001/jamasurgery.2013.409. PubMed PMID: 23324843.
32. Siddaiah-Subramanya M, Yunus RM, Khan S, Memon B, Memon MA. Anterior dor or posterior Toupet with Heller Myotomy for achalasia cardia: a systematic review and meta-analysis. World J Surg. 2019;43(6):1563–70. https://doi.org/10.1007/s00268-019-04945-9. PubMed PMID: 30756164.
33. Inoue H, Minami H, Kobayashi Y, Sato Y, Kaga M, Suzuki M, Satodate H, Odaka N, Itoh H, Kudo S. Peroral endoscopic myotomy (POEM) for esophageal achalasia. Endoscopy. 2010;42(4):265–71. https://doi.org/10.1055/s-0029-1244080. Epub 20100330. PubMed PMID: 20354937.

34. Evensen H, Kristensen V, Larssen L, Sandstad O, Hauge T, Medhus AW. Outcome of peroral endoscopic myotomy (POEM) in treatment-naive patients. A systematic review. Scand J Gastroenterol. 2019;54(1):1–7. https://doi.org/10.1080/00365521.2018.1549271. Epub 20190116. PubMed PMID: 30650313.
35. Swanström LL, Rieder E, Dunst CM. A stepwise approach and early clinical experience in peroral endoscopic myotomy for the treatment of achalasia and esophageal motility disorders. J Am Coll Surg. 2011;213(6):751–6. Epub 20111013. PubMed PMID: 21996484. https://doi.org/10.1016/j.jamcollsurg.2011.09.001.
36. Rassoul Abu-Nuwar M, Eriksson SE, Sarici IS, Zheng P, Hoppo T, Jobe BA, Ayazi S. GERD after peroral endoscopic myotomy: assessment of incidence and predisposing factors. J Am Coll Surg. 2023;236(1):58.
37. Kumbhari V, Familiari P, Bjerregaard NC, Pioche M, Jones E, Ko WJ, Hayee B, Cali A, Ngamruengphong S, Mion F, Hernaez R, Roman S, Tieu AH, El Zein M, Ajayi T, Haji A, Cho JY, Hazey J, Perry KA, Ponchon T, Kunda R, Costamagna G, Khashab MA. Gastroesophageal reflux after peroral endoscopic myotomy: a multicenter case-control study. Endoscopy. 2017;49(7):634–42. https://doi.org/10.1055/s-0043-105485. Epub 20170504. PubMed PMID: 28472834.
38. Repici A, Fuccio L, Maselli R, Mazza F, Correale L, Mandolesi D, Bellisario C, Sethi A, Khashab MA, Rösch T, Hassan C. GERD after per-oral endoscopic myotomy as compared with Heller's myotomy with fundoplication: a systematic review with meta-analysis. Gastrointest Endosc. 2018;87(4):934–43.e18. https://doi.org/10.1016/j.gie.2017.10.022. Epub 20171102. PubMed PMID: 29102729.
39. Nabi Z, Ramchandani M, Kotla R, Tandan M, Goud R, Darisetty S, Rao GV, Reddy DN. Gastroesophageal reflux disease after peroral endoscopic myotomy is unpredictable, but responsive to proton pump inhibitor therapy: a large, single-center study. Endoscopy. 2020;52(8):643–51. https://doi.org/10.1055/a-1133-4354. Epub 20200324. PubMed PMID: 32208499.
40. Ponds FA, Fockens P, Lei A, Neuhaus H, Beyna T, Kandler J, Frieling T, Chiu PWY, Wu JCY, Wong VWY, Costamagna G, Familiari P, Kahrilas PJ, Pandolfino JE, Smout A, Bredenoord AJ. Effect of peroral endoscopic myotomy vs pneumatic dilation on symptom severity and treatment outcomes among treatment-naive patients with achalasia: a randomized clinical trial. JAMA. 2019;322(2):134–44. https://doi.org/10.1001/jama.2019.8859. PubMed PMID: 31287522; PMCID: PMC6618792.
41. Nabi Z, Karyampudi A, Ramchandani M, Chavan R, Basha J, Inavolu P, Darisetty S, Goud R, Reddy DN. Predictors of long-term outcomes, recurrent dysphagia, and gastroesophageal reflux after per-oral endoscopic myotomy in esophageal motility disorders. J Gastrointest Surg. 2022;26(7):1352–61. https://doi.org/10.1007/s11605-022-05330-z. Epub 20220426. PubMed PMID: 35474561.
42. Teh JL, Tham HY, Soh AYS, Chee C, Kim G, Shabbir A, Wong RKM, So JBY. Gastroesophageal reflux disease (GERD) after peroral endoscopic myotomy (POEM). Surg Endosc. 2022;36(5):3308–16. https://doi.org/10.1007/s00464-021-08644-2. Epub 20210729. PubMed PMID: 34327547.
43. Smith CD, Stival A, Howell DL, Swafford V. Endoscopic therapy for achalasia before Heller myotomy results in worse outcomes than heller myotomy alone. Ann Surg. 2006;243(5):579–84; discussion 84–6. https://doi.org/10.1097/01.sla.0000217524.75529.2d. PubMed PMID: 16632991; PMCID: PMC1570551.
44. Patti MG, Feo CV, Arcerito M, De Pinto M, Tamburini A, Diener U, Gantert W, Way LW. Effects of previous treatment on results of laparoscopic Heller myotomy for achalasia. Dig Dis Sci. 1999;44(11):2270–6. https://doi.org/10.1023/a:1026660921776. PubMed PMID: 10573373.
45. Orenstein SB, Raigani S, Wu YV, Pauli EM, Phillips MS, Ponsky JL, Marks JM. Peroral endoscopic myotomy (POEM) leads to similar results in patients with and without prior

endoscopic or surgical therapy. Surg Endosc. 2015;29(5):1064–70. https://doi.org/10.1007/s00464-014-3782-5. Epub 20140924. PubMed PMID: 25249143.
46. Jones EL, Meara MP, Pittman MR, Hazey JW, Perry KA. Prior treatment does not influence the performance or early outcome of per-oral endoscopic myotomy for achalasia. Surg Endosc. 2016;30(4):1282–6. https://doi.org/10.1007/s00464-015-4339-y. Epub 20150627. PubMed PMID: 26123336.
47. Taft TH, Carlson DA, Triggs J, Craft J, Starkey K, Yadlapati R, Gregory D, Pandolfino JE. Evaluating the reliability and construct validity of the Eckardt symptom score as a measure of achalasia severity. Neurogastroenterol Motil. 2018;30(6):e13287. https://doi.org/10.1111/nmo.13287. Epub 20180108. PubMed PMID: 29315993; PMCID: PMC5992017.
48. Vaezi MF, Baker ME, Achkar E, Richter JE. Timed barium oesophagram: better predictor of long term success after pneumatic dilation in achalasia than symptom assessment. Gut. 2002;50(6):765–70. https://doi.org/10.1136/gut.50.6.765. PubMed PMID: 12010876; PMCID: PMC1773230.
49. Vaezi MF, Baker ME, Richter JE. Assessment of esophageal emptying post-pneumatic dilation: use of the timed barium esophagram. Am J Gastroenterol. 1999;94(7):1802–7. https://doi.org/10.1111/j.1572-0241.1999.01209.x. PubMed PMID: 10406238.
50. Nicodème F, de Ruigh A, Xiao Y, Rajeswaran S, Teitelbaum EN, Hungness ES, Kahrilas PJ, Pandolfino JE. A comparison of symptom severity and bolus retention with Chicago classification esophageal pressure topography metrics in patients with achalasia. Clin Gastroenterol Hepatol. 2013;11(2):131–7; quiz e15. https://doi.org/10.1016/j.cgh.2012.10.015. Epub 20121016. PubMed PMID: 23078890; PMCID: PMC3552153.
51. Ngamruengphong S, von Rahden BHA, Filser J, Tyberg A, Desai A, Sharaiha RZ, Lambroza A, Kumbhari V, El Zein M, Abdelgelil A, Besharati S, Clarke JO, Stein EM, Kalloo AN, Kahaleh M, Khashab MA. Intraoperative measurement of esophagogastric junction cross-sectional area by impedance planimetry correlates with clinical outcomes of peroral endoscopic myotomy for achalasia: a multicenter study. Surg Endosc. 2016;30(7):2886–94. https://doi.org/10.1007/s00464-015-4574-2.
52. Teitelbaum EN, Soper NJ, Pandolfino JE, Kahrilas PJ, Hirano I, Boris L, Nicodème F, Lin Z, Hungness ES. Esophagogastric junction distensibility measurements during Heller myotomy and POEM for achalasia predict postoperative symptomatic outcomes. Surg Endosc. 2015;29(3):522–8. https://doi.org/10.1007/s00464-014-3733-1.
53. Su B, Callahan ZM, Novak S, Kuchta K, Ujiki MB. Using Impedance planimetry (EndoFLIP) to evaluate myotomy and predict outcomes after surgery for Achalasia. J Gastrointest Surg. 2020;24(4):964–71. https://doi.org/10.1007/s11605-020-04513-w. Epub 20200114. PubMed PMID: 31939098.
54. Attaar M, Wong HJ, Wu H, Campbell M, Kuchta K, Denham W, Haggerty S, Linn J, Ujiki MB. Changes in impedance planimetry (EndoFLIP) measurements at follow-up after peroral endoscopic myotomy (POEM). Surg Endosc. 2022;36(12):9410–5. https://doi.org/10.1007/s00464-022-09286-8. Epub 20220503. PubMed PMID: 35505258.
55. Bredenoord AJ, Babaei A, Carlson D, Omari T, Akiyama J, Yadlapati R, Pandolfino JE, Richter J, Fass R. Esophagogastric junction outflow obstruction. Neurogastroenterol Motil. 2021;33(9):e14193. https://doi.org/10.1111/nmo.14193. Epub 20210612 PubMed PMID: 34120375
56. Clayton SB, Patel R, Richter JE. Functional and anatomic esophagogastric junction outflow obstruction: manometry, timed Barium esophagram findings, and treatment outcomes. Clin Gastroenterol Hepatol. 2016;14(6):907–11. https://doi.org/10.1016/j.cgh.2015.12.041. Epub 20160112. PubMed PMID: 26792374.
57. Carlson DA, Schauer JM, Kou W, Kahrilas PJ, Pandolfino JE. Functional lumen imaging probe panometry helps identify clinically relevant esophagogastric junction outflow obstruction per Chicago classification v4.0. Am J Gastroenterol. 2023;118(1):77–86. https://doi.org/10.14309/ajg.0000000000001980. Epub 20220823. PubMed PMID: 36002925; PMCID: PMC9822847.

58. Zikos TA, Triadafilopoulos G, Clarke JO. Esophagogastric junction outflow obstruction: current approach to diagnosis and management. Curr Gastroenterol Rep. 2020;22(2):9. https://doi.org/10.1007/s11894-020-0743-0. Epub 20200205. PubMed PMID: 32020310.
59. Visaggi P, Ghisa M, Del Corso G, Baiano Svizzero F, Mariani L, Tolone S, Frazzoni M, Buda A, Bellini M, Savarino V, Penagini R, Gyawali CP, Savarino EV, de Bortoli N. Chicago classification v4.0 protocol improves specificity and accuracy of diagnosis of oesophagogastric junction outflow obstruction. Aliment Pharmacol Ther. 2022;56(4):606–13. https://doi.org/10.1111/apt.17101. Epub 20220625. PubMed PMID: 35751633; PMCID: PMC9544646.
60. Sanchez MJ, Olivier S, Gedeklioglu F, Almeida M, Gaeta M, Nigro M, de la Rosa R, Nguyen M, Lalehzari M, Regala F, Njei B, Deng Y, Ciarleglio M, Masoud A. Chronic opioid use is associated with obstructive and spastic disorders in the esophagus. Neurogastroenterol Motil. 2022;34(3):e14233. https://doi.org/10.1111/nmo.14233. Epub 20210916. PubMed PMID: 34532898.
61. Beveridge CA, Triggs JR, Thanawala SU, Ahuja NK, Falk GW, Benitez AJ, Lynch KL. Can FLIP guide therapy in idiopathic esophagogastric junction outflow obstruction? Dis Esophagus. 2022;35(4):doab077. https://doi.org/10.1093/dote/doab077. PubMed PMID: 34864928; PMCID: PMC9016893.
62. DeLay K, Austin GL, Menard-Katcher P. Anatomic abnormalities are common potential explanations of manometric esophagogastric junction outflow obstruction. Neurogastroenterol Motil. 2016;28(8):1166–71. Epub 20160306. PubMed PMID: 26948429. https://doi.org/10.1111/nmo.12814.
63. Okeke FC, Raja S, Lynch KL, Dhalla S, Nandwani M, Stein EM, Chander Roland B, Khashab MA, Saxena P, Kumbhari V, Ahuja NK, Clarke JO. What is the clinical significance of esophagogastric junction outflow obstruction? Evaluation of 60 patients at a tertiary referral center. Neurogastroenterol Motil. 2017;29(6):e13061. https://doi.org/10.1111/nmo.13061. PubMed PMID: 28393437.
64. Liu A, Woo M, Nasser Y, Gupta M, Buresi MC, Curley M, Li DY, Wilsack L, Andrews CN. Esophagogastric junction outflow obstruction on manometry: outcomes and lack of benefit from CT and EUS. Neurogastroenterol Motil. 2019;31(12):e13712. https://doi.org/10.1111/nmo.13712. Epub 20190915. PubMed PMID: 31523911.
65. Sanagapalli S, McGuire J, Leong RW, Patel K, Raeburn A, Abdul-Razakq H, Plumb A, Banks M, Haidry R, Lovat L, Sehgal V, Graham D, Sami SS, Sweis R. The clinical relevance of manometric esophagogastric junction outflow obstruction can be determined using rapid drink challenge and solid swallows. Am J Gastroenterol. 2021;116(2):280–8. https://doi.org/10.14309/ajg.0000000000000988. PubMed PMID: 33136563
66. Schupack D, Katzka DA, Geno DM, Ravi K. The clinical significance of esophagogastric junction outflow obstruction and hypercontractile esophagus in high resolution esophageal manometry. Neurogastroenterol Motil. 2017;29(10):1–9. https://doi.org/10.1111/nmo.13105. Epub 20170523. PubMed PMID: 28544670.
67. Pérez-Fernández MT, Santander C, Marinero A, Burgos-Santamaría D, Chavarría-Herbozo C. Characterization and follow-up of esophagogastric junction outflow obstruction detected by high resolution manometry. Neurogastroenterol Motil. 2016;28(1):116–26. https://doi.org/10.1111/nmo.12708. Epub 20151030. PubMed PMID: 26517978.
68. Chen S, Liang M, Tan N, Zhang M, Lin Y, Cao P, Zhuang Q, Xiao Y. Upright integrated relaxation pressure predicts symptom outcome for esophagogastric junction outflow obstruction. J Neurogastroenterol Motil. 2021;27(3):363–9. https://doi.org/10.5056/jnm20106. PubMed PMID: 34210901; PMCID: PMC8266504.
69. Shahsavari D, Malik Z, Parkman HP. Management of the patient with esophagogastric junction outflow obstruction. Curr Opin Gastroenterol. 2021;37(4):397–407. https://doi.org/10.1097/mog.0000000000000747. PubMed PMID: 34059606.
70. Garbarino S, von Isenburg M, Fisher DA, Leiman DA. Management of functional esophagogastric junction outflow obstruction: a systematic review. J Clin Gastroenterol.

2020;54(1):35–42. https://doi.org/10.1097/mcg.0000000000001156. PubMed PMID: 30575636.
71. Porter RF, Gyawali CP. Botulinum toxin injection in dysphagia syndromes with preserved esophageal peristalsis and incomplete lower esophageal sphincter relaxation. Neurogastroenterol Motil. 2011;23(2):139–44, e27–8. https://doi.org/10.1111/j.1365-2982.2010.01604.x. Epub 20101001. PubMed PMID: 20939855.
72. Ribolsi M, Ghisa M, Savarino E. Nonachalasic esophageal motor disorders, from diagnosis to therapy. Expert Rev Gastroenterol Hepatol. 2022;16(3):205–16. Epub 20220302. PubMed PMID: 35220870. https://doi.org/10.1080/17474124.2022.2047648.
73. Behar J, Biancani P. Pathogenesis of simultaneous esophageal contractions in patients with motility disorders. Gastroenterology. 1993;105(1):111–8. https://doi.org/10.1016/0016-5085(93)90016-6. PubMed PMID: 8099885.
74. Roman S, Hebbard G, Jung KW, Katz P, Tutuian R, Wong R, Wu J, Yadlapati R, Sifrim D. Chicago classification update (v4.0): technical review on diagnostic criteria for distal esophageal spasm. Neurogastroenterol Motil. 2021;33(5):e14119. https://doi.org/10.1111/nmo.14119. Epub 20210305. PubMed PMID: 33666299.
75. Carlson DA, Baumann AJ, Prescott JE, Donnan EN, Yadlapati R, Khan A, Gyawali CP, Kou W, Kahrilas PJ, Pandolfino JE. Validation of secondary peristalsis classification using FLIP panometry in 741 subjects undergoing manometry. Neurogastroenterol Motil. 2022;34(1):e14192. https://doi.org/10.1111/nmo.14192. Epub 20210613. PubMed PMID: 34120383; PMCID: PMC8666463.
76. Khatami SS, Khandwala F, Shay SS, Vaezi MF. Does diffuse esophageal spasm progress to achalasia? A prospective cohort study. Dig Dis Sci. 2005;50(9):1605–10. https://doi.org/10.1007/s10620-005-2903-3.
77. Fontes LHS, Herbella FAM, Rodriguez TN, Trivino T, Farah JFM. Progression of diffuse esophageal spasm to achalasia: incidence and predictive factors. Dis Esophagus. 2013;26(5):470–4. https://doi.org/10.1111/j.1442-2050.2012.01377.x.
78. Roman S, Kahrilas PJ. Management of spastic disorders of the esophagus. Gastroenterol Clin North Am. 2013;42(1):27–43. Epub 20130104. PubMed PMID: 23452629; PMCID: PMC3618975. https://doi.org/10.1016/j.gtc.2012.11.002.
79. Vanuytsel T, Bisschops R, Farré R, Pauwels A, Holvoet L, Arts J, Caenepeel P, De Wulf D, Mimidis K, Rommel N, Tack J. Botulinum toxin reduces Dysphagia in patients with nonachalasia primary esophageal motility disorders. Clin Gastroenterol Hepatol. 2013;11(9):1115–21.e2. Epub 20130413. PubMed PMID: 23591282. https://doi.org/10.1016/j.cgh.2013.03.021.
80. Khashab MA, Messallam AA, Onimaru M, Teitelbaum EN, Ujiki MB, Gitelis ME, Modayil RJ, Hungness ES, Stavropoulos SN, El Zein MH, Shiwaku H, Kunda R, Repici A, Minami H, Chiu PW, Ponsky J, Kumbhari V, Saxena P, Maydeo AP, Inoue H. International multicenter experience with peroral endoscopic myotomy for the treatment of spastic esophageal disorders refractory to medical therapy (with video). Gastrointest Endosc. 2015;81(5):1170–7. https://doi.org/10.1016/j.gie.2014.10.011. Epub 20150126. PubMed PMID: 25634487.
81. Khashab MA, Familiari P, Draganov PV, Aridi HD, Cho JY, Ujiki M, Rio Tinto R, Louis H, Desai PN, Velanovich V, Albéniz E, Haji A, Marks J, Costamagna G, Devière J, Perbtani Y, Hedberg M, Estremera F, Martin Del Campo LA, Yang D, Bukhari M, Brewer O, Sanaei O, Fayad L, Agarwal A, Kumbhari V, Chen YI. Peroral endoscopic myotomy is effective and safe in non-achalasia esophageal motility disorders: an international multicenter study. Endosc Int Open. 2018;6(8):E1031–e6. https://doi.org/10.1055/a-0625-6288. Epub 20180810. PubMed PMID: 30105290; PMCID: PMC6086680.
82. Khan MA, Kumbhari V, Ngamruengphong S, Ismail A, Chen YI, Chavez YH, Bukhari M, Nollan R, Ismail MK, Onimaru M, Balassone V, Sharata A, Swanstrom L, Inoue H, Repici A, Khashab MA. Is POEM the answer for management of spastic esophageal disorders? A systematic review and meta-analysis. Dig Dis Sci. 2017;62(1):35–44. https://doi.org/10.1007/s10620-016-4373-1. Epub 20161117. PubMed PMID: 27858325.

83. Almansa C, Hinder RA, Smith CD, Achem SR. A comprehensive appraisal of the surgical treatment of diffuse esophageal spasm. J Gastrointest Surg. 2008;12(6):1133–45. https://doi.org/10.1007/s11605-007-0439-x. Epub 20071211. PubMed PMID: 18071832.
84. Chen JW, Savarino E, Smout A, Xiao Y, de Bortoli N, Yadlapati R, Cock C. Chicago classification update (v4.0): technical review on diagnostic criteria for hypercontractile esophagus. Neurogastroenterol Motil. 2021;33(6):e14115. https://doi.org/10.1111/nmo.14115. Epub 20210317. PubMed PMID: 33729642
85. Achem SR, Vazquez-Elizondo G, Fass R. Jackhammer esophagus: current concepts and dilemmas. J Clin Gastroenterol. 2021;55(5):369–79. https://doi.org/10.1097/mcg.0000000000001472. PubMed PMID: 33337637.
86. Mallet AL, Ropert A, Bouguen G, Siproudhis L, Boutroux D, Bretagne JF, Brochard C. Prevalence and characteristics of acid gastro-oesophageal reflux disease in jackhammer oesophagus. Dig Liver Dis. 2016;48(10):1136–41. https://doi.org/10.1016/j.dld.2016.06.030. Epub 20160709. PubMed PMID: 27453169.
87. Popescu AL, Costache RS, Costache DO, Balaban VD, Jinga M, Ionita-Radu F, Caruntu A, Fierbinteanu-Braticevici C. Manometric changes of the esophagus in morbidly obese patients. Exp Ther Med. 2021;21(6):604. https://doi.org/10.3892/etm.2021.10036. PubMed PMID: 33936261; PMCID: PMC8082643.
88. Kahn A, Al-Qaisi MT, Obeid RA, Katzka DA, Ravi KM, Ramirez FC, Crowell MD, Vela MF. Clinical features and long-term outcomes of lower esophageal sphincter-dependent and lower esophageal sphincter-independent jackhammer esophagus. Neurogastroenterol Motil. 2019;31(2):e13507. https://doi.org/10.1111/nmo.13507. Epub 20181115. PubMed PMID: 30443964.
89. de Bortoli N, Gyawali PC, Roman S, Tolone S, Sifrim D, Tutuian R, Penagini R, Pandolfino JE, Savarino EV. Hypercontractile esophagus from pathophysiology to management: proceedings of the Pisa symposium. Am J Gastroenterol. 2021;116(2):263–73. https://doi.org/10.14309/ajg.0000000000001061. PubMed PMID: 33273259.
90. Philonenko S, Roman S, Zerbib F, Gourcerol G, Gault N, Ropert A, Bruley Des Varannes S, Barret M, Vitton V, Bouchoucha M, Billard N, Gorbatchef C, Duboc H, Coffin B. Jackhammer esophagus: clinical presentation, manometric diagnosis, and therapeutic results-results from a multicenter French cohort. Neurogastroenterol Motil. 2020;32(11):e13918. https://doi.org/10.1111/nmo.13918. Epub 20200608. PubMed PMID: 32510747
91. Mion F, Marjoux S, Subtil F, Pioche M, Rivory J, Roman S, Zerbib F. Botulinum toxin for the treatment of hypercontractile esophagus: results of a double-blind randomized sham-controlled study. Neurogastroenterol Motil. 2019;31(5):e13587. https://doi.org/10.1111/nmo.13587. Epub 20190411. PubMed PMID: 30974039
92. Gyawali CP, Zerbib F, Bhatia S, Cisternas D, Coss-Adame E, Lazarescu A, Pohl D, Yadlapati R, Penagini R, Pandolfino J. Chicago classification update (V4.0): technical review on diagnostic criteria for ineffective esophageal motility and absent contractility. Neurogastroenterol Motil. 2021;33(8):e14134. https://doi.org/10.1111/nmo.14134. Epub 20210326. PubMed PMID: 33768698
93. Dao HV, Hoang LB, Luu HTM, Nguyen HL, Goldberg RJ, Allison J, Dao ATM, Van Nguyen HT, Matsumura T, Van Dao L. Clinical symptoms, endoscopic findings, and lower esophageal sphincter characteristics in patients with absent contractility. Medicine (Baltimore). 2022;101(43):e31428. https://doi.org/10.1097/md.0000000000031428. PubMed PMID: 36316894; PMCID: PMC9622690.
94. Kovacs B, Masuda T, Bremner RM, Mittal SK. Clinical spectrum and presentation of patients with absent contractility. Ann Gastroenterol. 2021;34(3):331–6. https://doi.org/10.20524/aog.2021.0583. Epub 20210125. PubMed PMID: 33948057; PMCID: PMC8079877.
95. Qureshi A, Jehangir A, Malik Z, Parkman HP. Rheumatologic disorders in patients undergoing esophageal manometry: prevalence, symptom characteristics, and manometric findings. Dis Esophagus. 2021;34(8):doaa135. https://doi.org/10.1093/dote/doaa135. PubMed PMID: 33558877.

96. Chan WW, Haroian LR, Gyawali CP. Value of preoperative esophageal function studies before laparoscopic antireflux surgery. Surg Endosc. 2011;25(9):2943–9. Epub 20110318. PubMed PMID: 21424193. https://doi.org/10.1007/s00464-011-1646-9.
97. Carlson DA, Crowell MD, Kimmel JN, Patel A, Gyawali CP, Hinchcliff M, Griffing WL, Pandolfino JE, Vela MF. Loss of peristaltic reserve, determined by multiple rapid swallows, is the most frequent esophageal motility abnormality in patients with systemic sclerosis. Clin Gastroenterol Hepatol. 2016;14(10):1502–6. https://doi.org/10.1016/j.cgh.2016.03.039. Epub 20160405. PubMed PMID: 27062902; PMCID: PMC5028229.
98. Carlson DA, Prescott JE, Germond E, Brenner D, Carns M, Correia CS, Tetreault MP, McMahan ZH, Hinchcliff M, Kou W, Kahrilas PJ, Perlman HR, Pandolfino JE. Heterogeneity of primary and secondary peristalsis in systemic sclerosis: a new model of "scleroderma esophagus". Neurogastroenterol Motil. 2022;34(7):e14284. https://doi.org/10.1111/nmo.14284. Epub 20211028. PubMed PMID: 34709690; PMCID: PMC9046463.
99. Sjogren RW. Gastrointestinal motility disorders in scleroderma. Arthritis Rheum. 1994;37(9):1265–82. https://doi.org/10.1002/art.1780370902. PubMed PMID: 7945489.
100. Rengarajan A, Rogers BD, Wong Z, Tolone S, Sifrim D, Serra J, Savarino E, Roman S, Remes-Troche JM, Ramos R, Perez De La Serna J, Pauwels A, Leguizamo AM, Lee YY, Kawamura O, Hayat J, Hani A, Gonlachanvit S, Cisternas D, Carlson D, Bor S, Bhatia S, Abrahao L, Pandolfino J, Gyawali CP. High-resolution manometry thresholds and motor patterns among asymptomatic individuals. Clin Gastroenterol Hepatol. 2022;20(3):e398–406. https://doi.org/10.1016/j.cgh.2020.10.052. Epub 20201102. PubMed PMID: 33144149.
101. Quader F, Rogers B, Sievers T, Mumtaz S, Lee M, Lu T, Gyawali CP. Contraction reserve with ineffective esophageal motility on esophageal high-resolution manometry is associated with lower acid exposure times compared with absent contraction reserve. Am J Gastroenterol. 2020;115(12):1981–8. https://doi.org/10.14309/ajg.0000000000000811. PubMed PMID: 32826576.
102. Aggarwal N, Thota PN, Lopez R, Gabbard S. A randomized double-blind placebo-controlled crossover-style trial of buspirone in functional dysphagia and ineffective esophageal motility. Neurogastroenterol Motil. 2018;30(2):1. https://doi.org/10.1111/nmo.13213. Epub 20170908. PubMed PMID: 28884884
103. Tran S, Gray R, Kholmurodova F, Thompson SK, Myers JC, Bright T, Irvine T, Watson DI. Laparoscopic fundoplication is effective treatment for patients with gastroesophageal reflux and absent esophageal contractility. J Gastrointest Surg. 2021;25(9):2192–200. https://doi.org/10.1007/s11605-021-05006-0. Epub 20210426. PubMed PMID: 33904061; PMCID: PMC8484087.
104. Watson DI, Jamieson GG, Bessell JR, Devitt PG. Laparoscopic fundoplication in patients with an aperistaltic esophagus and gastroesophageal reflux. Dis Esophagus. 2006;19(2):94–8. https://doi.org/10.1111/j.1442-2050.2006.00547.x. PubMed PMID: 16643177.
105. Nikolic M, Schwameis K, Kristo I, Paireder M, Matic A, Semmler G, Semmler L, Schoppmann SF. Ineffective esophageal motility in patients with GERD is no contraindication for Nissen fundoplication. World J Surg. 2020;44(1):186–93. https://doi.org/10.1007/s00268-019-05229-y. PubMed PMID: 31605176.
106. Tuan AW, Syed N, Panganiban RP, Lee RY, Dalessio S, Pradhan S, Zhu J, Ouyang A. Comparing patients diagnosed with ineffective esophageal motility by the Chicago classification version 3.0 and version 4.0 criteria. Gastroenterology Res. 2023;16(1):37–49. https://doi.org/10.14740/gr1563. Epub 20230228. PubMed PMID: 36895699; PMCID: PMC9990528.
107. Kurin M, Adil SA, Damjanovska S, Tanner S, Greer K. Clinical characteristics of patients with ineffective esophageal motility by Chicago classification version 4.0 compared to Chicago classification version 3.0. J Neurogastroenterol Motil. 2023;29(1):38–48. https://doi.org/10.5056/jnm21250. PubMed PMID: 36606435; PMCID: PMC9837536.
108. Boland K, Abdul-Hussein M, Tutuian R, Castell DO. Characteristics of consecutive esophageal motility diagnoses after a decade of change. J Clin Gastroenterol. 2016;50(4):301–6. https://doi.org/10.1097/mcg.0000000000000402. PubMed PMID: 26422715.

109. Kahrilas PJ, Bredenoord AJ, Fox M, Gyawali CP, Roman S, Smout AJ, Pandolfino JE. The Chicago Classification of esophageal motility disorders, v3.0. Neurogastroenterol Motil. 2015;27(2):160–74. Epub 20141203. PubMed PMID: 25469569; PMCID: PMC4308501. https://doi.org/10.1111/nmo.12477.
110. Rogers BD, Rengarajan A, Mauro A, Ghisa M, De Bortoli N, Cicala M, Ribolsi M, Penagini R, Savarino E, Gyawali CP. Fragmented and failed swallows on esophageal high-resolution manometry associate with abnormal reflux burden better than weak swallows. Neurogastroenterol Motil. 2020;32(2):e13736. https://doi.org/10.1111/nmo.13736. Epub 20191001. PubMed PMID: 31574208.
111. Gyawali CP, Sifrim D, Carlson DA, Hawn M, Katzka DA, Pandolfino JE, Penagini R, Roman S, Savarino E, Tatum R, Vaezi M, Clarke JO, Triadafilopoulos G. Ineffective esophageal motility: concepts, future directions, and conclusions from the Stanford 2018 symposium. Neurogastroenterol Motil. 2019;31(9):e13584. https://doi.org/10.1111/nmo.13584. Epub 20190411. PubMed PMID: 30974032; PMCID: PMC9380027
112. Shaker A, Stoikes N, Drapekin J, Kushnir V, Brunt LM, Gyawali CP. Multiple rapid swallow responses during esophageal high-resolution manometry reflect esophageal body peristaltic reserve. Am J Gastroenterol. 2013;108(11):1706–12. https://doi.org/10.1038/ajg.2013.289. PubMed PMID: 24019081; PMCID: PMC4091619.
113. Booth M, Stratford J, Dehn TC. Preoperative esophageal body motility does not influence the outcome of laparoscopic Nissen fundoplication for gastroesophageal reflux disease. Dis Esophagus. 2002;15(1):57–60. https://doi.org/10.1046/j.1442-2050.2002.00229.x. PubMed PMID: 12060044.
114. Rydberg L, Ruth M, Abrahamsson H, Lundell L. Tailoring antireflux surgery: a randomized clinical trial. World J Surg. 1999;23(6):612–8. https://doi.org/10.1007/pl00012356. PubMed PMID: 10227933.
115. Fibbe C, Layer P, Keller J, Strate U, Emmermann A, Zornig C. Esophageal motility in reflux disease before and after fundoplication: a prospective, randomized, clinical, and manometric study. Gastroenterology. 2001;121(1):5–14. https://doi.org/10.1053/gast.2001.25486. PubMed PMID: 11438489.
116. Addo A, George P, Zahiri HR, Park A. Patients with ineffective esophageal motility benefit from laparoscopic antireflux surgery. Surg Endosc. 2021;35(8):4459–68. https://doi.org/10.1007/s00464-020-07951-4. PubMed PMID: 32959180.
117. Ma Y, Cai R, Liu Z, Zou X, Qiao Z. Clinical efficacy and mechanism of transcutaneous neuromodulation on ineffective esophageal motility in patients with gastroesophageal reflux disease. Neurogastroenterol Motil. 2023;35(3):e14464. https://doi.org/10.1111/nmo.14464. Epub 20221018. PubMed PMID: 36256502
118. Patel DA, Yadlapati R, Vaezi MF. Esophageal motility disorders: current approach to diagnostics and therapeutics. Gastroenterology. 2022;162(6):1617–34. https://doi.org/10.1053/j.gastro.2021.12.289. PubMed PMID: 35227779; PMCID: PMC9405585.
119. Drossman DA. Functional gastrointestinal disorders: history, pathophysiology, clinical features and Rome IV. Gastroenterology. 2016;S0016–5085:00223–7. https://doi.org/10.1053/j.gastro.2016.02.032. PubMed PMID: 27144617.
120. Aziz Q, Fass R, Gyawali CP, Miwa H, Pandolfino JE, Zerbib F. Functional esophageal disorders. Gastroenterology. 2016;S0016-5085(16):00178–5. https://doi.org/10.1053/j.gastro.2016.02.012. PubMed PMID: 27144625.
121. Camilleri M, Chedid V, Ford AC, Haruma K, Horowitz M, Jones KL, Low PA, Park SY, Parkman HP, Stanghellini V. Gastroparesis. Nat Rev Dis Primers. 2018;4(1):41. https://doi.org/10.1038/s41572-018-0038-z. Epub 20181101. PubMed PMID: 30385743
122. Dilmaghani S, Zheng T, Camilleri M. Epidemiology and healthcare utilization in patients with gastroparesis: a systematic review. Clin Gastroenterol Hepatol. 2022;21:2239–2251.e2. https://doi.org/10.1016/j.cgh.2022.07.011. PubMed PMID: 35870768; PMCID: PMC9852358.

123. Camilleri M, Sanders KM. Gastroparesis. Gastroenterology. 2022;162(1):68–87.e1. https://doi.org/10.1053/j.gastro.2021.10.028. PubMed PMID: 34717924; PMCID: PMC8678360.
124. Bi D, Choi C, League J, Camilleri M, Prichard DO. Food residue during esophagogastroduodenoscopy is commonly encountered and is not pathognomonic of delayed gastric emptying. Dig Dis Sci. 2021;66(11):3951–9. https://doi.org/10.1007/s10620-020-06718-0. PubMed PMID: 33237388.
125. Vijayvargiya P, Jameie-Oskooei S, Camilleri M, Chedid V, Erwin PJ, Murad MH. Association between delayed gastric emptying and upper gastrointestinal symptoms: a systematic review and meta-analysis. Gut. 2019;68(5):804–13. https://doi.org/10.1136/gutjnl-2018-316405. PubMed PMID: 29860241.
126. Tougas G, Eaker EY, Abell TL, Abrahamsson H, Boivin M, Chen J, Hocking MP, Quigley EM, Koch KL, Tokayer AZ, Stanghellini V, Chen Y, Huizinga JD, Rydén J, Bourgeois I, McCallum RW. Assessment of gastric emptying using a low fat meal: establishment of international control values. Am J Gastroenterol. 2000;95(6):1456–62. https://doi.org/10.1111/j.1572-0241.2000.02076.x. PubMed PMID: 10894578
127. Stein E, Berger Z, Hutfless S, Shah L, Wilson LM, Haberl EB, Bass EB, Clarke JO. AHRQ comparative effectiveness reviews. Wireless motility capsule versus other diagnostic technologies for evaluating gastroparesis and constipation: a comparative effectiveness review. Rockville, MD: Agency for Healthcare Research and Quality (US); 2013.
128. Szarka LA, Camilleri M, Vella A, Burton D, Baxter K, Simonson J, Zinsmeister AR. A stable isotope breath test with a standard meal for abnormal gastric emptying of solids in the clinic and in research. Clin Gastroenterol Hepatol. 2008;6(6):635–43.e1. https://doi.org/10.1016/j.cgh.2008.01.009. PubMed PMID: 18406670; PMCID: PMC3739971.
129. Malik Z, Sankineni A, Parkman HP. Assessing pyloric sphincter pathophysiology using EndoFLIP in patients with gastroparesis. Neurogastroenterol Motil. 2015;27(4):524–31. https://doi.org/10.1111/nmo.12522. Epub 20150224. PubMed PMID: 25712043.
130. Snape WJ, Lin MS, Agarwal N, Shaw RE. Evaluation of the pylorus with concurrent intraluminal pressure and EndoFLIP in patients with nausea and vomiting. Neurogastroenterol Motil. 2016;28(5):758–64. https://doi.org/10.1111/nmo.12772. PubMed PMID: 26813266.
131. Vosoughi K, Ichkhanian Y, Jacques J, Aadam AA, Benias PC, Law R, Hasler WL, Canakis A, Ragi O, Triggs J, Bowers N, Brewer Gutierrez OI, Kumbhari V, Kalloo AN, Bulat RS, Pandolfino JE, Khashab MA. Role of endoscopic functional luminal imaging probe in predicting the outcome of gastric peroral endoscopic pyloromyotomy (with video). Gastrointest Endosc. 2020;91(6):1289–99. https://doi.org/10.1016/j.gie.2020.01.044. PubMed PMID: 32035074.
132. Pasricha PJ, Grover M, Yates KP, Abell TL, Bernard CE, Koch KL, McCallum RW, Sarosiek I, Kuo B, Bulat R, Chen J, Shulman RJ, Lee L, Tonascia J, Miriel LA, Hamilton F, Farrugia G, Parkman HP. Functional dyspepsia and gastroparesis in tertiary care are interchangeable syndromes with common clinical and pathologic features. Gastroenterology. 2021;160(6):2006–17. https://doi.org/10.1053/j.gastro.2021.01.230. PubMed PMID: 33548234; PMCID: PMC8547190.
133. Olausson EA, Alpsten M, Larsson A, Mattsson H, Andersson H, Attvall S. Small particle size of a solid meal increases gastric emptying and late postprandial glycaemic response in diabetic subjects with gastroparesis. Diabetes Res Clin Pract. 2008;80(2):231–7. https://doi.org/10.1016/j.diabres.2007.12.006. PubMed PMID: 18237818.
134. Olausson EA, Störsrud S, Grundin H, Isaksson M, Attvall S, Simrén M. A small particle size diet reduces upper gastrointestinal symptoms in patients with diabetic gastroparesis: a randomized controlled trial. Am J Gastroenterol. 2014;109(3):375–85. https://doi.org/10.1038/ajg.2013.453. PubMed PMID: 24419482.
135. Grover M, Farrugia G, Stanghellini V. Gastroparesis: a turning point in understanding and treatment. Gut. 2019;68(12):2238–50. https://doi.org/10.1136/gutjnl-2019-318712. PubMed PMID: 31563877; PMCID: PMC6874806.

136. Perkel MS, Moore C, Hersh T, Davidson ED. Metoclopramide therapy in patients with delayed gastric emptying: a randomized, double-blind study. Dig Dis Sci. 1979;24(9):662–6. https://doi.org/10.1007/bf01314461. PubMed PMID: 385260.
137. Snape WJ Jr, Battle WM, Schwartz SS, Braunstein SN, Goldstein HA, Alavi A. Metoclopramide to treat gastroparesis due to diabetes mellitus: a double-blind, controlled trial. Ann Intern Med. 1982;96(4):444–6. https://doi.org/10.7326/0003-4819-96-4-444. PubMed PMID: 7065559.
138. McCallum RW, Ricci DA, Rakatansky H, Behar J, Rhodes JB, Salen G, Deren J, Ippoliti A, Olsen HW, Falchuk K, et al. A multicenter placebo-controlled clinical trial of oral metoclopramide in diabetic gastroparesis. Diabetes Care. 1983;6(5):463–7. https://doi.org/10.2337/diacare.6.5.463. PubMed PMID: 6400707.
139. Patterson D, Abell T, Rothstein R, Koch K, Barnett J. A double-blind multicenter comparison of domperidone and metoclopramide in the treatment of diabetic patients with symptoms of gastroparesis. Am J Gastroenterol. 1999;94(5):1230–4. https://doi.org/10.1111/j.1572-0241.1999.00456.x. PubMed PMID: 10235199.
140. Erbas T, Varoglu E, Erbas B, Tastekin G, Akalin S. Comparison of metoclopramide and erythromycin in the treatment of diabetic gastroparesis. Diabetes Care. 1993;16(11):1511–4. https://doi.org/10.2337/diacare.16.11.1511. PubMed PMID: 8299441.
141. Loo FD, Palmer DW, Soergel KH, Kalbfleisch JH, Wood CM. Gastric emptying in patients with diabetes mellitus. Gastroenterology. 1984;86(3):485–94. PubMed PMID: 6693013
142. Parkman HP, Carlson MR, Gonyer D. Metoclopramide nasal spray is effective in symptoms of gastroparesis in diabetics compared to conventional oral tablet. Neurogastroenterol Motil. 2014;26(4):521–8. https://doi.org/10.1111/nmo.12296. PubMed PMID: 24372829.
143. Parkman HP, Carlson MR, Gonyer D. Metoclopramide nasal spray reduces symptoms of gastroparesis in women, but not men, with diabetes: results of a phase 2B randomized study. Clin Gastroenterol Hepatol. 2015;13(7):1256–63.e1. https://doi.org/10.1016/j.cgh.2014.12.030. PubMed PMID: 25576687.
144. Al-Saffar A, Lennernäs H, Hellström PM. Gastroparesis, metoclopramide, and tardive dyskinesia: risk revisited. Neurogastroenterol Motil. 2019;31(11):e13617. https://doi.org/10.1111/nmo.13617. Epub 20190502. PubMed PMID: 31050085.
145. Sarosiek I, Van Natta M, Parkman HP, Abell T, Koch KL, Kuo B, Shulman RJ, Farrugia G, Grover M, Hamilton FA, Pasricha PJ, Yates KP, Miriel L, Wilson L, Yamada G, Tonascia J, McCallum RW. Effect of domperidone therapy on gastroparesis symptoms: results of a dynamic cohort study by NIDDK gastroparesis consortium. Clin Gastroenterol Hepatol. 2022;20(3):e452–e64. https://doi.org/10.1016/j.cgh.2021.05.063. PubMed PMID: 34089855; PMCID: PMC8636553.
146. Farup CE, Leidy NK, Murray M, Williams GR, Helbers L, Quigley EM. Effect of domperidone on the health-related quality of life of patients with symptoms of diabetic gastroparesis. Diabetes Care. 1998;21(10):1699–706. https://doi.org/10.2337/diacare.21.10.1699. PubMed PMID: 9773734.
147. Camilleri M, McCallum RW, Tack J, Spence SC, Gottesdiener K, Fiedorek FT. Efficacy and safety of relamorelin in diabetics with symptoms of gastroparesis: a randomized, placebo-controlled study. Gastroenterology. 2017;153(5):1240–50.e2. https://doi.org/10.1053/j.gastro.2017.07.035. PubMed PMID: 28760384; PMCID: PMC5670003. Epub 20170729.
148. Lembo A, Camilleri M, McCallum R, Sastre R, Breton C, Spence S, White J, Currie M, Gottesdiener K, Stoner E. Relamorelin reduces vomiting frequency and severity and accelerates gastric emptying in adults with diabetic gastroparesis. Gastroenterology. 2016;151(1):87–96.e6. https://doi.org/10.1053/j.gastro.2016.03.038. PubMed PMID: 27055601. Epub 20160404.
149. Parkman HP, Van Natta ML, Abell TL, McCallum RW, Sarosiek I, Nguyen L, Snape WJ, Koch KL, Hasler WL, Farrugia G, Lee L, Unalp-Arida A, Tonascia J, Hamilton F, Pasricha PJ. Effect of nortriptyline on symptoms of idiopathic gastroparesis: the NORIG randomized clinical trial. JAMA. 2013;310(24):2640–9. https://doi.org/10.1001/jama.2013.282833. PubMed PMID: 24368464; PMCID: PMC4099968.

150. Lehmann S, Ferrie S, Carey S. Nutrition management in patients with chronic gastrointestinal motility disorders: a systematic literature review. Nutr Clin Pract. 2020;35(2):219–30. https://doi.org/10.1002/ncp.10273. Epub 20190415. PubMed PMID: 30989698.
151. Vosoughi K, Ichkhanian Y, Benias P, Miller L, Aadam AA, Triggs JR, Law R, Hasler W, Bowers N, Chaves D, Ponte-Neto AM, Draganov P, Yang D, El Halabi M, Sanaei O, Brewer Gutierrez OI, Bulat RS, Pandolfino J, Khashab M. Gastric per-oral endoscopic myotomy (G-POEM) for refractory gastroparesis: results from an international prospective trial. Gut. 2022;71(1):25–33. https://doi.org/10.1136/gutjnl-2020-322756. Epub 20210319. PubMed PMID: 33741641.
152. Dacha S, Mekaroonkamol P, Li L, Shahnavaz N, Sakaria S, Keilin S, Willingham F, Christie J, Cai Q. Outcomes and quality-of-life assessment after gastric per-oral endoscopic pyloromyotomy (with video). Gastrointest Endosc. 2017;86(2):282–9. https://doi.org/10.1016/j.gie.2017.01.031. Epub 20170201. PubMed PMID: 28161449.
153. Gonzalez JM, Benezech A, Vitton V, Barthet M. G-POEM with antro-pyloromyotomy for the treatment of refractory gastroparesis: mid-term follow-up and factors predicting outcome. Aliment Pharmacol Ther. 2017;46(3):364–70. https://doi.org/10.1111/apt.14132. Epub 20170515. PubMed PMID: 28504312.
154. Khashab MA, Ngamruengphong S, Carr-Locke D, Bapaye A, Benias PC, Serouya S, Dorwat S, Chaves DM, Artifon E, de Moura EG, Kumbhari V, Chavez YH, Bukhari M, Hajiyeva G, Ismail A, Chen YI, Chung H. Gastric per-oral endoscopic myotomy for refractory gastroparesis: results from the first multicenter study on endoscopic pyloromyotomy (with video). Gastrointest Endosc. 2017;85(1):123–8. https://doi.org/10.1016/j.gie.2016.06.048. PubMed PMID: 27354102. Epub 20160625.
155. Rodriguez JH, Haskins IN, Strong AT, Plescia RL, Allemang MT, Butler RS, Cline MS, El-Hayek K, Ponsky JL, Kroh MD. Per oral endoscopic pyloromyotomy for refractory gastroparesis: initial results from a single institution. Surg Endosc. 2017;31(12):5381–8. Epub 20170531. PubMed PMID: 28567693. https://doi.org/10.1007/s00464-017-5619-5.
156. Malik Z, Kataria R, Modayil R, Ehrlich AC, Schey R, Parkman HP, Stavropoulos SN. Gastric per oral endoscopic myotomy (G-POEM) for the treatment of refractory gastroparesis: early experience. Dig Dis Sci. 2018;63(9):2405–12. https://doi.org/10.1007/s10620-018-4976-9. Epub 20180222. PubMed PMID: 29468376.
157. Xu J, Chen T, Elkholy S, Xu M, Zhong Y, Zhang Y, Chen W, Qin W, Cai M, Zhou P. Gastric Peroral Endoscopic Myotomy (G-POEM) as a treatment for refractory gastroparesis: long-term outcomes. Can J Gastroenterol Hepatol. 2018;2018:6409698. https://doi.org/10.1155/2018/6409698. PubMed PMID: 30425974; PMCID: PMC6217887. Epub 20181022.
158. Jacques J, Pagnon L, Hure F, Legros R, Crepin S, Fauchais AL, Palat S, Ducrotté P, Marin B, Fontaine S, Boubaddi NE, Clement MP, Sautereau D, Loustaud-Ratti V, Gourcerol G, Monteil J. Peroral endoscopic pyloromyotomy is efficacious and safe for refractory gastroparesis: prospective trial with assessment of pyloric function. Endoscopy. 2019;51(1):40–9. https://doi.org/10.1055/a-0628-6639. PubMed PMID: 29895073.
159. Strong AT, Landreneau JP, Cline M, Kroh MD, Rodriguez JH, Ponsky JL, El-Hayek K. Per-oral pyloromyotomy (POP) for medically refractory post-surgical gastroparesis. J Gastrointest Surg. 2019;23(6):1095–103. https://doi.org/10.1007/s11605-018-04088-7. Epub 20190226. PubMed PMID: 30809781.
160. Ragi O, Jacques J, Branche J, Leblanc S, Vanbiervliet G, Legros R, Pioche M, Rivory J, Chaussade S, Barret M, Wallenhorst T, Barthet M, Kerever S, Gonzalez JM. One-year results of gastric peroral endoscopic myotomy for refractory gastroparesis: a French multicenter study. Endoscopy. 2021;53(5):480–90. https://doi.org/10.1055/a-1205-5686. Epub 20200721. PubMed PMID: 32575130.
161. Spadaccini M, Maselli R, Chandrasekar VT, Anderloni A, Carrara S, Galtieri PA, Di Leo M, Fugazza A, Pellegatta G, Colombo M, Palma R, Hassan C, Sethi A, Khashab MA, Sharma P, Repici A. Gastric peroral endoscopic pyloromyotomy for refractory gastroparesis: a system-

atic review of early outcomes with pooled analysis. Gastrointest Endosc. 2020;91(4):746–52.e5. https://doi.org/10.1016/j.gie.2019.11.039. PubMed PMID: 31809720.
162. Martinek J, Hustak R, Mares J, Vackova Z, Spicak J, Kieslichova E, Buncova M, Pohl D, Amin S, Tack J. Endoscopic pyloromyotomy for the treatment of severe and refractory gastroparesis: a pilot, randomised, sham-controlled trial. Gut. 2022;71(11):2170–8. https://doi.org/10.1136/gutjnl-2022-326904. PubMed PMID: 35470243; PMCID: PMC9554080.
163. Bai Y, Xu MJ, Yang X, Xu C, Gao J, Zou DW, Li ZS. A systematic review on intrapyloric botulinum toxin injection for gastroparesis. Digestion. 2010;81(1):27–34. Epub 20091222. doi: 10.1159/000235917. PubMed PMID: 20029206.
164. Abell T, McCallum R, Hocking M, Koch K, Abrahamsson H, Leblanc I, Lindberg G, Konturek J, Nowak T, Quigley EM, Tougas G, Starkebaum W. Gastric electrical stimulation for medically refractory gastroparesis. Gastroenterology. 2003;125(2):421–8. https://doi.org/10.1016/s0016-5085(03)00878-3. PubMed PMID: 12891544.
165. Abell TL, Johnson WD, Kedar A, Runnels JM, Thompson J, Weeks ES, Minocha A, Griswold ME. A double-masked, randomized, placebo-controlled trial of temporary endoscopic mucosal gastric electrical stimulation for gastroparesis. Gastrointest Endosc. 2011;74(3):496–503.e3. https://doi.org/10.1016/j.gie.2011.05.022. PubMed PMID: 21872708; PMCID: PMC5098698.
166. Ducrotte P, Coffin B, Bonaz B, Fontaine S, Bruley Des Varannes S, Zerbib F, Caiazzo R, Grimaud JC, Mion F, Hadjadj S, Valensi PE, Vuitton L, Charpentier G, Ropert A, Altwegg R, Pouderoux P, Dorval E, Dapoigny M, Duboc H, Benhamou PY, Schmidt A, Donnadieu N, Gourcerol G, Guerci B. Gastric electrical stimulation reduces refractory vomiting in a randomized crossover trial. Gastroenterology. 2020;158(3):506–14.e2. https://doi.org/10.1053/j.gastro.2019.10.018. Epub 20191021. PubMed PMID: 31647902.
167. McCallum RW, Snape W, Brody F, Wo J, Parkman HP, Nowak T. Gastric electrical stimulation with Enterra therapy improves symptoms from diabetic gastroparesis in a prospective study. Clin Gastroenterol Hepatol. 2010;8(11):947–54; quiz e116. https://doi.org/10.1016/j.cgh.2010.05.020. PubMed PMID: 20538073.
168. McCallum RW, Sarosiek I, Parkman HP, Snape W, Brody F, Wo J, Nowak T. Gastric electrical stimulation with Enterra therapy improves symptoms of idiopathic gastroparesis. Neurogastroenterol Motil. 2013;25(10):815–e636. https://doi.org/10.1111/nmo.12185. PubMed PMID: 23895180; PMCID: PMC4274014.
169. O'Grady G, Egbuji JU, Du P, Cheng LK, Pullan AJ, Windsor JA. High-frequency gastric electrical stimulation for the treatment of gastroparesis: a meta-analysis. World J Surg. 2009;33(8):1693–701. https://doi.org/10.1007/s00268-009-0096-1. PubMed PMID: 19506941; PMCID: PMC4127311.
170. Levinthal DJ, Bielefeldt K. Systematic review and meta-analysis: gastric electrical stimulation for gastroparesis. Auton Neurosci. 2017;202:45–55. https://doi.org/10.1016/j.autneu.2016.03.004. PubMed PMID: 27085627.
171. Shada AL, Dunst CM, Pescarus R, Speer EA, Cassera M, Reavis KM, Swanstrom LL. Laparoscopic pyloroplasty is a safe and effective first-line surgical therapy for refractory gastroparesis. Surg Endosc. 2016;30(4):1326–32. https://doi.org/10.1007/s00464-015-4385-5. Epub 20150821. PubMed PMID: 26293794.
172. Mohan BP, Chandan S, Jha LK, Khan SR, Kotagiri R, Kassab LL, Ravikumar NPG, Bhogal N, Chandan OC, Bhat I, Hewlett AT, Jacques J, Ponnada S, Asokkumar R, Adler DG. Clinical efficacy of gastric per-oral endoscopic myotomy (G-POEM) in the treatment of refractory gastroparesis and predictors of outcomes: a systematic review and meta-analysis using surgical pyloroplasty as a comparator group. Surg Endosc. 2020;34(8):3352–67. https://doi.org/10.1007/s00464-019-07135-9. Epub 20191003. PubMed PMID: 31583465.
173. Bharucha AE, Batey-Schaefer B, Cleary PA, Murray JA, Cowie C, Lorenzi G, Driscoll M, Harth J, Larkin M, Christofi M, Bayless M, Wimmergren N, Herman W, Whitehouse F, Jones K, Kruger D, Martin C, Ziegler G, Zinsmeister AR, Nathan DM. Delayed gastric emptying is associated with early and long-term hyperglycemia in type 1 diabetes mellitus.

Gastroenterology. 2015;149(2):330–9. https://doi.org/10.1053/j.gastro.2015.05.007. Epub 20150514. PubMed PMID: 25980755; PMCID: PMC4516593.
174. Calles-Escandón J, Koch KL, Hasler WL, Van Natta ML, Pasricha PJ, Tonascia J, Parkman HP, Hamilton F, Herman WH, Basina M, Buckingham B, Earle K, Kirkeby K, Hairston K, Bright T, Rothberg AE, Kraftson AT, Siraj ES, Subauste A, Lee LA, Abell TL, McCallum RW, Sarosiek I, Nguyen L, Fass R, Snape WJ, Vaughn IA, Miriel LA, Farrugia G. Glucose sensor-augmented continuous subcutaneous insulin infusion in patients with diabetic gastroparesis: an open-label pilot prospective study. PLoS One. 2018;13(4):e0194759. https://doi.org/10.1371/journal.pone.0194759. Epub 20180413. PubMed PMID: 29652893; PMCID: PMC5898706.
175. Bredenoord AJ, Weusten BL, Sifrim D, Timmer R, Smout AJ. Aerophagia, gastric, and supragastric belching: a study using intraluminal electrical impedance monitoring. Gut. 2004;53(11):1561–5. https://doi.org/10.1136/gut.2004.042945. PubMed PMID: 15479671; PMCID: PMC1774303.
176. Bredenoord AJ, Smout AJ. Physiologic and pathologic belching. Clin Gastroenterol Hepatol. 2007;5(7):772–5. https://doi.org/10.1016/j.cgh.2007.02.018. Epub 20070504. PubMed PMID: 17481963.
177. Koukias N, Woodland P, Yazaki E, Sifrim D. Supragastric belching: prevalence and association with gastroesophageal reflux disease and esophageal hypomotility. J Neurogastroenterol Motil. 2015;21(3):398–403. https://doi.org/10.5056/jnm15002. PubMed PMID: 26130635; PMCID: PMC4496903.
178. Hemmink GJ, Bredenoord AJ, Weusten BL, Timmer R, Smout AJ. Supragastric belching in patients with reflux symptoms. Am J Gastroenterol. 2009;104(8):1992–7. https://doi.org/10.1038/ajg.2009.203. Epub 20090519. PubMed PMID: 19455107.
179. Cigrang JA, Hunter CM, Peterson AL. Behavioral treatment of chronic belching due to aerophagia in a normal adult. Behav Modif. 2006;30:341–51. https://doi.org/10.1177/0145445504264746.
180. Chitkara DK, Bredenoord AJ, Talley NJ, Whitehead WE. Aerophagia and rumination: recognition and therapy. Curr Treat Options Gastroenterol. 2006;9(4):305–13. https://doi.org/10.1007/s11938-006-0012-9. PubMed PMID: 16836949.
181. Blondeau K, Boecxstaens V, Rommel N, Farré R, Depeyper S, Holvoet L, Boeckxstaens G, Tack JF. Baclofen improves symptoms and reduces postprandial flow events in patients with rumination and supragastric belching. Clin Gastroenterol Hepatol. 2012;10(4):379–84. Epub 20111109. PubMed PMID: 22079512. https://doi.org/10.1016/j.cgh.2011.10.042.
182. Pauwels A, Broers C, Van Houtte B, Rommel N, Vanuytsel T, Tack J. A randomized double-blind, placebo-controlled, cross-over study using baclofen in the treatment of rumination syndrome. Am J Gastroenterol. 2018;113(1):97–104. https://doi.org/10.1038/ajg.2017.441. PubMed PMID: 29206813. Epub 20171205.
183. Halland M, Pandolfino J, Barba E. Diagnosis and treatment of rumination syndrome. Clin Gastroenterol Hepatol. 2018;16(10):1549–55. https://doi.org/10.1016/j.cgh.2018.05.049. PubMed PMID: 29902642. Epub 20180612.
184. Murray HB, Juarascio AS, Di Lorenzo C, Drossman DA, Thomas JJ. Diagnosis and treatment of rumination syndrome: a critical review. Am J Gastroenterol. 2019;114(4):562–78. https://doi.org/10.14309/ajg.0000000000000060. PubMed PMID: 30789419; PMCID: PMC6492032.
185. Thompson WG, Irvine EJ, Pare P, Ferrazzi S, Rance L. Functional gastrointestinal disorders in Canada: first population-based survey using Rome II criteria with suggestions for improving the questionnaire. Dig Dis Sci. 2002;47(1):225–35. https://doi.org/10.1023/a:1013208713670. PubMed PMID: 11837727
186. Koloski NA, Talley NJ, Boyce PM. Epidemiology and health care seeking in the functional GI disorders: a population-based study. Am J Gastroenterol. 2002;97(9):2290–9. https://doi.org/10.1111/j.1572-0241.2002.05783.x. PubMed PMID: 12358247.

187. Palsson OS, Whitehead WE, van Tilburg MA, Chang L, Chey W, Crowell MD, Keefer L, Lembo AJ, Parkman HP, Rao SS, Sperber A, Spiegel B, Tack J, Vanner S, Walker LS, Whorwell P, Yang Y. Rome IV diagnostic questionnaires and tables for investigators and clinicians. Gastroenterology. 2016;S0016–5085(16):00180–3. https://doi.org/10.1053/j.gastro.2016.02.014. PubMed PMID: 27144634.
188. López-Colombo A, Morgan D, Bravo-González D, Montiel-Jarquín A, Méndez-Martínez S, Schmulson M. The epidemiology of functional gastrointestinal disorders in Mexico: a population-based study. Gastroenterol Res Pract. 2012;2012:606174. https://doi.org/10.1155/2012/606174. Epub 20120319. PubMed PMID: 22474443; PMCID: PMC3313569.
189. Rajindrajith S, Devanarayana NM, Crispus Perera BJ. Rumination syndrome in children and adolescents: a school survey assessing prevalence and symptomatology. BMC Gastroenterol. 2012;12:163. https://doi.org/10.1186/1471-230x-12-163. PubMed PMID: 23157670. PMCID: PMC3538663. Epub 20121116.
190. Hartmann AS, Poulain T, Vogel M, Hiemisch A, Kiess W, Hilbert A. Prevalence of pica and rumination behaviors in German children aged 7-14 and their associations with feeding, eating, and general psychopathology: a population-based study. Eur Child Adolesc Psychiatry. 2018;27(11):1499–508. https://doi.org/10.1007/s00787-018-1153-9. Epub 20180419. PubMed PMID: 29675593.
191. Murray HB, Thomas JJ, Hinz A, Munsch S, Hilbert A. Prevalence in primary school youth of pica and rumination behavior: the understudied feeding disorders. Int J Eat Disord. 2018;51(8):994–8. https://doi.org/10.1002/eat.22898. PubMed PMID: 30175409. Epub 20180902.
192. Chogle A, Velasco-Benitez CA, Koppen IJ, Moreno JE, Ramírez Hernández CR, Saps M. A population-based study on the epidemiology of functional gastrointestinal disorders in young children. J Pediatr. 2016;179:139–43.e1. https://doi.org/10.1016/j.jpeds.2016.08.095. Epub 20161007. PubMed PMID: 27726867.
193. Cai JX, Wong D, Lee DJH, Chan WW. Eating and psychiatric disorders are independent risk factors for rumination syndrome. J Clin Gastroenterol. 2022;56(3):228–33. https://doi.org/10.1097/mcg.0000000000001510. PubMed PMID: 33988353.
194. O'Brien MD, Bruce BK, Camilleri M. The rumination syndrome: clinical features rather than manometric diagnosis. Gastroenterology. 1995;108(4):1024–9. https://doi.org/10.1016/0016-5085(95)90199-x. PubMed PMID: 7698568.
195. Monagas J, Ritwik P, Kolomensky A, Acosta J, Kay D, Clendaniel L, Hyman PE. Rumination syndrome and dental erosions in children. J Pediatr Gastroenterol Nutr. 2017;64(6):930–2. https://doi.org/10.1097/mpg.0000000000001395. PubMed PMID: 27579694.
196. Barba E, Accarino A, Soldevilla A, Malagelada JR, Azpiroz F. Randomized, placebo-controlled trial of biofeedback for the treatment of rumination. Am J Gastroenterol. 2016;111(7):1007–13. https://doi.org/10.1038/ajg.2016.197. PubMed PMID: 27185077. Epub 20160517.
197. Barba E, Burri E, Accarino A, Malagelada C, Rodriguez-Urrutia A, Soldevilla A, Malagelada JR, Azpiroz F. Biofeedback-guided control of abdominothoracic muscular activity reduces regurgitation episodes in patients with rumination. Clin Gastroenterol Hepatol. 2015;13(1):100–6.e1. Epub 20140424. PubMed PMID: 24768808. https://doi.org/10.1016/j.cgh.2014.04.018.
198. Oelschlager BK, Chan MM, Eubanks TR, Pope CE 2nd, Pellegrini CA. Effective treatment of rumination with Nissen fundoplication. J Gastrointest Surg. 2002;6(4):638–44. https://doi.org/10.1016/s1091-255x(01)00068-3. PubMed PMID: 12127134.
199. Tucker E, Knowles K, Wright J, Fox MR. Rumination variations: aetiology and classification of abnormal behavioural responses to digestive symptoms based on high-resolution manometry studies. Aliment Pharmacol Ther. 2013;37(2):263–74. https://doi.org/10.1111/apt.12148.
200. Ford AC, Mahadeva S, Carbone MF, Lacy BE, Talley NJ. Functional dyspepsia. Lancet. 2020;396(10263):1689–702. https://doi.org/10.1016/s0140-6736(20)30469-4. Epub 20201010. PubMed PMID: 33049222.

Chapter 14
Quality in Lower Gastrointestinal Motility Disorders

Colleen H. Parker and David Rodrigues

Table of Quality Measures/Metrics

C. H. Parker (✉)
Division of Gastroenterology and Hepatology, University Health Network, Toronto, ON, Canada

Division of Gastroenterology and Hepatology, Department of Medicine, University of Toronto, Toronto, ON, Canada
e-mail: colleen.parker@uhn.ca

D. Rodrigues
Division of Gastroenterology, Department of Medicine, Queen's University, Kingston, ON, Canada
e-mail: davidmario.rodrigues@kingstonhsc.ca

J. D. Feuerstein, D. J. Stein (eds.), *Quality in Gastroenterology*,
https://doi.org/10.1007/978-3-031-58492-3_14

Key Points
- Irritable bowel syndrome is not a diagnosis of exclusion. A positive diagnosis can be made using appropriate clinical criteria and minimal investigations.
- The use of anorectal manometry in patients with chronic constipation should only be considered in patients who have a history/physical examination suspicious of dyssynergic defecation or in those with constipation symptoms refractory to conventional therapy.
- For the majority of patients with fecal incontinence, conservative measures such as regulating bowel habits and pelvic floor strengthening exercises are the mainstay of treatment.
- Opioid-induced bowel dysfunction is an important diagnostic consideration in patients with lower gastrointestinal symptoms that should not to be missed.

Introduction

Lower gastrointestinal motility disorders are a group of conditions that include alterations in both motor and sensory functions of the gut. These are among the most commonly encountered gastrointestinal conditions in both gastroenterology practice and primary care [1]. Currently, there is a lack of evidence-based quality indicators for the care of these patients. Despite the lack of quality indicators, it is important that quality care be provided to patients with lower gastrointestinal motility disorders given the impact of these conditions on a patient's quality of life and ability to function day to day. This chapter will review several common lower gastrointestinal motility disorders with a focus on performing appropriate workup of symptoms and providing high-quality therapies to these patients. Table 14.1 highlights the key messages from this chapter and potential quality indicators in the management of patients with lower gastrointestinal motility disorders.

Table 14.1 Quality metrics in lower gastrointestinal motility disorders

Ensure patients who are being evaluated for potential IBS are screened for anemia, celiac disease, hypothyroidism, hypercalcemia
In the absence of red flag symptoms, extensive and invasive investigations are not typically required in those presenting with symptoms suggestive of a lower gastrointestinal motility disorder
Medication history (particularly around opioid use) is necessary in those with lower gastrointestinal symptoms
In patients who present with diarrhea who undergo colonoscopy, random biopsies to rule out microscopic colitis are recommended if the colon mucosa appears macroscopically normal
A properly performed digital rectal examination is important in the evaluation of patients who present with constipation and fecal incontinence
An anorectal manometry is indicated in patients with constipation and fecal incontinence who do not respond to conservative or standard therapies

Irritable Bowel Syndrome

Irritable bowel syndrome (IBS) is a common disorder of gut-brain interaction that has a worldwide prevalence between 3% and 5% [2]. IBS has high personal [3], healthcare [4], and societal costs [4] associated with it. IBS affects a heterogeneous patient population with various pathophysiologic mechanisms that contribute to the development and severity of symptoms [5]. This highlights the need to have multiple treatment options for IBS and to consider combination therapy when appropriate.

Diagnosis of IBS

IBS is defined using the Rome IV criteria [6] and full criteria must be met for at least 3 months. This indicates that patients must have chronic, recurrent episodes of abdominal pain that occurs at least once per week. This pain is associated with at least two of the following three items; the pain changes with a bowel movement (can either get better or worse), change in stool frequency, and/or change in stool form. IBS subtype should be determined for all patients with a diagnosis of IBS. Subtype is defined by stool form on days when abnormal bowel movements are present [6]. To determine the stool form, the Bristol Stool Form Scale [7] should be used. IBS with constipation (IBS-C) occurs in patients who report having Bristol stool type 1 or 2 at least 25% of the time and Bristol stool type 6 or 7 less than 25% of the time. IBS with diarrhea (IBS-D) occurs in patients who report having Bristol stool type 6 or 7 bowel movements at least 25% of the time and Bristol stool type 1 or 2 less than 25% of the time. IBS mixed (IBS-M) occurs in patients with Bristol stool type 1 or 2 at least 25% of the time and Bristol stool type 6 or 7 at least 25% of the time. IBS unclassified (IBS-U) occurs in those patients who meet the Rome IV criteria but whose stool form does not fit in the categories defined above. It is necessary to accurately determine a patient's stool form as this will determine the most appropriate treatment options for that patient.

Appropriate Workup in Patients Presenting with IBS Symptoms

In all patients who present with IBS symptoms, a thorough history and physical exam must be performed to evaluate for red flag symptoms that should prompt further evaluation as they may indicate another diagnosis. Red flag signs and symptoms include new onset of symptoms over the age of 50, recent bowel habit change, overt signs of GI bleeding, iron-deficiency anemia, nocturnal symptoms, unintentional weight loss, family history of alternative GI diagnoses (i.e., colorectal cancer, inflammatory bowel disease, celiac disease, etc.), palpable abdominal mass, and/or

Table 14.2 Red flag or alarm symptoms in lower gastrointestinal symptoms

New onset of symptoms over age 50
Recent bowel habit change
Overt signs of gastrointestinal bleeding
Iron-deficiency anemia
Nocturnal symptoms
Unintentional weight loss
Constitutional symptoms such as fever, chills, night sweats
Family history of alternative gastrointestinal diagnoses
Abdominal mass or lymphadenopathy on physical examination
Crescendo symptoms
Imaging that demonstrates obstruction or bowel dilation

palpable lymphadenopathy (see Table 14.2). In patients who meet the Rome IV criteria and have an absence of red flag symptoms, a positive diagnosis of IBS can be made with the use of minimal investigations [8].

In all patients with IBS symptoms, a complete blood count should be performed at the time of presentation to rule out anemia which would prompt further investigations if present [8, 9]. In addition, all patients should be up-to-date with age-appropriate colorectal screening as per local guidelines. Celiac serology should be performed using immunoglobulin A (IgA) tissue transglutaminase and an IgA level to ensure the absence of IgA deficiency [8]. Upper endoscopy should be performed in those with positive serology. Given the overlap in symptoms between IBS-D and inflammatory bowel disease (IBD), fecal calprotectin or fecal lactoferrin and C-reactive protein can be considered [8]. While these tests do not confirm the diagnosis of either IBS or IBD, they can be helpful to determine which patients would benefit most from going on to more invasive testing to rule out IBD. In patients with IBS-C, anorectal manometry and/or balloon expulsion testing should be considered in patients with refractory symptoms or in whom a pelvic floor disorder is considered (see below) [8, 9].

The role of either glucose or lactulose breath testing to assess for small intestinal bacterial overgrowth (SIBO) in patients presenting with IBS remains somewhat controversial. Though there is evidence that SIBO may be more prevalent in patients who present with IBS symptoms, there is limited evidence that breath testing affects outcomes in patients with IBS [10]. There are some studies that have demonstrated the patients with a positive breath test have a higher rate of response to certain therapies such as rifaximin [11], but there is no data for the use of other antibiotics. Furthermore, lactulose breath testing is used to measure gastrointestinal transit and may be positive in the absence of SIBO [12].

Though IBS symptoms can develop after an enteric infection, there is currently no role for routine stool testing for enteric pathogens in patients with a diagnosis of IBS given the chronicity of symptoms involved [8]. Testing for specific pathogens, such as *Giardia*, can be considered in the correct clinical context.

Patients with IBS often report symptoms associated with ingestion of food and believe that food intake plays a role in their symptoms. Despite this, there is no role for food allergy testing in IBS [8].

The role of colonoscopy in patients with IBS symptoms and the absence of red flag symptoms are generally limited. The probability of finding an alternative diagnosis [13] or an advanced colonic lesion [14] is low in patients presenting with typical IBS symptoms. In addition, performing a colonoscopy is not associated with an increased feeling of reassurance or higher health-related quality of life in patients with IBS [15]. Colonoscopy should be performed in those presenting with red flag or alarm symptoms. In patients presenting with IBS-D symptoms who are at high risk for microscopic colitis (i.e., over age 60, female, severe diarrhea), a colonoscopy should be considered to perform random biopsies to rule out this diagnosis [9].

Management of IBS

To date, there are no clear indicators for providing quality care in the treatment of IBS. This is likely due to the heterogeneous nature of the IBS and the variable response to currently available therapies. There is a growing body of literature to support different treatment options in IBS. Treatments that are currently available and routinely used in clinical practice will be highlighted in this section. Choice of IBS therapy should be based on IBS subtype, severity of symptoms, and patient preference and understanding of their symptoms. Treatment often requires a multifaceted approach that targets pain, bowel habit, and disordered gut-brain interaction. In all patients, the first step in management should involve education around the diagnosis of IBS, the pathophysiologic mechanisms of IBS, and the treatment targets/options. In the initial stages of managing IBS, effective patient-provider communication and reasonable expectations regarding treatment outcomes should be established [16]. It should be discussed that the overall goal of treatment of IBS is reduction of symptoms and impact of symptoms on daily function rather than cure of symptoms entirely.

Dietary therapies have been studied and are often used in the management of IBS. The most well-studied diet in IBS is the low fermentable oligosaccharides, disaccharides, monosaccharides, and polyols (FODMAP) diet [17]. This diet has been shown to improve overall IBS symptom severity, bloating, and abdominal pain. Improvement in stool form is only seen in patients with IBS-D. It is important that patients follow both phases of the low FODMAP diet: avoidance of high FODMAP foods followed by reintroduction of food to determine potential triggers. Ideally, this should be done under the guidance of a trained dietitian where available. While the low FODMAP diet is considered to be a safe treatment option, prolonged food restriction (i.e., staying in the first phase of the low FODMAP) can lead to micronutrient deficiencies. In addition, this diet should be avoided in patients with a history of disordered eating as the restrictive phase can worsen disordered eating symptoms.

Soluble fiber can be used in any IBS subtype to improve overall IBS symptoms and stool consistency/form [10]. However, some forms of soluble fiber may cause bloating which may limit its use in the IBS patient population.

Peppermint oil has been shown to improve overall IBS symptom severity in all IBS subtypes [8, 10, 18, 19]. Overall, this seems to be a safe treatment, but there is a risk of worsening symptoms of gastroesophageal reflux disease due to the effect of peppermint on the function of the lower esophageal sphincter. It is believed that enteric-coated formulations may reduce this risk.

The role of antispasmodic medications such as dicyclomine, hyoscyamine, pinaverium, etc. in the management of IBS remains somewhat unclear though their use is currently recommended in IBS management guidelines [10, 18, 19]. The quality of evidence remains poor for their use and there is a risk for anticholinergic side effects with these medications.

The role of probiotics in the management of IBS also remains controversial. The use of probiotics may improve overall IBS symptom severity, abdominal pain, and bloating [10]. However, the ideal strain and combinations of strains remain unclear. There is some evidence that combination of *Lactobacillus* and *Bifidobacterium* may have the most benefit in IBS [10]. If patients are interested in trying a probiotic, one containing those strains can be considered. Patients should be counselled that the data regarding the use of probiotics remains unclear and there is a lack of rigorous trials regarding their use.

In patients with IBS-C, there are several medication options. Polyethylene glycol (PEG) is an osmotic laxative that improves stool form in patients with IBS [10, 18]. There is no evidence that it improves abdominal pain. Thus, PEG products are likely most helpful in IBS when used in combination with other medications that can target the abdominal pain component. Secretagogues are a growing category of medications for the treatment of IBS-C that targets various molecular mechanisms. Examples of secretagogues include chloride channel agonists (i.e., lubiprostone), guanylate cyclase C agonists (i.e., linaclotide, plecanatide), and sodium/hydrogen exchanger isoform 3 inhibitor (i.e., tenapanor). All these medication classes have demonstrated improvement in abdominal pain and stool frequency/form in IBS-C [10, 18]. Patients should be counselled that with all these medications, abdominal pain may take up to 12 weeks to show maximal improvement whereas the effect on bowel habit usually occurs in the first 1–2 weeks. For all these medications, the most common reported side effects are gastrointestinal in nature such as diarrhea. There are no studies to date to inform the place in therapy of these secretagogues, and choice of which medication to be used is generally based on patient preference. Finally, tegaserod is a 5-HT_4 that is indicated for treatment of IBS-C in women under the age of 65 with no more than one cardiovascular risk factor [18]. Given that this medication has been associated with cardiovascular ischemic events, it is currently contraindicated in patients with more than one cardiovascular risk factor.

In patients with IBS-D, the use of bile acid sequestrants has been shown to improve overall IBS symptoms in patients with evidence of bile acid malabsorption [20]. The lack of readily available testing for bile acid malabsorption may limit the regular use of bile acid sequestrants in patients. However, a trial can be considered in those patients with IBS-D who are at high risk for bile acid malabsorption based on history though its routine use remains somewhat debatable [10]. Rifaximin is a nonsystemic broad-spectrum antibiotic that has demonstrated an improvement in stool consistency, abdominal pain, and bloating in patients with

IBS-D [10, 19]. Rifaximin is given as a 14-day course and there is often the need for re-treatment. Eluxadoline is a μ-opioid agonists and δ-opioid antagonist that has been demonstrated to improve stool form and abdominal pain in IBS-D [10, 19]. Clinically, it can be particularly useful in patients who have significant urgency associated with bowel movements. In the initial clinical trials of eluxadoline, there was concern of an increased risk of pancreatitis in those receiving the medication. Subsequent analysis demonstrated that this occurred exclusively in patients who had a cholecystectomy. Thus, the use of eluxadoline is contraindicated in those with a cholecystectomy, previous bile duct obstruction, known history of sphincter of Oddi dysfunction, previous pancreatitis, and significant alcohol use (greater than three alcoholic beverages per day) [19]. Though loperamide is often used in the management of diarrhea, guidelines generally recommend against its routine use in IBS-D [10].

Neuromodulators are a group of medications that are designed to target the abdominal pain component of IBS [21]. The most well-studied neuromodulators in IBS are the tricyclic antidepressants [18, 19]. These have demonstrated evidence for improving abdominal pain in IBS. Caution should be taken in prescribing these to patients with IBS-C given their anticholinergic properties that can worsen constipation. While some IBS guidelines recommend the use of selective serotonin reuptake inhibitors (SSRIs) in IBS, others do not [10, 18, 19]. There is no evidence that SSRIs improve abdominal pain in IBS. SSRIs may be helpful to treat underlying anxiety or depression that may contribute to the severity of IBS symptoms. Serotonin norepinephrine reuptake inhibitors (SNRIs) may be considered for the management of abdominal pain in IBS [18, 19]. Though there are no studies of SNRIs in IBS, this group of medications has been studied in various other chronic pain conditions that likely share similar pathophysiologic mechanisms to IBS (i.e., fibromyalgia). SNRIs have the benefit that they do not worsen constipation and thus can be considered in IBS-C.

There is increasing evidence for the use of various psychological therapies in the management of IBS regardless of subtype [8, 10]. Cognitive behavioral therapy, hypnotherapy, and mindfulness-based stress reduction have the strongest levels of evidence for use in patients with IBS. Many of these therapies are designed to target triggers for IBS symptoms (i.e., stress management) or develop positive coping strategies for symptoms.

Chronic Constipation

Chronic constipation is one of the most common lower bowel disorders encountered in clinical practice with a worldwide prevalence estimated to be 11.7% [22]. Chronic constipation is associated with high healthcare costs and contributes to reduced quality of life in affected individuals [22]. The high prevalence and societal costs of chronic constipation highlight the importance of providing quality care in this patient group.

Signs and Symptoms of Chronic Constipation

The signs and symptoms of chronic constipation are defined by the Rome IV criteria [6] for functional constipation: straining more than 25% of bowel movements, Bristol Stool Form Scale type 1 or 2 stools more than 25% of bowel movements, sensation of incomplete evacuation more than 25% of bowel movements, sensation of anorectal blockage more than 25% of bowel movements, the use of manual maneuvers to facilitate a bowel movement more than 25% of the time, and/or less than three spontaneous bowel movements per week. Patients must have at least two of the listed symptoms to meet criteria for a diagnosis of functional constipation. Abdominal pain is not a predominant symptom in patients with functional constipation.

Subtypes of Chronic Constipation

There are three subtypes of chronic constipation including normal transit (the primary issue is a decrease in water content of stool), slow transit (there is objective evidence of prolonged transit time), and dyssynergic defecation or functional outlet obstruction [23].

Appropriate Workup of Patients Presenting with Constipation

The first step in evaluating a patient presenting with symptoms of constipation is a thorough history and physical examination [23]. The primary purpose of this is to assess for red flag symptoms (as discussed in Sect. "Irritable Bowel Syndrome" and in Table 14.2) and for potential secondary causes of constipation that should prompt targeted investigations.

Common secondary causes (see Table 14.3) of constipation that affect the motor function of the colon include medications (most commonly opioid medications and anticholinergics), metabolic (hypothyroidism, hypercalcemia, anorexia nervosa, cystic fibrosis) and neurological processes (Parkinson's disease, neuropathic processes, Hirschsprung's disease), smooth muscle myopathies (visceral myopathies), connective tissue disorders (Ehlers-Danlos syndrome, scleroderma, amyloidosis, sarcoidosis), and lifestyle factors such as immobility and poor diet. These may present on the spectrum of mild constipation to severe disease leading to intestinal pseudo-obstruction [24].

In patients presenting with red flag symptoms, structural or systemic causes for constipation should be considered. Structural causes that can lead to constipation include malignancy and inflammatory strictures (particularly in those with a history of inflammatory bowel disease). Fortunately, these are generally rare causes of constipation. The differential diagnoses in those patients that present with symptoms and risk factors suggestive of outlet obstruction (see Table 14.4) as a cause for

Table 14.3 Secondary causes of constipation

Metabolic causes – Diabetes mellitus – Hypercalcemia – Hypothyroidism – Anorexia nervosa
Structural – Obstructive lesion (i.e., malignancy, stricture) – Rectal prolapse – Rectocele – Intussusception
Neuropathic process – Neuropathies (genetic, acquired) – Hirschsprung's disease – Multiple sclerosis – Parkinson's disease – Spinal cord injury – Intestinal pseudo-obstruction
Myopathic – Scleroderma – Infiltrative disease (amyloidosis) – Smooth muscle myopathies
Medications – Opioids – Anticholinergics (antidepressants, antipsychotics, antispasmodics, antihistamines) – Calcium channel blockers – Iron supplements – Aluminum-containing medications – 5HT3 antagonists

Table 14.4 Symptoms and risk factors suggestive of possible obstructive defecation

Symptoms
Urgent bowel movements that require straining to pass
Requirement of digital disimpaction or maneuvers
Prolonged, excessive straining to pass bowel movement
Visible prolapse of tissue from the anal canal
Risk factors
Age
Female sex
Obesity
History of pelvic organ prolapse
Conditions predisposing to organ laxity (i.e., Ehlers-Danlos syndrome)
Pelvic trauma or pelvic surgery history (i.e., rectopexy, hysterectomy, hemorrhoidal intervention, etc.)
Obstetric history including operative vaginal delivery

constipation include functional outlet obstruction (such as dyssynergic defecation) and structural causes such as rectal prolapse, rectocele, anal stenosis, descending perineum syndrome, and intussusception [25].

In patients without red flag symptoms or symptoms suggestive of a secondary cause, investigations overall should be limited [23]. Blood work including complete blood count to rule out anemia, thyroid-stimulating hormone, and calcium level should all be sent. Screening for celiac disease using serology should be performed as it has been estimated that one in ten patients with celiac disease presents with constipation symptoms rather than diarrhea [26]. In female patients with new-onset symptoms, an abdominal/pelvic ultrasound should be performed to rule out ovarian pathology.

As in IBS, there is low diagnostic yield of colonoscopy in patients with constipation unless a structural cause is suspected. In those presenting with constipation as a primary complaint, it is no more likely to find significant pathology on the colonoscopy when compared to age-matched patients undergoing average-risk screening colonoscopies [27].

Abdominal X-ray may have a role in the evaluation of constipation, particularly in the acute phase, if obstruction is suspected. It may also aid in the diagnosis of ileus, chronic intestinal pseudo-obstruction, and Ogilvie's syndrome. Otherwise, it has poor diagnostic potential other than to confirm the presence of fecal loading and should not routinely be ordered for evaluation of chronic constipation [28, 29].

Cross-sectional imaging is generally not utilized in the evaluation of patients presenting with constipation as its resolution for luminal lesions is poor [30]. However, CT colonography may be utilized if the patient cannot tolerate endoscopic evaluation [31] in those whom colonoscopy is indicated. Furthermore, cross-sectional imaging, including abdominal CT scan, CT enterography, or MR/MR enterography, may be helpful in the presence of red flag symptoms to evaluate for structural or the severe motor disorders listed above. Outside of these clinical scenarios, it should not be routinely ordered for the evaluation of constipation.

Anorectal manometry in combination with balloon expulsion testing should only be considered in patients where a functional outlet obstruction or dyssynergic defecation is suspected based on history and physical exam or in those patients with an inadequate response to a trial of conventional therapy [23]. Elements of the history that can be used to help determine if dyssynergic defecation may be a contributor to a patient's constipation include prolonged straining times to have a bowel movement [32]. On physical examination, the digital rectal examination allows for assessment of potential structural secondary causes of constipation and for the evaluation of potential dyssynergic defecation (see Table 14.5). The digital rectal examination has a sensitivity of 75% and specificity of 87% for identifying dyssynergic defecation [33]. Dyssynergic defecation is diagnosed when there are a characteristic defecatory pattern on anorectal manometry and a prolonged balloon expulsion time [6]. In addition to examining anorectal coordination, anorectal manometry allows for the assessment of the rectoanal inhibitory reflex (RAIR). RAIR is an intrinsic reflex, mediated by the myenteric plexus, and is absent in patients with Hirschsprung's disease. The RAIR may also be absent due to numerous causes such as technical issues (air leakage, catheter displacement, artifact), other rectal pathologies

Table 14.5 Steps in a complete digital rectal examination

Explain rationale for exam and the steps involved with patient
Obtain consent from patient to proceed; offer a chaperone to be present if the patient wishes
Patient should be in the left lateral decubitus position and appropriately draped
Examine the perineal area
Examine for the anocutaneous reflex
Examine resting anal sphincter tone; patient may need a few seconds to minutes to relax to properly assess
Examine ability to squeeze the anal sphincter
Examine anorectal function with simulated defecation. Ask the patient to bear down, and they should contract the abdominal muscle walls (one hand should be on the abdomen for this maneuver) and relax the anal sphincter

(mega-rectum, prolapse, ileorectal anastomosis, etc.), and perhaps, most commonly, if a patient cannot relax completely during the procedure [34]. Therefore, the presence of RAIR can rule out Hirschsprung's disease, but its absence does not confirm Hirschsprung's disease. Care should be taken in sending patients with absent RAIR for invasive tissue diagnostic procedures if the clinical suspicion is low [35]. Symptoms that suggest possible Hirschsprung's disease include long-standing symptoms from early childhood, recurrent presentations with fecal impaction, and inadequate response to typical therapies for constipation. In patients with suspicious symptoms and absence of RAIR, full-thickness rectal biopsies are required to rule out Hirschsprung's disease.

Defecography is only considered if there is concern or high likelihood that a structural abnormality at the anorectum may be contributing to symptoms (see Table 14.4) [25]. Real-time images capture the dynamics of the defecation process and can comment on anatomic and/or structural abnormalities such as rectocele, enterocele, rectoanal intussusception, rectal prolapse, pelvic floor dysfunction, dyssynergic defecation, etc. [36].

In the majority of patients with chronic constipation, colonic transit studies, such as sitz marker studies, or wireless motility capsules are not indicated. This should only be considered in those with severe and refractory symptoms in whom potential surgical management is being considered as a last resort therapy [23]. In patients with evidence of dyssynergic defecation, consideration of colonic transit studies should be delayed until the patient has received adequate treatment of the dyssynergia [23]. In dyssynergic defecation, colonic transit studies may be altered due to issues with defecation rather than true slow transit.

Management of Functional Constipation

If a secondary cause of constipation is identified, the underlying issue should be treated. For instance, underlying medical conditions should be managed as best as possible, and offending medications should be substituted or titrated appropriately. But in the case of many processes such as neurological causes, the underlying pathology is irreversible and/or progressive. In these cases, many of the principles of management for functional constipation discussed below will also apply.

As with all lower gastrointestinal motility disorders, including functional constipation, establishing a productive patient-physician relationship and attainable therapeutic goals is a key first step in management. In chronic constipation, the next step should be a focus on lifestyle and dietary modifications particularly in those with mild to moderate symptoms. Supplemental soluble fiber should be first-line in patients with chronic constipation starting at a dose of 3–4 g/day and increasing as tolerated and to effect [37]. Regular and moderate exercise have been shown to improve chronic constipation and should be recommended in all patients with chronic constipation in whom it is safe to do so [38].

In patients who do not respond to lifestyle modifications, pharmacologic therapy is recommended. In many patients with chronic constipation, it is important to stress that symptoms are often better controlled with the use of medication on a regular basis instead of on an as-needed basis. Osmotic laxatives [23], such as polyethylene glycol (PEG), lactulose, and magnesium, are considered first-line pharmacologic therapy for chronic constipation. PEG has several benefits as it has less bloating compared to lactulose, is easily titratable, can be used in chronic renal insufficiency unlike magnesium, and has evidence for use in the older adults.

Stimulant laxatives [23] such as bisacodyl and senna can be considered in patients who do not adequately respond to osmotic laxatives or can be used as rescue therapy for transient worsening of constipation symptoms. The use of these medications is often limited by abdominal pain or cramping.

Secretagogues [23] such as the guanylate cyclase C agonists (linaclotide and plecanatide) and chloride channel agonist (lubiprostone) increase water content of stool. These medications are indicated for use in chronic constipation and should be used in patients who do not respond to the above therapies.

5-HT4 receptor agonists [23], such as prucalopride, decrease colonic transit times and improve frequency of bowel movements in patients with chronic constipation. It is generally well tolerated though side effects do include headache and nausea. Some patients will experience flu-like symptoms during the first week of therapy that typically resolve with continued use.

Patient with dyssynergic defecation often have a suboptimal response to typical pharmacotherapy. Biofeedback therapy involves real-time feedback using verbal commands and visual cues to retrain appropriate defecatory behaviors and improve anorectal coordination during defecation. This is very effective in clinical trials and should be considered first-line in patients with dyssynergic defecation [39].

Sacral nerve stimulation can be effective in those with chronic constipation that have failed management listed above and do not have a structural cause for their symptoms [40]. This procedure involves the temporary placement of a stimulation wire through the sacral foramen, where stimulation currents at varying doses and frequencies are delivered to the sacral nerve [41]. If patients have a positive response, a permanent stimulator is placed. Although there is not a large body of literature regarding the use of sacral nerve stimulation in constipation, most small studies suggest that it can be effective in improving frequency and consistency of stool [42].

The exact mechanism is unclear at this time but is thought to be mediated by modulation of sacral nerve function [43].

Lastly, patients with recalcitrant constipation may require a diverting colostomy/ileostomy or a colectomy [23]. Colectomy should only be considered in those with normal pelvic floor mechanics. The choice between a colostomy or ileostomy is unclear at this time, although a loop procedure may be helpful at triaging a patient to one procedure versus another.

Fecal Incontinence

Incontinence of stool is a common occurrence with North American prevalence noted at 16% and is more common in those over the age of 70 [44]. It is important to recognize that patients may not disclose stool incontinence to physicians, and the practitioner should specifically ask about this as part of a thorough review of systems [45].

Appropriate Workup of Fecal Incontinence

Similar to a constipation history, patients should be asked about relevant past medical and surgical history. Specific to stool incontinence, physicians should determine the frequency and timing of incontinence. The stool consistency should also be determined. With these historical clues, physicians can group incontinence into passive versus urge fecal incontinence [46]. Passive fecal incontinence usually involves seepage of small volumes of stool, but in some cases, patients may have a complete loss of their bowels without their knowledge. Passive incontinence may suggest issues of rectal compliance, rectal hyposensitivity, anal sphincter dysfunction, and/or cognitive impairment. Urge incontinence involves an urgent sensation to defecate with the inability to hold in the bowel movement. This suggests rectal hypersensitivity, poor rectal compliance, loose stool form, and/or anal sphincter dysfunction [47]. Physical exam should include a digital rectal exam with special attention paid to rectal tone and squeeze pressures. Routine blood work should assess for medical causes of diarrhea if present or signs of malignancy.

It is important to note that advanced investigations are usually not necessary for patients with incontinence because the existing treatments for incontinence can be initiated based on the history and physical exam alone [47]. Investigations should be reserved for those with red flag symptoms or for those who do not respond to conventional therapy.

For patients with a history of passive fecal incontinence, endoscopic evaluation should be considered to assess for potential causes of poor rectal compliance such as inflammation or a mass. An assessment for fecal overload using abdominal radiographs can also be helpful, as a cause for impaired rectal compliance.

For patients with a history of urge incontinence and chronic diarrhea, endoscopic evaluation should be considered to exclude inflammatory causes of diarrhea [48]. If underlying pathology is discovered, it should be treated with the aim that improving stool form will improve the incontinence.

Anorectal manometry with balloon expulsion can be utilized for patients with fecal incontinence. Important factors that are evaluated include external and internal anal sphincter function, squeeze duration, rectal sensitivity, and whether a patient was able to expel the balloon [49]. The findings on anorectal manometry can guide therapy and may allow for prognosticating the potential response to therapy.

Anal sphincter electromyography and pudendal nerve studies are uncommonly practiced forms of electromyography. It involves the insertion of sensors and EMG needles into areas of the anal sphincter and perineum. Nerve condition and stimulation are recorded [50]. This technique can help sort out the nature and location of neurologic lesions, but its use is limited by the lack of skilled practitioners and availability. Therefore, its use is not routinely recommended.

Endoscopic ultrasound has been utilized to determine whether there are deficits in the internal or external anal sphincter that may contribute to poor anal sphincter tone. It is the gold standard for assessing structural defect of the anal sphincter. EUS should be considered in patients with a history of anal trauma/surgery or a complex obstetric history with abnormalities on anorectal manometry and a failure of medical management [51]. EUS may also be considered in patients who have sustained an obstetric anal sphincter injury to risk stratify for further vaginal deliveries, but this area is currently under study.

Management of Fecal Incontinence

Initial therapies for management of fecal incontinence include treating underlying pathology that is contributing to diarrhea such as inflammatory bowel disease, or, in the case of suspected overflow incontinence, treating constipation. For most other patients, conservative medical management is often similar despite varying causes of incontinence [48]. Conservative management includes dietary modifications (avoiding triggers of bowel movements such as coffee [52]), avoidance of causative medications, bulking agents such as psyllium fiber [53], antidiarrheal medications [54], and pelvic floor physiotherapy/biofeedback [55].

Sacral nerve stimulation as described above has evidence in the treatment of stool incontinence. Its role is unclear in those with structural disruption of the anal sphincter or in those with suspected denervation of the anal sphincter. Randomized trial data suggests sacral nerve stimulation is more effective than medical management; however, there are a paucity of sham-controlled studies and few experienced surgeons that are available to provide this therapy [56, 57]. This should be considered only in those that have failed the conservative therapies described above.

Several other techniques have been studied including the use of radiofrequency energy [58] and injectable agents [59], but these are poorly studied, and guidance is not clear on their use. For these reasons, these interventions are not generally recommended for management of fecal incontinence.

Lastly, surgical management of fecal incontinence includes correction of obstructing deficits that may be contributing to incontinence (i.e., rectal prolapse, large rectoceles, etc.), colostomy, sphincteroplasty, or, less commonly, muscle transposition surgery [60]. Surgical management should be considered only after all other therapies have been exhausted. Sphincteroplasty has been best studied in the realm of external anal sphincter deficits, where the defect is repaired by overlapping the intact portions of the external anal sphincter [61]. Current data suggests this approach is effective; however, the effectiveness may decline over time [62].

Opioid-Induced Bowel Disorders

Opioids can have a profound effect on lower gastrointestinal motor and sensory function. Opioid-induced constipation [6] is diagnosed in patients presenting with signs and symptoms of constipation that are new or worsen with starting, changing, or increasing opioid therapy. Management of patients with opioid-induced constipation should include many of the therapies described above for functional constipation. Unfortunately, those therapies are often incompletely effective in opioid-induced constipation. In this patient group, an additional management consideration is the use of peripherally acting μ-opioid receptor antagonists (PAMORAs) [63]. PAMORAs have limited ability to cross the blood-brain barrier and thus act to reduce the effects of opioids in the periphery and have been demonstrated to improve constipation in opioid-induced constipation.

Narcotic bowel syndrome, also known as opioid-induced gastrointestinal hyperalgesia, is characterized by the presence of chronic abdominal pain that has been treated with high-dose or chronic opioids [64]. The abdominal pain in this condition does not resolve or worsens with increasing doses of opioids, worsens when opioid doses are decreased, and progressively worsens over time in terms of frequency, intensity, and duration. The mainstay of treatment of narcotic bowel syndrome is weaning and, ultimately, stopping the use of opioids. Treatment typically should involve a team approach including primary care physician, gastroenterologist, and addiction medicine physician/psychiatrist to work with patients to stop their opioid use.

Conclusion

Lower gastrointestinal motility disorders are common in clinical practice. Ensuring high-quality care of these patients is imperative to improve outcomes and has the potential to make significant impacts in the lives of patients with these conditions. Importantly, we suggest that high-quality care does not infer excessive diagnostic testing in the vast majority of patients.

References

1. Shivaji UN, Ford AC. Prevalence of functional gastrointestinal disorders among consecutive new patient referrals to a gastroenterology clinic. Frontline Gastroenterol. 2014;5(4):266–71.
2. Sperber AD, Bangdiwala SI, Drossman DA, Ghoshal UC, Simren M, Tack J, et al. Worldwide prevalence and burden of functional gastrointestinal disorders, results of Rome foundation global study. Gastroenterology. 2021;160(1):99–114.
3. Drossman DA, Morris CBB, Schneck S, Hu YJ, Norton NJ, Norton WF, et al. International survey of patients with IBS: symptom features and their severity, health status, treatments, and risk taking to achieve clinical benefit. J Clin Gastroenterol. 2009;43(6):541–50.
4. Fedorak RN, Vanner S, Paterson WG, Bridges RJ. Canadian Digestive Health Foundation public impact series 3: irritable bowel syndrome in Canada. Incidence, prevalence, and direct and indirect economic impact. Can J Gastroenterol. 2012;26(5):252–6.
5. Ford AC, Lacy BE, Talley NJ. Irritable bowel syndrome. N Engl J Med. 2017;376(26):2566–78.
6. Lacy BE, Mearin F, Chang L, Chey WD, Lembo AJ, Simren M, et al. Bowel disorders. Gastroenterology. 2016;150(6):1393–407.
7. Lewis SJ, Heaton KW. Stool form scale as a useful guide to intestinal transit time. Scand J Gastroenterol. 1997;32:920–4.
8. Lacy BE, Pimentel M, Brenner D, Chey WD, Keefer LA, Long MD, et al. ACG clinical guideline: management of irritable bowel syndrome. Am J Gastroenterol. 2021;116(1):17–44.
9. Chey WD, Kurlander J, Eswaran S. Irritable bowel syndrome: a clinical review. JAMA. 2015;313(9):949–58.
10. Moayyedi P, Andrews CN, MacQueen G, Korownyk C, Marsiglio M, Graff L, et al. Canadian Association of Gastroenterology Clinical Practice Guideline for the management of irritable bowel syndrome (IBS). JCAG. 2019;2(1):6–29.
11. Lembo A, Pimentel M, Rao SS. Repeat treatment with rifaximin is safe and effective in patients with diarrhea predominant irritable bowel syndrome. Gastroenterology. 2016;151:1113–21.
12. Yu D, Cheeseman F, Vanner S. Combined oro-caecal scintigraphy and lactulose hydrogen breath testing demonstrate that breath testing detects oro-caecal transit, not small intestinal bacterial overgrowth in patients with IBS. Gut. 2011;60(3):334–40.
13. Cash BD, Schoenfeld P, Chey WD. The utility of diagnostic tests in irritable bowel syndrome patients: a systematic review. Am J Gastroenterol. 2002;97(11):2812–9.
14. Rex DK. Colonoscopy: a review of its yield for cancers and adenomas by indication. Am J Gastroenterol. 1995;90(3):353–65.
15. Spiegel BMR, Gralnek IM, Bolus R, Chang L, Dulai GSBN, et al. Is a negative colonoscopy associated with reassurance or improved health-related quality of life in irritable bowel syndrome? Gastrointest Endosc. 2005;62(6):892–9.
16. Drossman DA, Ruddy J. Improving patient-provider relationships to improve health care. Clin Gastroenterol Hepatol. 2020;18(7):1417–26.
17. Halmos EP, Power VA, Shepher SJ, Gibson PR, Muir JG. A diet low in FODMAPs reduces symptoms of irritable bowel syndrome. Gastroenterology. 2014;146(1):67–75.
18. Chang L, Sultan S, Lembo A, Verne GN, Smalley W, Heidelbaugh JJ. AGA clinical practice guideline on the pharmacological management of irritable bowel syndrome with constipation. Gastroenterol. 2022;163(1):118–36.
19. Lembo A, Sultan S, Chang L, Heidelbaugh JJ, Smalley W, Verne GN. AGA clinical practice guideline on the pharmacological management of irritable bowel syndrome with diarrhea. Gastroenterology. 2022;163(1):137–51.
20. Wedlake L, A'Hern R, Russell D. Systematic review: the prevalence of idiopathic bile acid malabsorption as diagnosed by SeHCAT scanning in patients with diarrhea-predominant irritable bowel syndrome. Aliment Pharmacol Ther. 2009;30(7):707–17.
21. Drossman DA, Tack J, Ford AC, Szigethy E, Tornblom H, Van Oudenhove L. Neuromodulators for functional GI disorders (disorders of gut-brain interaction): a Rome Foundation Working Team report. Gastroenterology. 2018;154(4):1140–1171.

22. Suares NC, Ford AC. Prevalence of, and risk factors for, chronic idiopathic constipation in the community: systematic review and meta-analysis. Am J Gastroenterol. 2011;106(9):1582–91. quiz 1, 92
23. Aziz I, Whitehead WE, Palsson OS, Tornblom H, Simren M. An approach to the diagnosis and management of Rome IV functional disorders of chronic constipation. Expert Rev Gastroenterol Hepatol. 2020;14(1):39–49.
24. Andrews CN, Storr M. The pathophysiology of chronic constipation. Can J Gastroenterol. 2011;25:16B–21B.
25. Sharma A, Herekar A, Yan Y, Karunaratne T, Rao SSC. Dyssynergic defecation and other evacuation disorders. Gastroenterol Clin. 2022;51(1):55–69.
26. Spljkerman M, Tan IL, Kolkman JJ. A large variety of clinical features and concomitant disorders in celiac disease- a cohort study in The Netherlands. Dig Liver Dis. 2016;48(5):499–505.
27. Gupta M, Holub J, Knigge K, Eisen G. Constipation is not associated with an increased rate of findings on colonoscopy: results from a national endoscopy consortium. Endoscopy. 2010;42(3):208–12.
28. Hoskins B, Marek S. Things we do for no reason: obtaining an abdominal X-ray to assess for constipation in children. J Hosp Med. 2020;15(9):557–9.
29. Driver BE, Chittineni C, Kartha G, Cole JB, Klein LR, Rischall M. Utility of plain abdominal radiography in adult ED patients with suspected constipation. Am J Emerg Med. 2020;38(6):1092–6.
30. Lao IH, Chao H, Wang YJ, Mak CW, Tzeng WS, Wu RH, et al. Computed tomography has low sensitivity for the diagnosis of early colon cancer. Color Dis. 2013;15(7):807–77.
31. Plumb AA, Halligan S, Pendse DA, Taylor SA, Mallett S. Sensitivity and specificity of CT colonography for the detection of colonic neoplasia after positive faecal occult blood testing: systematic review and meta-analysis. Eur Radiol. 2014;24(5):1049–58.
32. Parker CH, Tomlinson GA, Correia AJ, Liu LW. Predictability of functional defecation disorder in patients with chronic constipation using a standardized constipation symptom questionnaire. Gastroenterology. 146(5):S-717.
33. Tantiphlachiva K, Rao P, Attaluri A, Rao SS. Digital rectal examination is a useful tool for identifying patients with dyssynergia. Clin Gastroenterol Hepatol. 2010;8(11):955–60.
34. Baaleman DF, Malamisura M, Benninga MA, Bali N, Vaz KH, Yacob D, et al. The not-so-rare absent RAIR: internal anal sphincter achalasia in a review of 1072 children with constipation undergoing high-resolution anorectal manometry. Neurogastroenterol Motil. 2021;33:e14028.
35. Bharucha AE, Basilisco G, Malcolm A, Lee TH, Hoy MB, Scott SM, et al. Review of the indications, methods, and clinical utility of anorectal manometry and the rectal balloon expulsion test. Neurogastroenterol Motil. 2022;34(9):e14335
36. Lalwani N, Khatri G, El Sayed RF, Ram R, Jambhekar K, Chernyak V, et al. MR defecography technique: recommendations of the society of abdominal radiology's disease-focused panel on pelvic floor imaging. Abdom Radiol. 2021;46(4):1351–61.
37. Suares NC, Ford AC. Systematic review: the effects of fibre in the management of chronic idiopathic constipation. Aliment Pharmacol Ther. 2011;33(8):895–901.
38. Gao R, Tao Y, Zhou C. Exercise therapy in patients with constipation: a systematic review and meta-analysis of randomized controlled trials. Scand J Gastroenterol. 2019;54(2):169–77.
39. Rao SS, Patcharatrakul T. Diagnosis and treatment of dyssynergic defecation. J Neurogastroenterol Motil. 2016;22(3):423–35.
40. Thomas GP, Dudding TC, Nicholls RJ, Vaizey CJ. Bilateral transcutaneous posterior tibial nerve stimulation for the treatment of fecal incontinence. Dis Colon Rectum. 2013;56(9):1075–9.
41. Matzel KE, Stadelmaier U, Hohenfellner M, Gall FP. Electrical stimulation of sacral spinal nerves for treatment of faecal incontinence. Lancet. 1995;346(8983):1124–7.
42. Kamm MA, Dudding TC, Melenhorst J, Jarrett ME, Wang Z, Buntzen S, et al. Sacral nerve stimulation for intractable constipation. Gut. 2010;59(3):333–40.
43. Norderval S, Rydningen M, Lindsetmo R, Lein D, Vonen B. Sacral nerve stimulation. Tidzzkr Nor Laegeforen. 2011;131(12):1190–3.

44. Ditah I, Devaki P, Luma HN, Ditah C, Njei B, Jaiyeoba C, et al. Prevalence, trends, and risk factors for fecal incontinence in United States adults, 2005-2010. Clin Gastroenterol Hepatol. 2014;12(4):636–43.
45. Frank C, Molnar F, Spencer M. Fecal incontinence in older adults. Can Fam Physician. 2020;66(4):264.
46. Knol ME, Snijders HS, van der Heyden JTM, Baeten CIM. Fecal incontinence: the importance of a structured pathophysiological model. J Anus Rectum Colon. 2022;6(1):58–66.
47. Guillaume A, Salem AE, Garcia P, Roland BC. Pathophysiology and therapeutic options for fecal incontinence. J Clin Gastroenterol. 2017;51(4):324–30.
48. Lazarescu A, Turnbull GK, Vanner S. Investigating and treating fecal incontinence: when and how. Can J Gastroenterol. 2009;23(4):301–8.
49. Scott SM, Carrington EV. The London classification: improving characterization and classification of anorectal function with anorectal manometry. Curr Gastroenterol Rep. 2020;22(11):55–67.
50. Podnar S, Vodusek DB, Stalberg E. Standardization of anal sphincter electromyography: normative data. Clin Neurophysiol. 2000;111(12):2200–7.
51. Albuquerque A. Endoanal ultrasonography in fecal incontinence: current and future perspectives. World J Gastroenterol Endosc. 2015;7(6):575–81.
52. Brown SR, Cann PA, Read NW. Effect of coffee on distal colon function. Gut. 1990;31(4):450–3.
53. Bliss DZ, Jung HJ, Savik K, Lowry A, LeMoine M, Jensen L, et al. Supplementation with dietary fiber improves fecal incontinence. Nurs Res. 2001;50(4):203–13.
54. Read M, Read NW, Barber DC, Duthie HL. Effects of loperamide on anal sphincter function in patients complaining of chronic diarrhea with fecal incontinence and urgency. Dig Dis Sci. 1982;27(9):807–14.
55. Ussing A, Dahn I, Due U, Sorensen M, Petersen J, Bandholm T. Efficacy of supervised pelvic floor muscle training and biofeedback vs attention-control treatment in adults with fecal incontinence. Clin Gastroenterol Hepatol. 2019;17(11):2253–61.
56. Kahlke V, Topic H, Peleikis H, Jongen J. Sacral nerve modulation for fecal incontinence: results of a prospective single-center randomized crossover study. Dis Colon Rectum. 2015;58(2):235–40.
57. Tan E, Ngo N, Darzi A, Shenouda M, Tekkis PP. Meta-analysis: sacral nerve stimulation versus conservative therapy in the treatment of faecal incontinence. Int J Color Dis. 2011;26(3):275–94.
58. Efron JE, Corman ML, Fleshman J, Barnett J, Nagle D, Birnbaum E, et al. Safety and effectiveness of temperature-controlled radio-frequency energy delivery to the anal canal (Secca procedure) for the treatment of fecal incontinence. Dis Colon Rectum. 2003;46(12):1606–16.
59. Tjandra JJ, Lim JF, Hiscock R, Rajendra P. Injectable silicone biomaterial for fecal incontinence caused by internal anal sphincter dysfunction is effective. Dis Colon Rectum. 2004;47(12):2138–46.
60. Forte ML, Andrade KE, Lowry AC, Butler M, Bliss DZ. Systematic review of surgical treatments for fecal incontinence. Dis Colon Rectum. 2016;53:443–69.
61. Dudding TC, Vaizey CJ, Kamm MA. Obstetric anal sphincter injury: incidence, risk factors, and management. Ann Surg. 2008;247(2):224–37.
62. Gutierrez AB, Madoff RD, Lowry AC, Parker SC, Buie WD, Baxter NN. Long-term results of anterior sphincteroplasty. Dis Colon Rectum. 2004;47(5):727–31.
63. Pergolizzi JV, Christo PJ, LeQuang JA, Magnusson P. The use of peripheral μ-opioid receptor antagonists (PAMORA) in the management of opioid-induced constipation: an update on their efficacy and safety. Drug Des Devel Ther. 2020;14:1009–25.
64. Keefer L, Drossman DA, Guthrie E, Simren M, Tillisch K, Olden K, et al. Centrally mediated disorders of gastrointestinal pain. Gastroenterology. 2016;150(6):1408–19.

Chapter 15
Pancreatic Diseases

Tarek Nammour and David X. Jin

Table of Quality Measures/Metrics

T. Nammour · D. X. Jin (✉)
Division of Gastroenterology, Hepatology and Endoscopy, Department of Medicine, Brigham and Women's Hospital, Boston, MA, USA
e-mail: djin@bwh.harvard.edu

J. D. Feuerstein, D. J. Stein (eds.), *Quality in Gastroenterology*,
https://doi.org/10.1007/978-3-031-58492-3_15

Key Points

- Diagnosis of acute pancreatitis requires at least two of the following three criteria: presence of characteristic abdominal pain, elevation in serum amylase and/or lipase >3× normal, and/or presence of characteristic changes on abdominal CT or MRI. Early imaging should be reserved for diagnostic uncertainty.
- Treatment of acute pancreatitis consists of goal-directed fluid resuscitation, early oral feeding as tolerated, analgesic support, and management of fluid collections.
- Chronic pancreatitis is characterized by abdominal pain and functional impairment. Treatment focuses on controlling symptoms and supporting endocrine and exocrine pancreatic insufficiency.
- Pancreatic cystic neoplasms are diagnosed with increasing frequency due to the widespread use of abdominal imaging. Accurate diagnosis is important for guiding subsequent management.

Introduction

Pancreatic diseases comprise a wide range of disorders that can significantly impact the lives of patients. We aim in this concise chapter to deliver an evidence-based update focused on three commonly encountered pancreatic disorders: acute pancreatitis, chronic pancreatitis, and pancreatic cystic neoplasms. Understanding key concepts in the management of these disorders is important to provide high-quality care and improve patient outcomes.

Acute Pancreatitis

Acute pancreatitis (AP) is an acute inflammatory condition of the pancreas characterized by abdominal pain and the occasional development of local and systemic complications. It is considered a leading cause of hospitalization and is associated with significant morbidity and mortality. The majority of patients will have a mild hospital course; however, 10–20% of patients can experience a more severe presentation characterized by organ failure and a mortality rate of up to 40% [1].

Incidence

The global incidence of AP is increasing in most western countries over the last 50 years. This increase has been attributed to an increased incidence of biliary disease [2]. In the USA, the incidence of AP is around 82 per 100,000 adults per year [3]. AP is responsible for more than 380,000 emergency department visits and

288,000 hospitalizations annually. The estimated median healthcare cost of every AP hospital admission is $26,434 [4].

Etiologies

The most common causes of AP are listed in Table 15.1. Determining the etiology of AP is important to prevent recurrence and/or progression to chronic pancreatitis as the majority of causes are treatable.

Gallstones and alcohol account for 70% of cases of AP in the USA [5]. Despite being the most common cause of AP, only 4–8% of patients with gallstones develop pancreatitis [6]. The mechanism is believed to be related to transient or complete obstruction of the ampulla during gallstones passage or reflux of bile into the pancreatic duct. Elevation in liver enzymes in the presence of AP is suggestive of a biliary etiology [7].

Alcohol-induced AP typically occurs after several years of heavy alcohol consumption (usually more than 20 g/day of alcohol) [8]. The risk is dose-dependent; however, only 10% of chronic alcohol abusers develop AP, suggesting the presence of other factors (genetics, tobacco) that increase the susceptibility to alcohol [9].

Table 15.1 Causes of acute pancreatitis

Alcohol
Autoimmune
Biliary (gallstones, microlithiasis/sludge)
Drugs
Iatrogenic (post-ERCP, postsurgical: common bile duct exploration, sphincterotomy, splenectomy, distal gastrectomy)
Idiopathic
Infection (viruses, e.g., mumps, hepatitis, coxsackievirus, cytomegalovirus, varicella-zoster virus. Bacteria, e.g., salmonella, mycoplasma, legionella, tuberculosis, *Mycobacterium avium* complex. Parasites, e.g., ascaris, *Clonorchis sinensis*)
Inherited (***PRSS1*** (cationic trypsinogen)-related hereditary pancreatitis mutations), ***CFTR*** (cystic fibrosis transmembrane conductance regulator) mutations, ***SPINK1*** (serine protease inhibitor Kazal type 1) mutations
Metabolic (hypercalcemia, hypertriglyceridemia)
Neoplastic (pancreatic or ampullary tumors)
Structural (e.g., pancreatic divisum, annular pancreas, sphincter of Oddi dysfunction, periampullary diverticula, duodenal duplication cysts, choledochocele, anomalous pancreaticobiliary junction)
Smoking
Toxin (e.g., organophosphates, scorpion venom)
Traumatic
Vascular disorders/vasculitis (e.g., hypotension, microscopic polyangiitis, Wegener's granulomatosis)

ERCP endoscopic retrograde cholangiopancreatography

Besides alcohol, smoking independently increases the risk of AP, recurrent AP, and chronic pancreatitis (CP).

High serum triglyceride levels can cause AP typically when levels exceed 1000 mg/dl. Hypercalcemia is a rare but treatable cause of AP. Several drugs have been implicated as a cause for AP. The diagnosis of drug-induced pancreatitis is challenging but may be considered when a temporal exposure to an offending agent is established and other common causes have been ruled out. Post-endoscopic retrograde cholangiopancreatography (ERCP) pancreatitis is the most common iatrogenic cause with an incidence rate of 3–10% in systematic reviews [10]. Other etiologies include various infections, exposure to certain toxins, anatomic variations, and trauma. In 15–20% of patients, no cause is found even after a thorough evaluation [11]. Despite being labeled as idiopathic AP, a significant proportion of these cases are caused by biliary sludge (microlithiasis) not evident on the initial abdominal US. Endoscopic ultrasound (EUS) and magnetic resonance cholangiopancreatography (MRCP) examinations after resolution of symptoms can be used for the evaluation of biliary sludge, pancreatic neoplasia, and anatomic variations. In a young patient with recurrent idiopathic pancreatitis or with a family history of pancreatitis, testing for genetic mutations in *PRSS1*, *SPINK1*, and *CFTR*, among others, is appropriate.

Clinical Features

AP is characterized by an acute onset of severe persistent abdominal pain, localized to the epigastrium, and radiating to the back in 50% of cases. Patients often have accompanied nausea, vomiting, and anorexia. In severe AP, patients may have associated signs and symptoms related to systemic inflammatory response syndrome (SIRS) and organ failure. Physical examination typically reveals abdominal tenderness and may also show guarding and rebound tenderness. Other signs include abdominal distention, hypoactive bowel sounds secondary to ileus, fever, tachypnea, tachycardia, and hypotension. Rarely, patients may develop ecchymosis in the flanks (Grey-Turner's sign) or periumbilical areas (Cullen's sign). They occur in less than 3% of patients due to retroperitoneal bleeding and are associated with a high mortality rate [12].

Diagnosis

The diagnosis of AP depends on the presence of two of the following three criteria: characteristic abdominal pain, elevation in serum amylase and/or lipase to three times or greater the upper limit of normal, and characteristic imaging findings of AP on contrast-enhanced CT or magnetic resonance imaging (MRI) [13]. In the vast majority of cases, the diagnosis can be made without the need for imaging. Early imaging (CT or MRI) is reserved for cases where the diagnosis of AP is uncertain, or when an alternative life-threatening condition needs to be ruled out [14]. After the diagnosis has been determined, a complete history (prior episodes, known gallstones, alcohol intake, medication usage, recent procedure, family history of pancreatic disease), physical examination, laboratory tests (liver enzymes, calcium, triglycerides), and imaging (right upper quadrant US) should be carried out to investigate the etiology of AP.

Imaging

Abdominal US is recommended as the initial imaging of a patient with suspected AP. The aim is to investigate the presence of cholelithiasis, choledocholithiasis, or signs of extrahepatic biliary tract obstruction.

Despite various guidelines discouraging the use of routine early CT imaging in AP, it remains overutilized [14]. At presentation, CT imaging should be reserved for cases of diagnostic uncertainty. Following 72–96 h after the onset of symptoms, CT imaging may be considered to evaluate for local complications such as necrosis or fluid collection in the setting of clinical deterioration or persistent abdominal pain [15].

MRI can similarly be used to assess for complications. The advantages of MRI include improved sensitivity for detection of biliary pathology, a lack of radiation, a lower risk of nephrotoxicity compared to iodinated CT contrast, and the ability to use non-enhanced MRI to identify necrosis in patients who cannot receive IV contrast [16]. The use of MRI may be limited to local availability and expertise. In addition, it requires a longer scanning time, limiting its use for critically ill patients.

Classification of Severity and Prediction Models

Severity assessment is important for appropriate triage and management. While the majority of patients will develop a mild course, up to 15% of patients may have severe disease with mortality reaching 30–60% in some cases [17].

The 2012 revised Atlanta Classification categorizes AP into mild, moderately severe, and severe disease based on the presence (or absence) of organ failure and local/systemic complications (Table 15.2) [13]. Organ failure is defined as a score of

Table 15.2 Classification of acute pancreatitis

Classification	Organ failure	Local complications	Systemic complications
Mild	None	None	None
Moderately severe	Transient (≤48 h)	Yes (without persistent organ failure)	Yes (without persistent organ failure)
Severe	Persistent organ failure (>48 h) involving one or more organs	Yes	Yes

Source: adapted from Banks et al. [13]

2 or above for at least one of the three organ systems (respiratory, cardiovascular, and renal) using the modified Marshall scoring system [18]. Persistent organ failure (more than 48 hours) is considered one of the strongest determinants of mortality in AP. In addition, persistent multiple organ failure is associated with higher mortality rate compared to single persistent organ failure [19]. Local complications refer to fluid collections that develop in the acute setting (acute (peri)pancreatic fluid collection and acute necrotic collections) as well as those that develop after 4 weeks (pancreatic pseudocyst and walled-off necrosis). Other local complications include gastric outlet dysfunction, splanchnic vein thrombosis, and colonic necrosis. Systemic complications represent an exacerbation of preexisting comorbid conditions, such as coronary artery disease, congestive heart failure, or chronic lung disease.

Several clinical models have been validated for the prediction of poor outcomes in AP and should be utilized at presentation. Of these, SIRS and the Bedside Index of Severity in Acute Pancreatitis (BISAP) are commonly used and easy to calculate. One study showed that nearly 50% of patients who fulfilled all four SIRS criteria (temperature <36 °C or >38 °C, heart rate >90/min, respiratory rate >20/min, white blood cells $<4 \times 10^6$/mL or $>12 \times 10^6$/mL, or >10% immature bands) on presentation needed intensive care unit (ICU) admission within the first week [20]. BISAP considers five criteria: BUN >25 mg/dL, impaired mental status, presence of SIRS, age >50, and the presence of a pleural effusion. One point is given for each, and a score of more than 3 is associated with an increased risk of developing organ failure, pancreatic necrosis, and increased mortality [21].

The Pancreatitis Activity Scoring System (PASS) is a more recent clinical model that comprises five weighted parameters: organ failure, SIRS, abdominal pain, analgesics requirement, and diet tolerance [22]. An elevated admission PASS score is associated with higher disease severity, SIRS development, ICU admission, local complications, and prolonged length of stay. An elevated PASS score on discharge is associated with early readmission rates [23].

Other factors that have been shown to predict severity in AP include older age (>60 years), obesity, comorbid disease, the presence of hemoconcentration on admission (hematocrit >44%), and rise in BUN during the initial resuscitation period.

Treatment

The basis of treatment includes early evaluation of severity, appropriate triage, fluid resuscitation, symptomatic support, and treatment of the underlying etiology.

Patients with AP should be observed closely in the first few days of presentation. This includes monitoring vital signs, daily fluid balance, urine output, and serum electrolytes. Those with, or predicted to develop, organ failure should be monitored in the ICU.

Intravenous fluid resuscitation is considered the basis of therapy in AP. The goal is to replace the lost circulatory fluids secondary to inflammation, vascular permeability, and fluid sequestration. In addition, fluid replacement helps maintain oxygenation and perfusion of organ systems. Lactated Ringer's solution is preferred over normal saline as the crystalloid fluid of choice with studies suggesting a decreasing rate of SIRS, hospital stay, and ICU admissions [24].

There is controversy regarding the appropriate rate and volume of resuscitation. Most society guidelines have recommended aggressive fluid resuscitation on the basis that prior studies have shown poor outcomes in AP patients who were under-resuscitated. Recently, the WATERFALL study (the Early Weight-Based Aggressive vs. Nonaggressive Goal-Directed Fluid Resuscitation in the Early Phase of Acute Pancreatitis: an Open-Label Multicenter Randomized Controlled Trial) showed that early aggressive fluid resuscitation (bolus of 20 ml/kg body weight and then infusion 3 ml/kg/h) was associated with higher incidence of fluid overload with no improvement in clinical outcomes [25]. The results favored a moderate resuscitation protocol with an initial rate of no more than 1.5 ml/kg/h. with a bolus of 10 ml/kg only if there are signs of hypovolemia. Regardless of rate, volume, or type of fluids, clinical and hemodynamic parameters such as heart rate, blood pressure, urine output, hematocrit, and BUN should be carefully monitored. Patients with fluid overload can benefit from diuresis in the first few days of resuscitation.

Analgesia should be offered in the early stage. A stepped approach is recommended for pain medication. Non-opioid analgesics can be used for mild AP. Opioid medications are considered for patients with constant and/or severe pain not controlled on non-opioid analgesics. An enhanced recovery strategy encouraging non-opioid analgesia, patient-directed early initiation of oral feeding, and early ambulation was shown to be safe and effective in patients hospitalized with AP and was associated with earlier time to refeeding [26].

In addition to treating pancreatic inflammation, it is essential to address the underlying causative factors. For cases of mild biliary pancreatitis, a same admission cholecystectomy should be performed prior to discharge as it has been shown to be a cost-effective method to prevent readmission due to biliary complications [27]. Surgery can be postponed for moderately severe and severe cases until symptoms resolve. For drug-induced pancreatitis, the offending agents should be discontinued. For patients with hypertriglyceridemia-induced pancreatitis, infusions of insulin and/or plasmapheresis may be used. For hypercalcemia-induced pancreatitis, treatment is directed at normalizing serum calcium and determining the underlying etiology.

Most (peri)pancreatic fluid collections, including sterile necrosis, will not need intervention. However, sterile collections that cause symptoms such as pain, nausea, vomiting, early satiety, weight loss, or jaundice secondary to mass effect will require drainage.

Another indication for intervention is the development of infected pancreatic necrosis (IPN). Infected necrosis should be suspected when patients with necrotizing pancreatitis clinically deteriorate or fail to improve after 7 days of hospitalization. It can be confirmed by the presence of gas within a fluid collection on imaging or with a positive gram stain or culture via percutaneous aspiration. Antibiotics should be started once a diagnosis of IPN is made. When indicated, drainage or debridement should ideally be deferred for at least 4 weeks until necrotic collections have consolidated with the development of "walled-off necrosis." Recent evidence showed that a postponed drainage strategy as compared to immediate drainage (within 24 h) results in fewer invasive interventions without affecting mortality or adverse events [28]. The choice of intervention depends on the location and extension of the cyst, the presence of necrosis, and the status of the patient. In general, an endoscopic step-up approach is recommended [29]. Percutaneous drainage is used if endoscopy is unsuccessful or unfeasible. Surgery is reserved for patients who failed endoscopic and/or percutaneous interventions.

Nutrition

Early oral feeding is important in AP. It should be allowed as soon as the patients are hungry and ideally when they are not vomiting with improved nausea and abdominal pain. Initiating a low-fat solid diet is safe, does not increase adverse events, and is associated with decreased hospital stay [30]. If patients develop oral feeding intolerance, defined as relapse of symptoms after initiating oral feeding, enteral nutrition can be started with either nasogastric or nasojejunal tubes as both have similar efficacy and safety. Enteral feeding can be delayed for 72 h in patients with mild and moderately severe AP to assess if they can tolerate oral feeding. However, it should not be delayed more than 48 h in severe AP. Parenteral nutrition should be reserved for patients intolerant of enteral feeding.

Role of Antibiotics and Endoscopic Retrograde Cholangiopancreatography

Prophylactic antibiotics have no role in preventing IPN or decreasing mortality [31]. Antibiotics should be used in the setting of cholangitis, if there is evidence of extra-pancreatic infection, or once the diagnosis of IPN is made.

ERCP with sphincterotomy should be performed urgently (within 24 hours) in patients with gallstones pancreatitis and concomitant cholangitis. Otherwise, elective ERCP can be scheduled for patients with persistent biliary obstruction. EUS or MRCP can be performed to assess the need for ERCP in patients with persistently elevated liver enzymes and/or dilation of the common bile duct without clinical cholangitis.

Prognosis

An episode of AP is associated with an increased long-term risk of exocrine and endocrine insufficiency. In a systematic review, diabetes mellitus was found in 23% of patients following AP episodes. Fifteen percent developed new-onset diabetes mellitus within 1 year after the first AP event [32]. The prevalence of exocrine insufficiency following AP can reach 27%, especially in patients with severe presentation [33]. Screening for exocrine and endocrine insufficiency is recommended even after a single AP episode.

Patients are at increased risk of developing recurrent pancreatitis and progression to chronic pancreatitis (CP) following their first AP event. The risk is highest among smokers, alcohol abusers, and those with necrosis.

Multiple studies have demonstrated an association between AP and pancreatic cancer. The risk appears to be highest during the 5 years following AP. Patients who are older than 40 years, especially those with associated risk factors such as smoking, alcohol, diabetes, and obesity, should be monitored for concerning symptoms [34].

Chronic Pancreatitis

CP is a disorder of progressive pancreatic inflammation and fibrosis characterized by abdominal pain, exocrine and endocrine insufficiency, and detectable damage on imaging studies. In the USA, the reported incidence is around 5–12 per 100,000 and the prevalence is 50 per 100,000 [34].

Etiologies

The etiologies of CP are classified using the "Toxic-metabolic, Idiopathic, Genetic, Autoimmune, Recurrent and severe acute pancreatitis and Obstructive" (TIGAR-O) system and summarized in Table 15.3 [35].

Chronic alcohol use and tobacco smoking are considered the most common causes of CP. Most patients need to consume more than 80 g of alcohol/day for more than 6 years to develop CP. The more alcohol is consumed, the greater the risk of disease developing. However, only a minority of heavy alcohol abusers develop CP suggesting the presence of other contributing factors. Smoking can cause CP in an independent and dose-dependent manner.

Autoimmune pancreatitis is a distinct inflammatory condition affecting the pancreas among other organs that dramatically respond to steroid therapy. Two subtypes of autoimmune pancreatitis exist. Type 1 is associated with elevated IgG4 levels and other organ involvement. Type 2 or idiopathic duct-centric pancreatitis (IDCP) is associated with inflammatory bowel disease in approximately 15% of cases.

Chronic obstruction of the pancreatic duct by malignancy, stones, cysts, or strictures can lead to upstream inflammation and atrophy. It is controversial whether pancreatic divisum and sphincter of Oddi dysfunction can be considered primary causes of CP. Other causes include genetic mutations and polymorphisms, hypertriglyceridemia, and hypercalcemia. If an extensive workup (including genetic studies) fails to determine a cause for CP, the disease is labeled idiopathic.

Table 15.3 Causes of chronic pancreatitis

Toxic-metabolic	Alcohol
	Smoking
	Hypercalcemia
	Hypertriglyceridemia
	Medications
	Toxins (chronic kidney disease, oxidative stress)
	Metabolic (diabetes mellitus, obesity, diet)
Idiopathic	Early onset (<35 years of age)
	Late onset (>35 years of age)
Genetic	Suspected (no or limited genotyping available)
	Autosomal dominant (*PRSS1* mutation (hereditary pancreatitis), CEL—MODY8 phenotype)
	Autosomal recessive (*CFTR, SPINK1*)
	Complex genetics (non-Mendelian, genotype ± environment)
	Modifier genes (pathogenic genetic variants)
	Hypertriglyceridemia syndromes
Autoimmune	Autoimmune pancreatitis type 1 (IgG4-related disease)
	Autoimmune pancreatitis type 2
Recurrent acute pancreatitis and severe acute pancreatitis	Acute pancreatitis (single episode)
	Biliary pancreatitis
	Post-ERCP
	Traumatic
	Ischemic
	Infectious
	Recurrent acute pancreatitis
Obstructive	Pancreatic divisum
	Ampullary stenosis
	Main duct pancreatic stones
	Widespread pancreatic calcifications
	Main pancreatic duct strictures
	Localized mass causing duct obstruction
	Mass effect

Source: adapted from Whitcomb [35]
ERCP endoscopic retrograde cholangiopancreatography

Clinical Features

Abdominal pain is the most common clinical presentation. The pattern varies from intermittent to constant with periods of severe exacerbation. The presence and severity of pain do not necessarily correlate with the extent of CP as some patients may be free of any pain. Other related symptoms include nausea, vomiting, anorexia, and weight loss.

Exocrine pancreatic insufficiency may present as bloating, weight loss, and steatorrhea. At least 90% of the gland's exocrine function needs to be damaged for steatorrhea to manifest. Patients may develop osteopenia and osteoporosis and are at increased risk of bone fractures. Endocrine insufficiency manifesting as type 3c diabetes mellitus is usually a late presentation.

Diagnosis and Imaging Techniques

The diagnosis of CP is based on a thorough history and physical examination, followed by cross-sectional imaging and functional testing. History-taking focuses on the presence of clinical symptoms and signs (abdominal pain, steatorrhea, weight loss), alcohol and smoking, medications, and family history of pancreatic diseases. Physical examination may elicit signs of malnutrition (edema, cachexia) and vitamin or mineral deficiencies. Laboratory workup includes basic chemistry, liver enzymes, inflammatory markers, and screening for iron and vitamin deficiencies. Additional tests can be ordered to target specific underlying etiologies (autoimmune and genetic studies).

Cross-sectional imaging using CT and MRI/MRCP is frequently used as the initial diagnostic test for CP. CT with a pancreas protocol has a sensitivity of 80–90% for CP changes [36]. The sensitivity and specificity increase with the duration of the disease. Findings include parenchymal atrophy, ductal dilatation, and calcifications. MRI combined with MRCP can similarly evaluate for CP changes with the added benefits of a detailed assessment of pancreatic ductal anatomy and lack of radiation compared to CT. While MRI may have better sensitivity for detecting early CP compared to CT, subtle abnormalities may be missed with both imaging modalities. EUS allows for detailed examination of both the pancreatic parenchyma and ductal system and may detect features not evident on other CT or MRI. Diagnosis is made using the Rosemont classification, an international consensus-based criteria for EUS features of CP [37]. A major limitation is that EUS is operator dependent. Mild EUS changes are nonspecific, can be observed in multiple conditions, and are subject to significant interobserver variability in their interpretation.

Exocrine pancreatic function testing is most useful at identifying early stages of CP when imaging studies are equivocal. After administration of stimulatory hormones such as secretin or cholecystokinin, pancreatic secretions can be aspirated using a luminal tube and analyzed periodically for bicarbonate concentration. A peak bicarbonate level of <80 mEq/l is consistent with chronic pancreatitis [38]. Indirect assessment of pancreatic functioning can be made by measuring fecal elastase (FE-1). Using a random stool sample that should be solid or semisolid, a level >200 mcg/g of stool is considered normal, and a level <100 mcg/g indicates exocrine pancreatic insufficiency [39].

Management

General management of CP includes treatment of the underlying etiology, including alcohol and smoking cessation counseling, treatment of pancreatic insufficiency, and management of symptoms.

Malnutrition is common in patients with CP due to a combination of factors such as pain, decreased oral intake, vomiting, and exocrine insufficiency. Patients are advised to consume low-fat meals rich in antioxidants. Smaller, more frequent meals may be better tolerated than larger portions. Patients should be screened for nutritional deficiencies (iron, vitamins A, D, E, K, and B12), sarcopenia, osteopenia, and osteoporosis.

Exocrine pancreatic insufficiency will develop in the majority of patients 10–12 years after diagnosis [40]. Pancreatic enzyme replacement therapy is the mainstay of treatment. Enteric-coated preparations protect enzymes from acidic degradation and allow them to reach the duodenum. Non-enteric-coated preparations should be given with acid suppression medications. The effectiveness of therapy is measured by the resolution of steatorrhea. Pancreatogenic (type 3c) diabetes should be screened for with fasting glucose and HbA1c.

Pain is one of the important and most difficult components of CP management that requires a dedicated multidisciplinary approach. A step-up strategy can be implemented starting with pancreatic enzyme replacement therapy, antioxidants, non-opioid, and opioid analgesics. Adjunctive agents such as tricyclic antidepressants, serotonin reuptake inhibitors, and gabapentinoids can be added. Celiac plexus blockade can be performed for refractory pain. Endoscopic therapy consists of stent placement and/or stone extraction and should be mainly considered for patients with obstructing stones/strictures and ductal dilation. Surgical treatment is another treatment modality for refractory pain providing long-term benefits when indicated [41]. Surgical drainage procedures like the modified Puestow operation (lateral pancreaticojejunostomy) can be performed to improve ductal flow in patients with a dilated pancreatic duct. Surgical resection procedures such as the Whipple procedure and partial or total resection with islet cell autotransplantation are options for patients with limited or diffuse parenchymal fibrosis without ductal dilation.

Prognosis and Complications

The natural history of CP is variable depending on the nature and extent of the disease. It negatively impacts the quality of life independent of risk factors and coexistent medical comorbidity. Patients frequently need healthcare services and hospital admission with significant associated medical costs. The overall mortality is two- to fourfold higher than the general population [42].

Complications of CP include pseudocyst formation which can develop in around 10% of patients. Biliary and duodenal obstruction may develop secondary to compressing pseudocysts, tissue inflammation, fibrosis, and strictures. Vascular complications include pseudoaneurysms and splenic vein thrombosis. CP patients have an increased risk of pancreatic cancer compared to the general population. The risk depends on the duration and etiology of the disease as well as the presence of contributing factors such as smoking.

Pancreatic Cystic Neoplasms

Classification

Pancreatic cysts include a group of congenital, inflammatory, and neoplastic cysts that are often detected incidentally on abdominal imaging. The prevalence has been increasing over the last few decades due to the widespread use of cross-sectional imaging and the increasing sensitivity of imaging modalities. The prevalence has been reported to be as high as 50% in older patients.

Pancreatic cystic neoplasms (PCNs) account for more than 50% of all pancreatic cysts [43, 44]. The clinical manifestations range from benign to malignant disease. Accurate diagnosis and differentiating those at highest risk of malignancy are clinically important. PCNs include four subtypes: serous cystadenomas (SCAs), mucinous cystic neoplasm (MCN), intraductal papillary mucinous neoplasms (IPMNs), and solid pseudopapillary neoplasms (SPNs). Table 15.4 summarizes the key clinical features of PCNs.

Table 15.4 Features of pancreatic cystic neoplasms

	Serous cystic neoplasm	Mucinous cystic neoplasm	Intraductal papillary mucinous neoplasm	Solid pseudopapillary neoplasm
Age	Fifth to seventh decade	Fifth to seventh decade	Fifth to seventh decade	Second to third decade
Sex	F > M	F > M	F = M	F > M
Imaging appearance	Microcystic, honeycomb	Unilocular or septated, calcifications	Dilated ducts (main or branches)	Solid and cystic mass
CEA	Low	High	High	Low
Amylase	Low	Low	High	Low
Cytology	Cuboidal cells, glycogen-positive stain	Columnar cells, mucin-positive stain	Columnar cells, mucin-positive stain	Characteristic branching papillae with myxoid stroma
Malignant potential	No	Yes	Yes	Yes
Treatment	Resection if symptomatic	Resection	Resection for main duct IPMN, surveillance or resection for branch duct IPMN	Resection

Source: adapted from Khalid and Brugge [50]

F female, *M* male, *CEA* carcinoembryonic antigen, *IPMN* intraductal papillary mucinous neoplasm

Diagnostic Approach

The vast majority of PCNs are found incidentally on cross-sectional imaging with MRI/MRCP or CT. Worrisome features include dilated main pancreatic duct >5 mm, change in main duct caliber with upstream atrophy, cyst size >3 cm, and presence of a mural nodule or solid component. The development of jaundice, acute pancreatitis secondary to the cyst, or elevated serum CA 19–9 are also considered high-risk characteristics [45].

EUS-guided fine needle aspirate may aid in diagnosis and risk stratification. The aspirated fluid is analyzed for cytology, chemistry, tumor, and molecular markers. Cytological analysis for high-grade dysplasia or cancer is specific but not sensitive. Carcinoembryonic antigen (CEA) level > 192 ng/ml has been shown to differentiate between mucinous cysts (MCNs and IPMNs) and non-mucinous cysts with greatest diagnostic accuracy [46]. DNA analysis and molecular markers such as *KRAS* and *GNAS* mutations can also help in cyst differentiation and risk stratification. Next-generation sequencing of pancreatic cyst fluid was shown to be highly sensitive and specific in determining the etiology of pancreatic cysts and the malignant potential of mucinous cysts [47].

Serous Cystadenomas

SCAs are almost always benign. They are usually diagnosed incidentally and have an indolent course. Patients are usually females in their seventh decade of life. They can occur anywhere in the pancreas, but typically they are located in the body and tail of the pancreas. On imaging, they may have a microcystic honeycomb appearance with central scar. Cyst fluid analysis shows a low CEA level. Surgical resection is only needed in symptomatic cases.

Mucinous Cystic Neoplasms

MCNs are mucinous cysts that are diagnosed almost exclusively in females, usually in their fifth decade of life. They are located predominantly in the body and tail of the pancreas and do not communicate with the pancreatic duct. They can be macrocystic and have projections, septations, and wall calcifications. Fluid analysis shows an elevated CEA level. On histology, they demonstrate an ovarian-like stroma. The presence of mural nodules and large size (>4 cm) are risk factors for malignancy [48]. Surgical resection is usually recommended. Prognosis is excellent if MCNs are removed entirely.

Intraductal Papillary Mucinous Neoplasms

IPMNs are mucin-producing papillary neoplasms which communicate with the pancreatic ductal system. They have an equal sex distribution and are typically diagnosed in patients over the age of 60. IPMNs are divided into three subtypes: main duct, branch duct, and mixed types. Cyst fluid CEA is elevated in all subtypes.

While branch duct IPMNs generally have low malignant potential, presence of the aforementioned worrisome features should prompt further assessment with EUS and referral to a multidisciplinary pancreas center. Main duct and mixed-type IPMNs have a high malignant potential, with up to 70% risk of high-grade dysplasia or carcinoma depending on the degree of main duct dilation [49].

Surgical resection is recommended for main duct IPMNs (duct ≥10 or 5–9 mm with suspicious features) in patients who are surgical candidates with reasonable life expectancy. In asymptomatic patients with branch duct IPMN without worrisome features or patients who are not candidates for surgery, surveillance is recommended.

Solid Pseudopapillary Neoplasms

SPNs are rare neoplasms that occur almost exclusively in young females. They are commonly detected in the body and tail of the pancreas. Imaging can show solid and cystic components. SCAs have malignant potential but most exhibit a benign indolent course even in the presence of metastasis. Surgical resection is typically curative.

References

1. Padhan RK, Jain S, Agarwal S, Harikrishnan S, Vadiraja P, Behera S, et al. Primary and secondary organ failures cause mortality differentially in acute pancreatitis and should be distinguished. Pancreas. 2018;47(3):302–7.
2. Iannuzzi JP, King JA, Leong JH, Quan J, Windsor JW, Tanyingoh D, et al. Global incidence of acute pancreatitis is increasing over time: a systematic review and meta-analysis. Gastroenterology. 2022;162(1):122–34.
3. Gapp J, Hall AG, Walters RW, Jahann D, Kassim T, Reddymasu S. Trends and outcomes of hospitalizations related to acute pancreatitis: epidemiology from 2001 to 2014 in the United States. Pancreas. 2019;48(4):548–54.
4. Peery AF, Crockett SD, Murphy CC, Jensen ET, Kim HP, Egberg MD, et al. Burden and cost of gastrointestinal, liver, and pancreatic diseases in the United States: update 2021. Gastroenterology. 2022;162(2):621–44.
5. Forsmark CE, Baillie J. AGA Institute technical review on acute pancreatitis. Gastroenterology. 2007;132(5):2022–44.

6. EASL Clinical Practice Guidelines on the prevention, diagnosis and treatment of gallstones. J Hepatol. 2016;65(1):146–81.
7. Tenner S, Dubner H, Steinberg W. Predicting gallstone pancreatitis with laboratory parameters: a meta-analysis. Am J Gastroenterol. 1994;89(10):1863–6.
8. Kume K, Masamune A, Ariga H, Shimosegawa T. Alcohol consumption and the risk for developing pancreatitis: a case-control study in Japan. Pancreas. 2015;44(1):53–8.
9. Rebours V, Vullierme MP, Hentic O, Maire F, Hammel P, Ruszniewski P, et al. Smoking and the course of recurrent acute and chronic alcoholic pancreatitis: a dose-dependent relationship. Pancreas. 2012;41(8):1219–24.
10. Kochar B, Akshintala VS, Afghani E, Elmunzer BJ, Kim KJ, Lennon AM, et al. Incidence, severity, and mortality of post-ERCP pancreatitis: a systematic review by using randomized, controlled trials. Gastrointest Endosc. 2015;81(1):143–9.e9
11. Tenner S, Baillie J, DeWitt J, Vege SS. American College of Gastroenterology guideline: management of acute pancreatitis. Am J Gastroenterol. 2013;108(9):1400–15. 16
12. Mookadam F, Cikes M. Images in clinical medicine. Cullen's and Turner's signs. N Engl J Med. 2005;353(13):1386.
13. Banks PA, Bollen TL, Dervenis C, Gooszen HG, Johnson CD, Sarr MG, et al. Classification of acute pancreatitis—2012: revision of the Atlanta classification and definitions by international consensus. Gut. 2013;62(1):102–11.
14. Jin DX, McNabb-Baltar JY, Suleiman SL, Wu BU, Khorasani R, Bollen TL, et al. Early abdominal imaging remains over-utilized in acute pancreatitis. Dig Dis Sci. 2017;62(10):2894–9.
15. IAP/APA evidence-based guidelines for the management of acute pancreatitis. Pancreatology. 2013;13(4 Suppl 2):e1–e15.
16. Stimac D, Miletić D, Radić M, Krznarić I, Mazur-Grbac M, Perković D, et al. The role of nonenhanced magnetic resonance imaging in the early assessment of acute pancreatitis. Am J Gastroenterol. 2007;102(5):997–1004.
17. Jin DX, Banks PA, McNabb-Baltar J. Chapter 3: Definitions of Complications and Severity of Acute Pancreatitis for Clinical Practise. In: JE Dominguez-Muñoz editor. Clinical Pancreatology for Practising Gastroenterologists and Surgeons 2nd Ed. John Wiley & Sons Ltd; 2021. p. 25–29.
18. Marshall JC, Cook DJ, Christou NV, Bernard GR, Sprung CL, Sibbald WJ. Multiple organ dysfunction score: a reliable descriptor of a complex clinical outcome. Crit Care Med. 1995;23(10):1638–52.
19. Machicado JD, Gougol A, Tan X, Gao X, Paragomi P, Pothoulakis I, et al. Mortality in acute pancreatitis with persistent organ failure is determined by the number, type, and sequence of organ systems affected. United European Gastroenterol J. 2021;9(2):139–49.
20. Singh VK, Wu BU, Bollen TL, Repas K, Maurer R, Mortele KJ, et al. Early systemic inflammatory response syndrome is associated with severe acute pancreatitis. Clin Gastroenterol Hepatol. 2009;7(11):1247–51.
21. Singh VK, Wu BU, Bollen TL, Repas K, Maurer R, Johannes RS, et al. A prospective evaluation of the bedside index for severity in acute pancreatitis score in assessing mortality and intermediate markers of severity in acute pancreatitis. Am J Gastroenterol. 2009;104(4):966–71.
22. Wu BU, Batech M, Quezada M, Lew D, Fujikawa K, Kung J, et al. Dynamic measurement of disease activity in acute pancreatitis: the pancreatitis activity scoring system. Am J Gastroenterol. 2017;112(7):1144–52.
23. Buxbaum J, Quezada M, Chong B, Gupta N, Yu CY, Lane C, et al. The pancreatitis activity scoring system predicts clinical outcomes in acute pancreatitis: findings from a prospective cohort study. Am J Gastroenterol. 2018;113(5):755–64.
24. Lee A, Ko C, Buitrago C, Hiramoto B, Hilson L, Buxbaum J. Lactated ringers vs normal saline resuscitation for mild acute pancreatitis: a randomized trial. Gastroenterology. 2021;160(3):955–7.e4.
25. de-Madaria E, Buxbaum JL, Maisonneuve P, García García de Paredes A, Zapater P, Guilabert L, et al. Aggressive or moderate fluid resuscitation in acute pancreatitis. N Engl J Med. 2022;387(11):989–1000.

26. Dong E, Chang JI, Verma D, Butler RK, Villarin CK, Kwok KK, et al. Enhanced recovery in mild acute pancreatitis: a randomized controlled trial. Pancreas. 2019;48(2):176–81.
27. da Costa DW, Bouwense SA, Schepers NJ, Besselink MG, van Santvoort HC, van Brunschot S, et al. Same-admission versus interval cholecystectomy for mild gallstone pancreatitis (PONCHO): a multicentre randomised controlled trial. Lancet (London, England). 2015;386(10000):1261–8.
28. Boxhoorn L, van Dijk SM, van Grinsven J, Verdonk RC, Boermeester MA, Bollen TL, et al. Immediate versus postponed intervention for infected necrotizing pancreatitis. N Engl J Med. 2021;385(15):1372–81.
29. Bang JY, Arnoletti JP, Holt BA, Sutton B, Hasan MK, Navaneethan U, et al. An endoscopic transluminal approach, compared with minimally invasive surgery, reduces complications and costs for patients with necrotizing pancreatitis. Gastroenterology. 2019;156(4):1027–40.e3
30. Moraes JM, Felga GE, Chebli LA, Franco MB, Gomes CA, Gaburri PD, et al. A full solid diet as the initial meal in mild acute pancreatitis is safe and result in a shorter length of hospitalization: results from a prospective, randomized, controlled, double-blind clinical trial. J Clin Gastroenterol. 2010;44(7):517–22.
31. Villatoro E, Mulla M, Larvin M. Antibiotic therapy for prophylaxis against infection of pancreatic necrosis in acute pancreatitis. Cochrane Database Syst Rev. 2010;2010(5):Cd002941.
32. Das SL, Singh PP, Phillips AR, Murphy R, Windsor JA, Petrov MS. Newly diagnosed diabetes mellitus after acute pancreatitis: a systematic review and meta-analysis. Gut. 2014;63(5):818–31.
33. Hollemans RA, Hallensleben NDL, Mager DJ, Kelder JC, Besselink MG, Bruno MJ, et al. Pancreatic exocrine insufficiency following acute pancreatitis: systematic review and study level meta-analysis. Pancreatology. 2018;18(3):253–62.
34. Yadav D, Lowenfels AB. The epidemiology of pancreatitis and pancreatic cancer. Gastroenterology. 2013;144(6):1252–61.
35. Whitcomb DC. Pancreatitis: TIGAR-O version 2 risk/etiology checklist with topic reviews, updates, and use primers. Clin Transl Gastroenterol. 2019;10(6):e00027.
36. Issa Y, Kempeneers MA, van Santvoort HC, Bollen TL, Bipat S, Boermeester MA. Diagnostic performance of imaging modalities in chronic pancreatitis: a systematic review and meta-analysis. Eur Radiol. 2017;27(9):3820–44.
37. Catalano MF, Sahai A, Levy M, Romagnuolo J, Wiersema M, Brugge W, et al. EUS-based criteria for the diagnosis of chronic pancreatitis: the Rosemont classification. Gastrointest Endosc. 2009;69(7):1251–61.
38. Kothari D, Ketwaroo G, Sawhney MS, Freedman SD, Sheth SG. Comparison of combined endoscopic ultrasonography and endoscopic secretin testing with the traditional secretin pancreatic function test in patients with suspected chronic pancreatitis: a prospective crossover study. Pancreas. 2017;46(6):770–5.
39. Vanga RR, Tansel A, Sidiq S, El-Serag HB, Othman MO. Diagnostic performance of measurement of fecal Elastase-1 in detection of exocrine pancreatic insufficiency: systematic review and meta-analysis. Clin Gastroenterol Hepatol. 2018;16(8):1220–8.e4
40. Machicado JD, Chari ST, Timmons L, Tang G, Yadav D. A population-based evaluation of the natural history of chronic pancreatitis. Pancreatology. 2018;18(1):39–45.
41. Strand DS, Law RJ, Yang D, Elmunzer BJ. AGA clinical practice update on the endoscopic approach to recurrent acute and chronic pancreatitis: expert review. Gastroenterology. 2022;163(4):1107–14.
42. Yadav D, Timmons L, Benson JT, Dierkhising RA, Chari ST. Incidence, prevalence, and survival of chronic pancreatitis: a population-based study. Am J Gastroenterol. 2011;106(12):2192–9.
43. Fernández-del Castillo C, Targarona J, Thayer SP, Rattner DW, Brugge WR, Warshaw AL. Incidental pancreatic cysts: clinicopathologic characteristics and comparison with symptomatic patients. Arch Surg. 2003;138(4):427–3. discussion 33-4
44. Spinelli KS, Fromwiller TE, Daniel RA, Kiely JM, Nakeeb A, Komorowski RA, et al. Cystic pancreatic neoplasms: observe or operate. Ann Surg. 2004;239(5):651–7. discussion 7-9

45. Elta GH, Enestvedt BK, Sauer BG, Lennon AM. ACG clinical guideline: diagnosis and management of pancreatic cysts. Am J Gastroenterol. 2018;113(4):464–79.
46. Brugge WR, Lewandrowski K, Lee-Lewandrowski E, Centeno BA, Szydlo T, Regan S, et al. Diagnosis of pancreatic cystic neoplasms: a report of the cooperative pancreatic cyst study. Gastroenterology. 2004;126(5):1330–6.
47. Paniccia A, Polanco PM, Boone BA, Wald AI, McGrath K, Brand RE, et al. Prospective, multi-institutional, real-time next-generation sequencing of pancreatic cyst fluid reveals diverse genomic alterations that improve the clinical management of pancreatic cysts. Gastroenterology. 2023;164(1):117–33.e7
48. Crippa S, Fernández-Del Castillo C, Salvia R, Finkelstein D, Bassi C, Domínguez I, et al. Mucin-producing neoplasms of the pancreas: an analysis of distinguishing clinical and epidemiologic characteristics. Clin Gastroenterol Hepatol. 2010;8(2):213–9.
49. Crippa S, Aleotti F, Longo E, Belfiori G, Partelli S, Tamburrino D, et al. Main duct thresholds for malignancy are different in Intraductal papillary mucinous neoplasms of the pancreatic head and body-tail. Clin Gastroenterol Hepatol. 2022;20(2):390–9.e7
50. Khalid A, Brugge W. ACG practice guidelines for the diagnosis and management of neoplastic pancreatic cysts. Am J Gastroenterol. 2007;102(10):2339–49.

Chapter 16
Quality in Endoscopic Sedation

Otto S. Lin

Table of Quality Measures/Metrics

Abbreviations

ACLS	Advanced Cardiac Life Support
ASA	American Society of Anesthesiologists
ASGE	American Society for Gastrointestinal Endoscopy
CAPS	Computer-assisted propofol sedation
EGD	Esophagogastroduodenoscopy
GI	Gastrointestinal
M&M	Morbidity and mortality
MAC	Monitored anesthesia care
MF	Midazolam fentanyl
NAPCIS	Nurse-administered propofol continuous infusion sedation
NAPS	Nurse-administered propofol sedation
QA	Quality assurance

O. S. Lin (✉)
Center for Digestive Health, Virginia Mason Medical Center, Seattle, WA, USA

Gastroenterology Division, University of Washington School of Medicine, Seattle, WA, USA
e-mail: Otto.Lin@vmmc.org

J. D. Feuerstein, D. J. Stein (eds.), *Quality in Gastroenterology*,
https://doi.org/10.1007/978-3-031-58492-3_16

Key Points

- High-quality sedation is a prerequisite of high-quality endoscopy, so it is critical to define, measure, and improve endoscopic sedation quality.
- Based on patient risk assessment, predicted ease of sedation, and procedural requirements, a decision must be made between moderate sedation and monitored anesthesia care.
- Pre-procedural sedation quality issues include sedation training and certification for endoscopic personnel, accurate assessment of patient risk and sedation requirements, and formulation of a suitable sedation plan (moderate sedation versus monitored anesthesia care).
- Intra-procedural sedation quality issues include informed consent, the procedural pause, comprehensive procedural monitoring and effective management of complications, and an efficient and safe recovery and discharge process.
- Post-procedural sedation quality issues include the management of delayed sedation-related complications, systematic adverse event tracking, and quality improvement measures on a unit and individual level (morbidity and mortality conferences, personal improvement plans, equipment upgrades, and/or protocol changes).

Introduction

In most developed countries, the majority of gastrointestinal (GI) endoscopic procedures are performed with sedation or anesthesia [1]. Due to abdominal pain, cramping, and bloating during colonoscopy [2], and gagging, retching, and choking during esophagogastroduodenoscopy (EGD), endoscopy is an inherently uncomfortable procedure. The use of sedation permits a more thorough and relaxed procedure, resulting in higher procedural completion and (for colonoscopy) polyp detection rates [3]. A sedated, comfortable patient is not only associated with higher endoscopist satisfaction [4], but leads to the patient being more willing to undergo the procedure again.

High-quality sedation is a prerequisite of high-quality endoscopy, which is why endoscopy guidelines include quality metrics related to sedation, such as patient risk assessment, intra-procedural monitoring, adverse event tracking and analysis, training and certification for sedation privileges, and proper informed consent [5, 6]. In the past, most endoscopic procedures were performed with moderate sedation using midazolam and fentanyl (MF), but the past decade has seen a marked increase in the use of propofol for routine outpatient endoscopy in low-risk patients [7–10]. In the USA, propofol is almost always administered by anesthesia professionals; thus, quality in endoscopic sedation is an issue of interest to both gastroenterologists and anesthesia professionals [11, 12].

Quality Aspects of Endoscopic Sedation

Sedation quality issues can be broadly separated into three categories: pre-procedural, intra-procedural, and post-procedural.

Pre-Procedural Issues

Pre-procedural sedation quality issues encompass all preparatory measures that occur before the day of the actual procedure. These include sedation training and certification of involved personnel, assessment of patient risk and ease of sedation, and formulation of an individualized sedation plan based on predetermined criteria and clinical judgment. These preparations have a critical bearing on sedation success and safety on the day of the procedure.

Sedation Training and Certification

For cases where the sedation is to be administered by non-anesthesia professionals, endoscopists and endoscopy nurses who administer sedative medications must have undergone formal training and be certified in conscious sedation; they should also be Advanced Cardiac Life Support certified [13].

The sedation training and certification process can vary between endoscopy units but typically includes online or in-person courses, assessment tests, and a proctorship period. For example, at the Virginia Mason Medical Center (VMMC) endoscopy unit, all endoscopy nurses must: (1) complete a multi-modular online course that covers the properties of relevant sedative medications, the endoscopy unit-specific sedation protocol, and pre-planned strategies for rescuing patients who inadvertently lapse into a deeper than intended level of sedation [14]; (2) attend an in-person 2-h lecture taught by an anesthesiologist or certified registered nurse anesthetist; (3) pass an online assessment test to ensure understanding of sedation principles; and (4) lastly, new nurses are paired with an experienced nurse for an "apprenticeship" period, so that the former can learn on the job under supervision. At the end of the apprenticeship period, the preceptor nurse must certify that the new nurse is competent to perform sedation independently. Endoscopists, all of whom must already be board-certified gastroenterologists or surgeons, must complete the online course, attend the 2-h live course, pass the online examination, and finally be proctored during three procedures by an experienced endoscopist before being certified for endoscopic sedation.

Assessment of Patient Risk and Sedation Requirements

A comprehensive history and focused physical examination are essential for patient risk assessment. Key components of the history include patient age, comorbidities, body mass index, list of medications (with special attention to potential interactions

Table 16.1 The American Society of Anesthesiologists classification system for patient health and risk

Class	
I	Normal, healthy patient
II	Patient with mild systemic disease
III	Patient with severe systemic disease
IV	Patient with severe, life-threatening systemic disease

with procedural sedatives), and any history of medication allergies and side effects, previous difficulties with sedation or anesthesia, and substance abuse. The physical examination should focus on a targeted assessment of the cardiopulmonary system, airway (including Mallampati class), and dentition. Based on these factors, an American Society of Anesthesiologists (ASA) score can be determined for the patient (Table 16.1) [15, 16], which can serve as the basis for estimation of procedural risk. In addition to risk of complications, the risk of procedural failure due to inability to adequately sedate the patient must also be considered. Patients who are likely to be more difficult to sedate include regular opiate abusers [17–20], heavy marijuana users [21, 22], and those with post-traumatic stress disorders [19, 23]. Patients taking opiate antagonists, such as Suboxone or naloxone, can also pose challenges to sedation and may require more potent forms of sedation (such as the use of propofol over MF sedation) [24].

Except in emergency situations, the patient's history should ideally be assessed before the day of the procedure through a review of the medical records, but the physical examination may not be possible until the day of the procedure. This may pose a particular issue with open-access endoscopies (endoscopic procedures that are scheduled without the patient being previously seen by the endoscopist or any member of the GI department), which are becoming more and more common, especially for screening or surveillance purposes [25]. There have been concerns that open-access endoscopy may increase the risk of endoscopic complications, but this has not been borne out by the limited data available. In fact, studies have generally shown that pre-procedural screening protocols can correctly identify patients suitable for open-access EGD and colonoscopy [26–28].

Formulation of Sedation Plan

A sedation plan should then be formulated, based on an assessment of: (1) patient risk; (2) predicted ease (or difficulty) of sedation; and (3) procedure duration, complexity, and type (longer, more complex, and/or upper as opposed lower endoscopic procedures are more likely to require the involvement of an anesthesia professional). In fact, colonoscopies often can be completed with only light or no sedation [29, 30], while it is unlikely that EGDs can be completed without sedation unless ultrathin transnasal endoscopes are used [31].

In most cases, the main dichotomous choice is between targeting moderate versus deep sedation, as defined by the ASA (Table 16.2). Specifically, at the level of

Table 16.2 Definition of American Society of Anesthesiologists levels of sedation and anesthesia [92]

	Minimal sedation (anxiolysis)	Moderate sedation (conscious sedation)	Deep sedation	General anesthesia
Responsiveness	Normal response to verbal stimuli	Purposeful response to verbal or tactile stimuli	Purposeful response to noxious stimuli or insistent verbal stimuli	Unarousable
Airway	Normal	No intervention needed	Intervention may be needed	Airway support needed
Spontaneous ventilation	Normal	Adequate	Usually inadequate	Ventilatory support usually needed
Cardiovascular function	Normal	Usually maintained	Usually maintained	May be impaired

Table 16.3 Properties of commonly used sedative agents for gastrointestinal endoscopy

Agent	Onset of action, min	Peak effect, min	Duration of effect, min	Metabolism	Excretion	Reversal agent
Midazolam	1–2.5	3–4	15–80	Hepatic	Renal	Flumazenil
Fentanyl	1–2	3–5	30–60	Hepatic	Renal	Naloxone
Propofol	0.5–1	1–2	4–8	Hepatic	Renal	None

"moderate sedation," the patient maintains ventilatory and cardiovascular function and is able to make purposeful responses to verbal or tactile stimuli, while at "deep sedation," patients cannot be easily aroused but are still able to respond to noxious or insistent stimuli. The involvement of an anesthesia professional is usually required for deep sedation.

Moderate Sedation

Traditionally, moderate sedation is used for most endoscopic procedures, induced by combining a benzodiazepine sedative with an opioid analgesic, as the two classes have complementary and synergistic effects with each other. Intravenous midazolam (a benzodiazepine) and fentanyl (an opioid) are the most commonly used sedation agents in the USA [32] and many other countries [33]. Both agents have a favorable pharmacokinetic profile, i.e., fast onset of action and short duration of effect (Table 16.3). Effective reversal agents, naloxone for opioids and flumazenil for benzodiazepines, are readily available. MF sedation has been found to be effective for routine endoscopy in many studies [34], while cardiopulmonary complication rates are generally low [35, 36].

Although MF sedation is the most common method of moderate sedation in the USA, alternative approaches such as nurse-administered propofol sedation

(NAPS) [37], computer-assisted propofol sedation (CAPS), nurse-administered propofol continuous infusion sedation (NAPCIS), and patient-controlled sedation (PCS) have been investigated. In NAPS, specially trained nurses administer small boluses of propofol at frequent intervals to achieve moderate sedation [38]. Numerous studies have shown NAPS to be feasible and safe in appropriately selected patients [39–44]. In fact, an exhaustive review of worldwide safety data involving 646,080 NAPS procedures reported only 11 emergent intubations, no permanent neurological injuries, and four deaths; only 0.1% of patients required transient mask ventilation [40]. European and American GI guidelines endorse the use of NAPS for low-risk procedures [45–47], a position which is at odds with ASA guidelines [16]. Currently, NAPS is rarely used in the USA for various reasons, including financial incentives, Food and Drug Administration labeling issues, Center for Medical Services policies, insurance regulations, hospital credentialing rules, and medicolegal concerns [48, 49].

CAPS was FDA approved to allow non-anesthesiologists to administer propofol sedation for ASA class I and II patients undergoing routine EGD and colonoscopy. The SEDASYS® CAPS system (Ethicon Endo-Surgery, Cincinnati, Ohio, USA) continuously monitors capnography, oxygen saturation, EKG, blood pressure, and patient alertness [50]. Hypoventilation, oxygen desaturation, hypotension, or unresponsiveness can cause the CAPS system to decrease or discontinue the propofol infusion and trigger alerts to the provider team. Despite favorable data on effectiveness, endoscopist and patient satisfaction, procedure and recovery time, and endoscopy unit efficiency and safety from both clinical trials [50] and real-world studies [51–53], CAPS was withdrawn from the market by its manufacturer in 2016 due to financial reasons [54, 55]. Currently, there are significant financial incentives for endoscopy practices to continue using anesthesia-administered propofol [56, 57], thereby limiting the number of providers willing to invest in a CAPS system.

After the withdrawal of CAPS, NAPCIS was developed at VMMC as a propofol delivery method that replicates the capabilities of CAPS by using programmable intravenous fluid infusion pumps commonly available in the hospital (Alaris® pump module, Becton, Dickinson and Company, Franklin Lakes, New Jersey, USA). NAPCIS delivers propofol as a continuous infusion after an optional loading dose of fentanyl, using a dosing and safety protocol identical to that in CAPS. Specifically, NAPCIS is based on a rigid, detailed, and explicit written protocol to which all doctors and nurses must adhere (see Fig. 16.1). The protocol contains three parts:

1. Patient selection: The protocol specifies the type of patients who are suitable for NAPCIS, typically healthy patients undergoing uncomplicated, elective EGDs and/or colonoscopies.
2. Dosing: The protocol specifies the maximum weight-based starting infusion rate, the time interval that must elapse before the infusion rate can be increased, the magnitude of each infusion rate increase, the absolute maximum ("ceiling") infusion rate, the dose of each bolus, and the "lockout" period between boluses.
3. Safety: The protocol specifies the capnography, oxygen saturation, blood pressure, and heart rate and rhythm parameters that will lead to the propofol infusion being manually shut off.

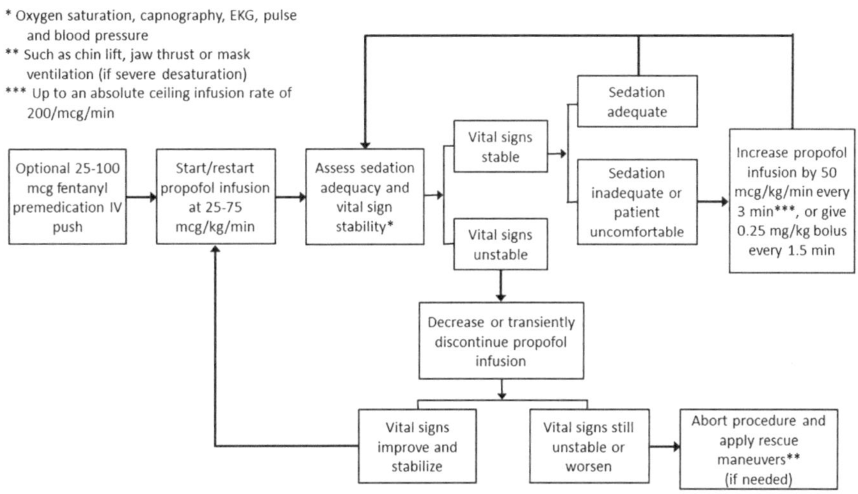

Fig. 16.1 Sedation protocol for nurse-administered propofol continuous infusion sedation (NAPCIS) at Virginia Mason Medical Center

Since NAPCIS (like CAPS) is geared toward the attainment of moderate (not deep) sedation, the total propofol dose given is typically smaller than that delivered by anesthesia professionals during monitored anesthesia care (MAC).

Published studies showed very low complication rates, no serious complications, and high patient and endoscopist satisfaction with NAPCIS [58]; NAPCIS was also effective for patients who are challenging to sedate with MF sedation [59]. Currently, NAPCIS is only available at VMMC. If bundled payment for screening and surveillance colonoscopy were to become a reality [60–63], NAPCIS has the potential to become more widely adopted.

The final option, PCS, is analogous to the patient-controlled analgesia that allows hospitalized patients to control their own pain medications. PCS has been found to be effective compared against MAC [64] and conventional MF sedation [65–67]. However, PCS is not widely used because most patients are reluctant to take charge of their own sedation.

Monitored Anesthesia Care and General Anesthesia

In the USA, over the past decade, there has been a dramatic increase in the prevalence of anesthesia involvement in endoscopic procedures, including routine EGDs and colonoscopies on low-risk patients [7, 8, 68]. Sedation provided by anesthesia professionals (anesthesiologists and certified registered nurse anesthetists) generally takes the form of MAC, whereby a combination of medications, primarily propofol, is administered intravenously at the discretion of the anesthesia provider. Generally, propofol is extremely effective at inducing deep sedation, with high procedural success rates, rapid recovery times, and low complication rates [34, 69–71].

However, the use of MAC has resulted in significant increases in endoscopy costs [72, 73], leading to concerns that these substantial anesthesia costs are not justified by any improvement in clinical outcomes [56, 74–76]. For example, the use of MAC does not increase the adenoma detection rate during colonoscopy [77–79], and anesthesia-administered propofol sedation is not necessarily safer than non-anesthesiologist-administered MF sedation. In fact, available data on MAC show either similar complication rates [70, 78, 80] or higher complication rates compared with MF sedation [81–83]. Nevertheless, in the USA the use of MAC for routine endoscopy continues to increase [10].

For certain patients at high risk of aspiration or airway compromise (e.g., those with a history of oropharyngeal surgery or radiation treatment) or for complex and protracted procedures (such as endoscopic ultrasound), full general anesthesia may be required; this involves endotracheal intubation of the patient, positive pressure ventilation, and the use of anesthetic agents such as nitrous oxide or ketamine. Furthermore, if airway or ventilation difficulties are encountered during an endoscopy that was originally started with MAC, the anesthesia provider may decide to perform intubation halfway through the procedure in order to deliver more effective ventilatory support.

Intra-Procedural Issues

Intra-procedural issues include everything that occurs on the day of the procedure, ranging from obtaining a proper informed consent to ensuring appropriate recovery and discharge of the patient following the endoscopy.

Informed Consent

Informed consent is a critical part of the entire endoscopic process [84]; unless the procedure is emergent, complete informed consent must always be obtained. Since sedation-related complications constitute a major component of the overall procedural risk, informed consent obtained by the endoscopy team (either the endoscopist or a representative such as a physician assistant, nurse practitioner, or trainee [84]) should explicitly address sedation issues. If an anesthesia professional will be administering MAC, then the anesthesia team will usually have a separate discussion with the patient as well. The informed consent should involve a detailed discussion of the sedation plan, potential intra-procedural changes to the sedation plan (e.g., transitioning from MAC to intubated anesthesia during the procedure), and the risk of adverse events. The reasons for the use of sedation, including patient comfort and higher probability of successful procedure completion, should be explained. Possible sedation-related adverse events that should be addressed include hypoxia, hypotension, cardiac arrhythmias, aspiration, and post-operative somnolence; some older patients may be particularly concerned about long-term memory loss from exposure to sedative medications. The patient should be given ample opportunity to ask questions and express concerns. The informed consent process should then end with provider and patient signatures on the informed consent form, witnessed by appropriate personnel.

Procedural Pause

Immediately prior to starting the sedation, a formal procedural pause, otherwise known as a "safety pause" or "time-out," is an important safety and quality measure. This is mandated by the Joint Commission on Accreditation of Healthcare Organizations and the Centers for Medicare & Medicaid Services [11]. The pause consists of an oral checklist confirming the identification of the patient (using at least two forms of identification), the planned procedure, patient allergies and medications, any special equipment or antibiotics needed, and plans after discharge (e.g., whether or not overnight hospitalization is anticipated) [85].

Procedural Monitoring and Complication Management

American Society for Gastrointestinal Endoscopy (ASGE) guidelines recommend intra-procedural monitoring of blood pressure, pulse oximetry, and patient responsiveness [86]. ASA guidelines additionally recommend the monitoring of EKG and capnography tracings [16]. Studies have shown that capnography is useful for ventilation monitoring during endoscopic procedures, because capnographic changes occur before drops in oxygen saturation [87–89]. Experimental methods such as bispectral index monitoring, a form of electroencephalography, are not widely available as yet. The patient's vital signs should be recorded throughout the entire procedure and recovery period. Routine administration of supplemental oxygen by nasal cannula is recommended for all patients.

The procedure team may have to take measures to deal with minor cardiopulmonary issues such as oxygen desaturation, hypotension, or partial obstruction of the airway. Common interventions include temporary interruption of sedative administration, airway maneuvers such as a jaw thrust or chin lift, and/or verbal and tactile stimulation of the patient to increase the consciousness level. These common interventions should not be considered complications. However, in more severe cases of cardiopulmonary decompensation, additional interventions may be needed, such as mask ventilation, emergent intubation, the use of reversal agents, or even calling for the assistance of a "code" team. These interventions should be recorded as adverse events and tracked for post hoc analysis. Complications such as aspiration and phlebitis also need to be noted.

Recovery and Discharge

Discharge criteria vary from unit to unit. At the minimum, patients need to exhibit stable vital signs, absence of severe abdominal pain, and an adequate level of consciousness. Some units use more formal scoring systems, such as the Aldrete score or Modified Post-Anesthesia Discharge Scoring System (Tables 16.4 and 16.5) [14], for determining suitability for discharge. It is standard to require that the patient be accompanied by an escort when leaving, because of the unpredictable delayed effects of sedation.

All patients need to be given an oral summary of procedural findings from the endoscopist or recovery nurse, as well as written discharge instructions. These should include dietary and activity restrictions (e.g., no driving) and signs and symptoms of delayed adverse events and what to do in response (e.g., returning to the emergency room or calling the hospital). Since the patient typically has impaired memory, if there are critical instructions or findings, it may be helpful to communicate these to the patient's escort (assuming that the patient has given permission for medical information to be divulged). Many endoscopy units also give the patient a printed copy of the procedure note or procedural finding summary.

Post-Procedural Issues

Post-procedural issues include management of delayed sedation-related complications, systematic adverse event tracking and post hoc analysis, and quality assessment and improvement.

Table 16.4 Aldrete score [14]

Respiration	
Can cough and breathe deeply	2
Short of breath	1
Apneic	0
Blood pressure	
20% of pre-sedation level	2
20–50% of pre-sedation level	1
>50% of pre-sedation level	0
Oxygen saturation	
O_2 saturation > 92%	2
Needs oxygen to maintain O_2 saturation > 90%	1
Oxygen saturation < 90% with supplemental oxygen	0
Consciousness	
Awake and oriented ×3	2
Arousable to command	1
Nonresponsive	0
Activity	
Can move all four extremities on command	2
Can move two extremities on command	1
Cannot move extremities on command	0
Total score of 8 or more for 2 consecutive measurements needed for discharge	0–10

Table 16.5 Modified Post Anesthesia Discharge Score [14]

Vital signs	
BP and HR ±20% of pre-sedation level	2
BP and HR ±20–40% of pre-sedation level	1
BP and HR ±40% of pre-sedation level	0
Activity	
Meets pre-sedation level	2
Requires assistance	1
Unable to ambulate	0
Nausea and vomiting	
None or minimal (oral medication treatment)	2
Moderate (IV medication treatment)	1
Severe or recalcitrant	0
Pain	
None or minimal	2
Moderate	1
Severe	0
Surgical bleeding	
None or minimal	2
Moderate	1
Severe	0
Total score of 9 or more for 2 consecutive measurements needed for discharge	0–10

Delayed Sedation-Related Complications

Delayed adverse events, which typically manifest themselves after the patient has already left the endoscopy unit, are usually procedure-related (such as post-polypectomy bleeding) rather than sedation-related, but there are occasional instances of delayed side effects of sedation (e.g., persistent post-sedation confusion or nausea). These typically resolve spontaneously within 1 or 2 days and do not require specific treatment, although sometimes patients may need a temporary allocation of anti-nausea medications.

Adverse Event Tracking and Analysis

Data collected during the procedure will need to be stored indefinitely and analyzed periodically in order to identify any quality problems on a unit as well as individual level. Adverse event data can be obtained through two primary channels: proactive self-reporting and retrospective chart review. Self-reporting of intra-procedural adverse events by the physician or nurse is efficient and logistically straightforward but may suffer from under-reporting issues because intentional or unintentional under-reporting may occur. Chart review, usually in the form of automated download of information collected from electronic medical record systems, such as Provation® (Provation Inc., Minneapolis, Minnesota, USA), is also highly efficient but requires the participation of personnel knowledgeable in the process of data extraction from electronic medical records. Furthermore, the reliability of the extracted data depends on accurate input during the procedure. These two methods are of course not mutually exclusive, and in fact should be used concurrently in order to ensure collection of adverse event data in a comprehensive manner. Because of its labor-intensive nature, manual review of charts is only feasible in selected cases (e.g., when there is already a known complication). Comparison of adverse event data against national and local benchmarks helps to reassure quality or, in cases where quality is below par, can guide quality improvement initiatives.

Sedation-related adverse event endpoints that should be recorded and analyzed include, but are not limited to, the following: (1) patient injury or death; (2) unanticipated hospitalization; (3) "codes" called for cardiopulmonary reasons; (4) use of reversal agents or pressors; (5) and procedure abortion due to severe desaturation, hypotension, arrhythmias, or patient agitation.

Lastly, there should be systematic attempts to monitor patient satisfaction by offering a validated questionnaire, such as the GHAA-9 survey, to patients either in the recovery unit or subsequently by mail or online [90]. Although patient satisfaction is affected by many different aspects of the endoscopy experience, sedation quality is a major variable. Satisfaction survey scores need to be interpreted cautiously because of bias issues associated with data collection methods [91].

Quality Improvement Measures

Every endoscopy unit should have a designated Quality Assurance (QA) Director, ideally an experienced and respected physician who performs endoscopy on a regular basis and is well versed in quality metrics. In smaller units, quality assurance duties can be performed by the endoscopy unit chief. The QA Director should be responsible for monitoring the unit's quality metrics (see Table 16.6) and for executing the following initiatives: First, in every (academic or nonacademic) hospital endoscopy unit, a formal morbidity and mortality (M&M) conference should be held at periodic intervals (typically monthly to quarterly) to review notable cases of adverse events in detail. It is not necessary to include every single adverse event in the M&M conference, but all cases of sedation-related deaths, emergent intubations, codes, and unanticipated hospitalizations, as well as cases of educational merit in the opinion of the QA Director, should be presented and subjected to peer review. To encourage attendance and frank discussion, M&M conferences should be held in a spirit of educational advancement and quality improvement, and should not be used as a vehicle for punitive sanctions.

Second, with the help of computer support personnel, the QA Director should periodically review quality metrics for all endoscopists in the unit, including adenoma detection rates, mean withdrawal times, colonoscopy completion rates, and adverse events. From a sedation perspective, the relevant quality metrics are

Table 16.6 Quality metrics pertinent to endoscopic sedation

Quality metric	Notes
Procedures aborted due to sedation reasons (%)	No validated national benchmarks; compare to local variance
Sedation-related deaths (%)	
Sedation-related injuries (%)	
Sedation-related codes (%)	
Use of reversal agents or pressors (%)	
Designated QA director (yes/no)	All endoscopy units should have a designated QA Director
Formal sedation training and certification process (yes/no)	All endoscopy units should have a formal sedation training and certification process for staff
Sedation plan guidelines (yes/no)	Sedation plans are usually based on clinical judgment, with some objective parameters (e.g., patients with BMI >50 must be done with MAC)
Procedural pause (yes/no)	All procedures should be preceded by a procedural pause
Informed consent (yes/no)	All procedures should be preceded by proper informed consent
Formal intra-procedural monitoring protocol (yes/no)	The protocol specifies how frequently vital signs are measured
Formal sedation protocol (yes/no)	Required for non-anesthesiologist-administered sedation
Formal discharge protocol (yes/no)	Some units may use the Aldrete score or other validated scoring systems
Regular M&M conferences (yes/no)	Frequency should range from monthly to quarterly
Tracking and analysis of adverse events (yes/no)	Typically performed by the QA Director or associated staff

BMI body mass index, *MAC* monitored anesthesia care, *M&M* morbidity and mortality, *QA* quality assurance

sedation-related adverse events and proportion of procedures aborted due to sedation reasons. If there appears to be a signal, then the data should be parsed to determine if the issue is particular to the unit, equipment, or an individual nurse, anesthesia professional, or endoscopist. If a quality issue is identified with an individual, e.g., if an individual endoscopist is associated with a particularly high incidence of sedation complications when compared with peers and benchmarks, then further investigation should be carried out, and the individual in question may benefit from a personal improvement plan, usually involving constructive feedback, additional training and proctoring, and remeasurement of quality metrics. To sustain morale, the entire process will need to be carried out in a sensitive and impartial manner, with measurable and (if possible) objective metrics and goals. Equipment defects, such as faulty capnography units, can be corrected by upgrading the equipment. Finally, protocol changes are required when a systemic issue is identified, e.g., when the sedative titration protocol needs to be modified.

Conclusion

Quality assurance and improvement of endoscopic sedation are an integral component of high-quality endoscopy. Pre-procedural aspects of endoscopic sedation include a comprehensive sedation training and certification program for all involved personnel, accurate assessment of patient risk and sedation requirements, and formulation of a suitable sedation plan (moderate sedation versus monitored anesthesia care). Intra-procedural aspects include the obtaining of proper informed consent, a methodical procedural pause, careful procedural monitoring with timely management of complications, and a safe recovery and discharge process. Post-procedural aspects include the competent management of delayed sedation-related complications, systematic adverse event tracking, and effective quality improvement measures, such as regular M&M conferences and, if needed, personal improvement plans, equipment upgrades, and protocol changes.

Conflict of Interest Otto Lin served as a consultant for SEDASYS Inc. up to 2016.

Author Contributions Otto Lin: Contributions include drafting of the manuscript and final approval of the article.

Guarantor of the Article Otto Lin, M.D.

Financial Support No funding sources were involved in the execution of this paper.

References

1. Standards of Practice Committee of the American Society for Gastrointestinal E, Lichtenstein DR, Jagannath S, Baron TH, Anderson MA, Banerjee S, et al. Sedation and anesthesia in GI endoscopy. Gastrointest Endosc. 2008;68(5):815–26.
2. Ghanouni A, Plumb A, Hewitson P, Nickerson C, Rees CJ, von Wagner C. Patients' experience of colonoscopy in the English bowel cancer screening Programme. Endoscopy. 2016;48(3):232–40.
3. Radaelli F, Meucci G, Sgroi G, Minoli G. Italian Association of Hospital G. Technical performance of colonoscopy: the key role of sedation/analgesia and other quality indicators. Am J Gastroenterol. 2008;103(5):1122–30.
4. Cohen LB, Wecsler JS, Gaetano JN, Benson AA, Miller KM, Durkalski V, et al. Endoscopic sedation in the United States: results from a nationwide survey. Am J Gastroenterol. 2006;101(5):967–74.
5. Rizk MK, Sawhney MS, Cohen J, Pike IM, Adler DG, Dominitz JA, et al. Quality indicators common to all GI endoscopic procedures. Gastrointest Endosc. 2015;81(1):3–16.
6. Allen JI. Quality assurance for gastrointestinal endoscopy. Curr Opin Gastroenterol. 2012;28(5):442–50.
7. Inadomi JM, Gunnarsson CL, Rizzo JA, Fang H. Projected increased growth rate of anesthesia professional-delivered sedation for colonoscopy and EGD in the United States: 2009 to 2015. Gastrointest Endosc. 2010;72(3):580–6.

8. Liu H, Waxman DA, Main R, Mattke S. Utilization of anesthesia services during outpatient endoscopies and colonoscopies and associated spending in 2003-2009. JAMA. 2012;307(11):1178–84.
9. Krigel A, Chen L, Wright JD, Lebwohl B. Substantial increase in anesthesia assistance for outpatient colonoscopy and associated cost Nationwide. Clin Gastroenterol Hepatol. 2019;17(12):2489–96.
10. Predmore Z, Nie X, Main R, Mattke S, Liu H. Anesthesia service use during outpatient gastroenterology procedures continued to increase from 2010 to 2013 and potentially discretionary spending remained high. Am J Gastroenterol. 2017;112(2):297–302.
11. Harris ZP, Liu J, Saltzman JR. Quality assurance in the endoscopy suite: sedation and monitoring. Gastrointest Endosc Clin N Am. 2016;26(3):553–62.
12. Zebris J, Maurer W. Quality assurance in the endoscopy suite: sedation and monitoring. Gastrointest Endosc Clin N Am. 2004;14(2):415–29.
13. Despott EJ, Schreiber F. Advanced cardiac life support training. Digestion. 2010;82(2):113–4.
14. American Association for Study of Liver Diseases, American College of Gastroenterology, American Gastroenterological Association Institute, American Society for Gastrointestinal Endoscopy, Society for Gastroenterology Nurses and Associates, et al. Multisociety sedation curriculum for gastrointestinal endoscopy. Gastrointest Endosc. 2012;76(1):e1–e25.
15. Committee on Standards and Practice Parameters, Apfelbaum JL, Connis RT, Nickinovich DG, American Society of Anesthesiologists Task Force on Preanesthesia Evaluation, et al. Practice advisory for preanesthesia evaluation: an updated report by the American Society of Anesthesiologists Task Force on Preanesthesia evaluation. Anesthesiology. 2012;116(3):522–38.
16. American Society of Anesthesiologists Task Force on S, Analgesia by N-A. Practice guidelines for sedation and analgesia by non-anesthesiologists. Anesthesiology. 2002;96(4):1004–17.
17. Patel R, Clayton S, Quintero E, Gill J. Chronic opioid users are more difficult to sedate than alcoholics and controls. South Med J. 2015;108(12):744–7.
18. Papachristou GI, Gleeson FC, Papachristou DJ, Petersen BT, Baron TH. Endoscopist administered sedation during ERCP: impact of chronic narcotic/benzodiazepine use and predictive risk of reversal agent utilization. Am J Gastroenterol. 2007;102(4):738–43.
19. Braunstein ED, Rosenberg R, Gress F, Green PH, Lebwohl B. Development and validation of a clinical prediction score (the SCOPE score) to predict sedation outcomes in patients undergoing endoscopic procedures. Aliment Pharmacol Ther. 2014;40(1):72–82.
20. McCain JD, Stancampiano FF, Bouras EP, DeVault KR, Gilbert EL, Ryan T, et al. Creation of a score to predict risk of high conscious sedation requirements in patients undergoing endoscopy. Gastrointest Endosc. 2020;91(3):595–605. e3
21. Twardowski MA, Link MM, Twardowski NM. Effects of cannabis use on sedation requirements for endoscopic procedures. J Am Osteopath Assoc. 2019;15
22. Woo M, Andrews CN. Implications of cannabis use on sedation for endoscopic procedures. Gastrointest Endosc. 2019;90(4):656–8.
23. Pena LR, Mardini HE, Nickl NJ. Development of an instrument to assess and predict satisfaction and poor tolerance among patients undergoing endoscopic procedures. Dig Dis Sci. 2005;50(10):1860–71.
24. Delegge MH. The difficult-to-sedate patient in the endoscopy suite. Gastrointest Endosc Clin N Am. 2008;18(4):679–93. viii
25. Committee ASoP, Chandrasekhara V, Eloubeidi MA, Bruining DH, Chathadi K, Faulx AL, et al. Open-access endoscopy. Gastrointest Endosc. 2015;81(6):1326–9.
26. Kothari D, Feuerstein JD, Moss L, D'Souza J, Montanaro K, Leffler DA, et al. An open-access endoscopy screen correctly and safely identifies patients for conscious sedation. Gastroenterol Rep. 2016;4(4):281–6. Pubmed Central PMCID: 5193065
27. Rainis T, Keren D, Goldstein O, Stermer E, Lavy A. Diagnostic yield and safety of colonoscopy in Israeli patients in an open access referral system. J Clin Gastroenterol. 2007;41(4):394–9.

28. Keren D, Rainis T, Stermer E, Lavy A. A nine-year audit of open-access upper gastrointestinal endoscopic procedures: results and experience of a single Centre. Can J Gastroenterol. 2011;25(2):83–8. Pubmed Central PMCID: 3043009
29. Leung FW. Water-aided colonoscopy. Gastroenterol Clin N Am. 2013;42(3):507–19.
30. Rex DK, Imperiale TF, Portish V. Patients willing to try colonoscopy without sedation: associated clinical factors and results of a randomized controlled trial. Gastrointest Endosc. 1999;49(5):554–9.
31. Sami SS, Subramanian V, Ortiz-Fernandez-Sordo J, Saeed A, Singh S, Guha IN, et al. Performance characteristics of unsedated ultrathin video endoscopy in the assessment of the upper GI tract: systematic review and meta-analysis. Gastrointest Endosc. 2015;82(5):782–92.
32. Childers RE, Williams JL, Sonnenberg A. Practice patterns of sedation for colonoscopy. Gastrointest Endosc. 2015;82(3):503–11. Pubmed Central PMCID: 4540687
33. Riphaus A, Macias-Gomez C, Deviere J, Dumonceau JM. Propofol, the preferred sedation for screening colonoscopy, is underused. Results of an international survey. Dig Liver Dis. 2012;44(5):389–92.
34. McQuaid KR, Laine L. A systematic review and meta-analysis of randomized, controlled trials of moderate sedation for routine endoscopic procedures. Gastrointest Endosc. 2008;67(6):910–23.
35. Waring JP, Baron TH, Hirota WK, Goldstein JL, Jacobson BC, Leighton JA, et al. Guidelines for conscious sedation and monitoring during gastrointestinal endoscopy. Gastrointest Endosc. 2003;58(3):317–22.
36. Wadhwa V, Issa D, Garg S, Lopez R, Sanaka MR, Vargo JJ. Similar risk of cardiopulmonary adverse events between Propofol and traditional anesthesia for gastrointestinal endoscopy: a systematic review and meta-analysis. Clin Gastroenterol Hepatol. 2017;15(2):194–206.
37. Vargo JJ. Big NAPS, little NAPS, mixed NAPS, computerized NAPS: what is your flavor of propofol? Gastrointest Endosc. 2007;66(3):457–9.
38. Rex DK, Overley CA, Walker J. Registered nurse-administered propofol sedation for upper endoscopy and colonoscopy: Why? When? How? Rev Gastroenterol Disord. 2003;3(2):70–80.
39. Sieg A, bng Study G, Beck S, Scholl SG, Heil FJ, Gotthardt DN, et al. Safety analysis of endoscopist-directed propofol sedation: a prospective, national multicenter study of 24 441 patients in German outpatient practices. J Gastroenterol Hepatol. 2014;29(3):517–23.
40. Rex DK, Deenadayalu VP, Eid E, Imperiale TF, Walker JA, Sandhu K, et al. Endoscopist-directed administration of propofol: a worldwide safety experience. Gastroenterology. 2009;137(4):1229–37. quiz 518-9
41. Rex DK, Heuss LT, Walker JA, Qi R. Trained registered nurses/endoscopy teams can administer propofol safely for endoscopy. Gastroenterology. 2005;129(5):1384–91.
42. Sathananthan D, Young E, Nind G, George B, Ashby A, Drummond S, et al. Assessing the safety of physician-directed nurse-administered propofol sedation in low-risk patients undergoing endoscopy and colonoscopy. Endosc Int Open. 2017;5(2):E110–E5. Pubmed Central PMCID: 5305421
43. Sipe BW, Rex DK, Latinovich D, Overley C, Kinser K, Bratcher L, et al. Propofol versus midazolam/meperidine for outpatient colonoscopy: administration by nurses supervised by endoscopists. Gastrointest Endosc. 2002;55(7):815–25.
44. Walker JA, McIntyre RD, Schleinitz PF, Jacobson KN, Haulk AA, Adesman P, et al. Nurse-administered propofol sedation without anesthesia specialists in 9152 endoscopic cases in an ambulatory surgery center. Am J Gastroenterol. 2003;98(8):1744–50.
45. Dumonceau JM, Riphaus A, Beilenhoff U, Vilmann P, Hornslet P, Aparicio JR, et al. European curriculum for sedation training in gastrointestinal endoscopy: position statement of the European Society of Gastrointestinal Endoscopy (ESGE) and European Society of Gastroenterology and Endoscopy Nurses and Associates (ESGENA). Endoscopy. 2013;45(6):496–504.
46. Dumonceau JM, Riphaus A, Schreiber F, Vilmann P, Beilenhoff U, Aparicio JR, et al. Non-anesthesiologist administration of propofol for gastrointestinal endoscopy: European Society

of Gastrointestinal Endoscopy, European Society of Gastroenterology and Endoscopy Nurses and Associates Guideline—updated June 2015. Endoscopy. 2015;47(12):1175–89.
47. Vargo JJ, Cohen LB, Rex DK, Kwo PY, American Association for the Study of Liver D, American College of G, et al. Position statement: nonanesthesiologist administration of propofol for GI endoscopy. Gastroenterology. 2009;137(6):2161–7.
48. Rex DK. Effect of the Centers for Medicare & Medicaid Services policy about deep sedation on use of propofol. Ann Intern Med. 2011;154(9):622–6.
49. Aisenberg J, Cohen LB, Piorkowski JD Jr. Propofol use under the direction of trained gastroenterologists: an analysis of the medicolegal implications. Am J Gastroenterol. 2007;102(4):707–13.
50. Pambianco DJ, Vargo JJ, Pruitt RE, Hardi R, Martin JF. Computer-assisted personalized sedation for upper endoscopy and colonoscopy: a comparative, multicenter randomized study. Gastrointest Endosc. 2011;73(4):765–72.
51. Lin OS, Kozarek RA, Tombs D, La Selva D, Weigel W, Beecher R, et al. The first US clinical experience with computer-assisted propofol sedation: a retrospective observational comparative study on efficacy, safety, efficiency, and endoscopist and patient satisfaction. Anesth Analg. 2017;125(3):804–11.
52. Lin OS, La Selva D, Kozarek RA, Tombs D, Weigel W, Beecher R, et al. Computer-assisted Propofol sedation for esophagogastroduodenoscopy is effective, efficient, and safe. Dig Dis Sci. 2019;64(12):3549–56.
53. Lin OS, La Selva D, Kozarek RA, Tombs D, Weigel W, Beecher R, et al. One year experience with computer-assisted propofol sedation for colonoscopy. World J Gastroenterol. 2017;23(16):2964–71. Pubmed Central PMCID: 5413791
54. Martin JF, Niklewski PJ, White JD. The rise, fall, and future direction of computer-assisted personalized sedation. Curr Opin Anaesthesiol. 2019;32(4):480–7.
55. Lin OS. Sedation for routine gastrointestinal endoscopic procedures: a review on efficacy, safety, efficiency, cost and satisfaction. Intest Res. 2017;15(4):456–66. Pubmed Central PMCID: 5683976
56. Rex DK, Vargo JJ. Anesthetist-directed sedation for colonoscopy: a safe haven or Siren's song? Gastroenterology. 2016;150(4):801–3.
57. Dumonceau JM. Nonanesthesiologist administration of propofol: it's all about money. Endoscopy. 2012;44(5):453–5.
58. Lin OS, La Selva D, Kozarek RA, Weigel W, Beecher R, Gluck M, et al. Nurse-administered propofol continuous infusion sedation: a new paradigm for gastrointestinal procedural sedation. Am J Gastroenterol. 2021;116(4):710–6.
59. Lee HS, Nagra N, La Selva D, Kozarek RA, Ross A, Weigel W, et al. Nurse-administered propofol continuous infusion sedation for gastrointestinal endoscopy in patients who are difficult to sedate. Clin Gastroenterol Hepatol. 2021;19(1):180–8.
60. Brill JV, Jain R, Margolis PS, Kosinski LR, Holt WS Jr, Ketover SR, et al. A bundled payment framework for colonoscopy performed for colorectal cancer screening or surveillance. Gastroenterology. 2014;146(3):849–53 e9.
61. Patel K, Presser E, George M, McClellan M. Shifting away from fee-for-service: alternative approaches to payment in gastroenterology. Clin Gastroenterol Hepatol. 2016;14(4):497–506.
62. Dorn SD. The road ahead 3.0: changing payments, changing practice. Clin Gastroenterol Hepatol. 2016;14(6):785–9.
63. Adams MA. Putting the horse back in the barn: right-sizing use of anesthesia assistance for routine gastrointestinal endoscopy. Clin Gastroenterol Hepatol. 2019;17(12):2434–6.
64. Mandel JE, Lichtenstein GR, Metz DC, Ginsberg GG, Kochman ML. A prospective, randomized, comparative trial evaluating respiratory depression during patient-controlled versus anesthesiologist-administered propofol-remifentanil sedation for elective colonoscopy. Gastrointest Endosc. 2010;72(1):112–7.
65. Kulling D, Orlandi M, Inauen W. Propofol sedation during endoscopic procedures: how much staff and monitoring are necessary? Gastrointest Endosc. 2007;66(3):443–9.

66. Roseveare C, Seavell C, Patel P, Criswell J, Kimble J, Jones C, et al. Patient-controlled sedation and analgesia, using propofol and alfentanil, during colonoscopy: a prospective randomized controlled trial. Endoscopy. 1998;30(9):768–73.
67. Liu SY, Poon CM, Leung TL, Wong CW, Chan YL, Leung TC, et al. Nurse-administered propofol-alfentanil sedation using a patient-controlled analgesia pump compared with opioid-benzodiazepine sedation for outpatient colonoscopy. Endoscopy. 2009;41(6):522–8.
68. Khiani VS, Soulos P, Gancayco J, Gross CP. Anesthesiologist involvement in screening colonoscopy: temporal trends and cost implications in the medicare population. Clin Gastroenterol Hepatol. 2012;10(1):58–64. e1. Pubmed Central PMCID: 3214600
69. Qadeer MA, Vargo JJ, Khandwala F, Lopez R, Zuccaro G. Propofol versus traditional sedative agents for gastrointestinal endoscopy: a meta-analysis. Clin Gastroenterol Hepatol. 2005;3(11):1049–56.
70. Wang D, Chen C, Chen J, Xu Y, Wang L, Zhu Z, et al. The use of propofol as a sedative agent in gastrointestinal endoscopy: a meta-analysis. PLoS One. 2013;8(1):e53311. Pubmed Central PMCID: 3540096
71. Tsai HC, Lin YC, Ko CL, Lou HY, Chen TL, Tam KW, et al. Propofol versus midazolam for upper gastrointestinal endoscopy in cirrhotic patients: a meta-analysis of randomized controlled trials. PLoS One. 2015;10(2):e0117585. Pubmed Central PMCID: 4315567
72. Inadomi JM. Editorial: endoscopic sedation: who, which, when? Am J Gastroenterol. 2017;112(2):303–5.
73. Hassan C, Rex DK, Cooper GS, Benamouzig R. Endoscopist-directed propofol administration versus anesthesiologist assistance for colorectal cancer screening: a cost-effectiveness analysis. Endoscopy. 2012;44(5):456–64.
74. Agrawal D, Rockey DC. Propofol for screening colonoscopy in low-risk patients: are we paying too much? JAMA Intern Med. 2013;173(19):1836–8.
75. Repici A, Hassan C. The endoscopist, the anesthesiologists, and safety in GI endoscopy. Gastrointest Endosc. 2017;85(1):109–11.
76. Rex DK. The science and politics of propofol. Am J Gastroenterol. 2004;99(11):2080–3.
77. Metwally M, Agresti N, Hale WB, Ciofoaia V, O'Connor R, Wallace MB, et al. Conscious or unconscious: the impact of sedation choice on colon adenoma detection. World J Gastroenterol. 2011;17(34):3912–5. Pubmed Central PMCID: 3198020
78. Dominitz JA, Baldwin LM, Green P, Kreuter WI, Ko CW. Regional variation in anesthesia assistance during outpatient colonoscopy is not associated with differences in polyp detection or complication rates. Gastroenterology. 2013;144(2):298–306. Pubmed Central PMCID: 3622787
79. Paspatis GA, Tribonias G, Manolaraki MM, Konstantinidis K, Chainaki I, Theodoropoulou A, et al. Deep sedation compared with moderate sedation in polyp detection during colonoscopy: a randomized controlled trial. Color Dis. 2011;13(6):e137–44.
80. Lubarsky DA, Guercio JR, Hanna JW, Abreu MT, Ma Q, Uribe C, et al. The impact of anesthesia providers on major morbidity following screening colonoscopies. J Multidiscip Healthc. 2015;8:255–70. Pubmed Central PMCID: 4454218
81. Wernli KJ, Brenner AT, Rutter CM, Inadomi JM. Risks associated with anesthesia services during colonoscopy. Gastroenterology. 2016;150(4):888–94.
82. Cooper GS, Kou TD, Rex DK. Complications following colonoscopy with anesthesia assistance: a population-based analysis. JAMA Intern Med. 2013;173(7):551–6. Pubmed Central PMCID: 3987111
83. Vargo JJ, Niklewski PJ, Williams JL, Martin JF, Faigel DO. Patient safety during sedation by anesthesia professionals during routine upper endoscopy and colonoscopy: an analysis of 1.38 million procedures. Gastrointest Endosc. 2017;85(1):101–8.
84. Committee ASoP, Storm AC, Fishman DS, Buxbaum JL, Coelho-Prabhu N, Al-Haddad MA, et al. American Society for Gastrointestinal Endoscopy guideline on informed consent for GI endoscopic procedures. Gastrointest Endosc. 2022;95(2):207–15. e2

85. Matharoo M, Thomas-Gibson S, Haycock A, Sevdalis N. Implementation of an endoscopy safety checklist. Frontline Gastroenterol. 2014;5(4):260–5. Pubmed Central PMCID: 4173736
86. Force AESitGEUT, Calderwood AH, Chapman FJ, Cohen J, Cohen LB, Collins J, et al. Guidelines for safety in the gastrointestinal endoscopy unit. Gastrointest Endosc. 2014;79(3):363–72. Pubmed Central PMCID: 3980655
87. Beitz A, Riphaus A, Meining A, Kronshage T, Geist C, Wagenpfeil S, et al. Capnographic monitoring reduces the incidence of arterial oxygen desaturation and hypoxemia during propofol sedation for colonoscopy: a randomized, controlled study (ColoCap study). Am J Gastroenterol. 2012;107(8):1205–12.
88. Qadeer MA, Vargo JJ, Dumot JA, Lopez R, Trolli PA, Stevens T, et al. Capnographic monitoring of respiratory activity improves safety of sedation for endoscopic cholangiopancreatography and ultrasonography. Gastroenterology. 2009;136(5):1568–76. quiz 819-20
89. Nelson DB, Freeman ML, Silvis SE, Cass OW, Yakshe PN, Vennes J, et al. A randomized, controlled trial of transcutaneous carbon dioxide monitoring during ERCP. Gastrointest Endosc. 2000;51(3):288–95.
90. Harewood GC, Wiersema MJ, de Groen PC. Utility of web-based assessment of patient satisfaction with endoscopy. Am J Gastroenterol. 2003;98(5):1016–21.
91. Lin OS, Schembre DB, Ayub K, Gluck M, McCormick SE, Patterson DJ, et al. Patient satisfaction scores for endoscopic procedures: impact of a survey-collection method. Gastrointest Endosc. 2007;65(6):775–81.
92. Gross JB, Bachenberg KL, Benumof JL, Caplan RA, Connis RT, Cote CJ, et al. Practice guidelines for the perioperative management of patients with obstructive sleep apnea: a report by the American Society of Anesthesiologists Task Force on perioperative management of patients with obstructive sleep apnea. Anesthesiology. 2006;104(5):1081–93. quiz 117-8

Index

J. D. Feuerstein, D. J. Stein (eds.), *Quality in Gastroenterology*, https://doi.org/10.1007/978-3-031-58492-3

MIX
Papier aus verantwortungsvollen Quellen
Paper from responsible sources
FSC® C105338

If you have any concerns about our products,
you can contact us on
ProductSafety@springernature.com

In case Publisher is established outside the EU,
the EU authorized representative is:
Springer Nature Customer Service Center GmbH
Europaplatz 3, 69115 Heidelberg, Germany

Printed by Libri Plureos GmbH
in Hamburg, Germany